TRANSESOPHAGEAL
ECHOCARDIOGRAPHY

TRANSESOPHAGEAL ECHOCARDIOGRAPHY

EDITOR

Gerald Maurer, M.D.

Professor of Medicine
Director, Department of Cardiology
University of Vienna Medical School
Vienna, Austria
Formerly Associate Professor of Medicine
UCLA School of Medicine
Director, Cardiac Noninvasive Laboratory
Cedars-Sinai Medical Center
Los Angeles, California

McGraw-Hill, Inc.
HEALTH PROFESSIONS DIVISION

New York   St. Louis   San Francisco   Auckland   Bogotá   Caracas   Lisbon   London   Madrid
Mexico City   Milan   Montreal   New Delhi   Paris   San Juan   Singapore   Sydney   Tokyo   Toronto

TRANSESOPHAGEAL ECHOCARDIOGRAPHY

Copyright © 1994 McGraw-Hill, Inc. All rights reserved. Printed in the United States of America. Except as permitted under the United States Copyright Act of 1976, no part of this publication may be reproduced or distributed in any form or by any means, or stored in a data or retrieval system, without the prior written permission of the publisher.

1234567890   KGPKGP   9876543

ISBN 0-07-040988-9

This book was set in Caslon by Monotype, Inc.
The editors were Michael J. Houston and Lester A. Sheinis;
the production supervisor was Clare Stanley;
the cover designer was N.S.G. Design;
the indexer was Barbara Littlewood.
Arcata Graphics/Kingsport was printer and binder.

Library of Congress Cataloging-in-Publication Data

Transesophageal echocardiography/[edited by] Gerald Maurer.
    p. cm.
  Includes bibliographical references and index.
  ISBN 0-07-040988-9
  1. Transesophageal echocardiography. I. Maurer, Gerald.
  [DNLM: 1. Echocardiography—methods. 2. Heart Diseases-
-diagnosis. WG 141.5.E2 T7717 1994]
  RC683.5.T83T732 1994
  616.1'207543—dc20
  DNLM/DC
  for Library of Congress   32–31255
                               CIP

Contents

Contributors

The numbers in brackets following the contributors' names refer to the chapters written or co-written by the contributors.

Siva Arunasalam, M.D. [11]
Clinical Fellow
Division of Cardiology
Cedars-Sinai Medical Center
Los Angeles, California

Helmut Baumgartner, M.D. [6, 8]
Associate Professor of Medicine
University of Vienna
Director, Echocardiography Laboratory
Krankenhaus der Barmherzigen Schwestern
Linz, Austria

John S. Child, M.D. [10]
Professor of Medicine
Division of Cardiology
Department of Medicine
UCLA School of Medicine
Los Angeles, California

Lawrence S. C. Czer, M.D. [13]
Medical Director
Heart Transplantation Program
Cedars-Sinai Medical Center
Associate Professor of Medicine
UCLA School of Medicine
Los Angeles, California

Frederick A. Dressler, M.D. [7]
Assistant Professor
Department of Internal Medicine
Division of Cardiology
St. Louis University Health Sciences Center
St. Louis, Missouri

Julius M. Gardin, M.S., F.A.C.C. [5]
Professor of Medicine
College of Medicine
University of California, Irvine
Director, Cardiology Noninvasive Laboratory

University of California Irvine Medical Center
Orange, California

Tsui-Lieh Hsu, M.D. [2]
Visiting Scholar
Cardiovascular Imaging and Hemodynamic
  Laboratory
New England Medical Center
Instructor in Medicine
Tufts University School of Medicine
Boston, Massachusetts

Jui-Sung Hung, M.D., F.A.C.C. [12]
Professor of Medicine
Department of Cardiology
Chang Gung Medical College
Taipei, Taiwan

Steven Khan, M.D. [6]
Professor
UCLA School of Medicine
Associate Cardiologist
Cedars-Sinai Medical Center
Los Angeles, California

Toshiki Kobayashi, M.D. [12]
Assistant Professor of Cardiology
Instructor of Pediatric Cardiology
Department of Cardiology
Saitama Medical School
Saitama, Japan

Kazuyuki Koike, M.D. [12]
Professor of Pediatric Cardiology
Department of Pediatrics
Saitama Medical School
Saitama, Japan

Shunei Kyo, M.D. [12]
Associate Professor of Surgery
Department of Surgery
Saitama Medical School
Saitama, Japan

Arthur J. Labovitz, M.D., F.A.C.C. [7]
Professor of Medicine
Department of Internal Medicine
Division of Cardiology
St. Louis University Health Sciences Center
St. Louis, Missouri

Yuk Kong Lau, M.D. [13]
Cardiology Fellow
Cedars-Sinai Medical Center
Los Angeles, California

Ariane J. Marelli, M.D. [10]
Assistant in Medicine
Massachusetts General Hospital
Harvard Medical School
Boston, Massachusetts

Gerald Maurer, M.D. [1,3,4,6,8,11]
Professor of Medicine
Director, Department of Cardiology
University of Vienna Medical School
Vienna, Austria
Formerly Associate Professor of Medicine
UCLA School of Medicine
Director, Cardiac Noninvasive Laboratory
Cedars-Sinai Medical Center
Los Angeles, California

Naomasa Miyamoto, M.D. [12]
Instructor of Cardiology
Department of Cardiology
Saitama Medical School
Saitama, Japan

Takeshi Mototyama, M.D. [12]
Assistant Professor of Cardiology
Department of Cardiology
Saitama Medical School
Saitama, Japan

Navin C. Nanda, M.D., F.A.C.C. [4,9]
Professor of Medicine
Director, Heart Station/Echocardiography-
   Graphics Laboratories
The Kirklin Clinic
University of Alabama Health Services
   Foundation
Birmingham, Alabama

**Elizabeth O. Ofili, M.D., M.P.H.,
   F.A.C.C. [9]**
Assistant Professor of Medicine
St. Louis University Medical Center
St. Louis, Missouri

Yasu Oka, M.D. [14]
Professor
Director of Cardiothoracic Anesthesia
Department of Anesthesiology Albert Einstein
   College of Medicine
Montefiore Medical Center
Bronx, New York

Ryozo Omoto, M.D. [12]
Chairman and Professor of Surgery
Department of Surgery
Saitama Medical School
Saitama, Japan

Natesa G. Pandian, M.D. [2]
Director
Cardiovascular Imaging and Hemodynamic
   Laboratory
New England Medical Center
Associate Professor of Medicine and
   Radiology
Tufts University School of Medicine
Boston, Massachusetts

Jack Panopoulos, M.D. [14]
Instructor
Department of Anesthesiology
Albert Einstein College of Medicine
Montefiore Medical Center
Bronx, New York

Luiz Pinheiro, M.D. [4]
Echocardiographic Associate
Cardiovascular Associates, Inc.
Birmingham, Alabama

Formerly Research Fellow and
   Echocardiographic Associate
Heart Station/Echocardiography-Graphics
   Laboratories
University of Alabama Health Services
   Foundation
Birmingham, Alabama

Cheryl L. Reid, M.D., F.A.C.C. [5]
Associate Professor of Medicine
Director, Interventional Echocardiography
Department of Medicine/Cardiology
University of California Irvine Medical Center
Orange, California

Rajat S. Sanyal, M.D. [4]
Echocardiographic Associate
University of Alabama Hospital
Associate/Fellow
Division of Cardiovascular Disease
University of Alabama at Birmingham
Birmingham, Alabama

Steven L. Schwartz, M.D. [2]
Associate Director
Cardiovascular Imaging and Hemodynamic
   Laboratory
New England Medical Center
Assistant Professor of Medicine
Tufts University School of Medicine
Boston, Massachusetts

Edward J. Share, M.D. [3]
Attending Physician
Division of Gastroenterology
Cedars-Sinai Medical Center
Los Angeles, California

Robert J. Siegel, M.D. [11]
Associate Cardiologist
Cedars-Sinai Medical Center
Professor of Medicine
UCLA School of Medicine
Los Angeles, California

Octavia Storey [4]
Diagnostic Medical Sonographer Supervisor
University of Alabama Hospital
Echocardiography Laboratory
Birmingham, Alabama

Jean-Claude Tardif, M.D. [2]
Research Fellow
Cardiovascular Imaging and Hemodynamic
   Laboratory
New England Medical Center
Instructor in Medicine
Tufts University School of Medicine
Boston, Massachusetts

Hiroshi Watanabe, M.D. [14]
Research Associate
Department of Anesthesiology
Albert Einstein College of Medicine
Montefiore Medical Center
Bronx, New York

Shiro Yamachika, M.D. [5]
Visiting Research Physician
University of Nagasaki
Nagasaki, Japan
Visiting Postgraduate Researcher
University of California Irvine Medical Center
Orange, California

Preface

The rise of transesophageal echocardiography (TEE) has had a profound impact on the diagnosis of cardiovascular function. Cardiologists, anesthesiologists, and cardiac surgeons are challenged with the need to keep up with the growing list of TEE applications. This book is designed to be a practical reference source for practitioners and residents wishing to gain an understanding of the theory and technique of transesophageal imaging. The book provides a clear summary of the current state of the field with single-plane and biplane probes and also points to new developments such as multiplane TEE and its impact on the diagnosis and assessment of cardiovascular disorders.

The opening chapters focus on the latest instrumentation, including multiplane, panoramic TEE, 3D reconstruction, and intravascular and intracardiac echo. The test then provides a detailed description of upper gastrointestinal anatomy, endoscopic techniques, and safety precautions. Authorities on the clinical applications of TEE then proceed to provide practical information on the procedure with the aid of a large number of figures and illustrations.

TRANSESOPHAGEAL
ECHOCARDIOGRAPHY

1

Introduction

Gerald Maurer

It seems that every few years some skeptics suspect that echocardiography has reached its peak and that no new developments are on the horizon. Fortunately, such notions have so far always quickly been dispelled by groundbreaking new developments. One of the most significant, and perhaps the one with the most profound impact on clinical practice, has been the rise of transesophageal echocardiography (TEE). Interestingly, this approach was first proposed more than 20 years ago but did not gain widespread acceptance until the late 1980s. This acceptance was most likely triggered by technological developments that resulted in improved echocardiographic image quality, in the ability to visualize flow by Doppler color flow mapping, and also by advances in probe design that allow us to easily examine the heart in multiple image planes.

The first endeavors to use transesophageal ultrasound for assessment of cardiovascular function were reported in the early 1970s, when attempts were made to obtain Doppler measurements of aortic flow velocity[1,2] and to measure pulsatile changes in the diameter of the thoracic aorta.[3] These early devices were truly prototypes, which were difficult to use

and which did not provide information in an easily understood, graphic display format. The first utilization of a TEE device that promised to have clinical utility was reported in 1976 by Frazin and coworkers,[4] who described the application of transesophageal M-mode echocardiography. The use of this technology was subsequently reported for continuous intraoperative monitoring of left ventricular performance[5] and for the evaluation of ventricular function during supine exercise.[6]

The next major breakthrough was the development of real-time, two-dimensional TEE imaging, as first described in 1980 by Hisanaga,[7] who developed a wide-angle mechanical sector scanner, while in 1982 Schlüter[8] reported on the use of transesophageal phased-array two-dimensional echocardiography. Further milestones were the development of pulsed Doppler[9,10] and perhaps most importantly, the incorporation of color flow mapping into a TEE device, which was first reported by investigators from Saitama Medical School in Japan.[11] The same group was instrumental in the early development and clinical validation of standard biplane, matrix phased-array biplane, and small pediatric probes.[12,13] The future, how-

1

ever, seems to belong to multiplane TEE, [14–16] which allows us to view the heart in an almost unlimited number of planes, and which is rapidly becoming the state of the art of transesophageal imaging.

Other exciting transesophageal techniques are on the horizon but might still be considered largely investigational. They include widefield, or panoramic, TEE,[17,18] which was actually already used by Hisanaga in 1980.[7] The panoramic approach contributes to better understanding of cardiovascular anatomy but may have a particular impact on the detection of extracardiac abnormalities. Three-dimensional transesophageal echocardiographic imaging[19] promises to offer improved spatial understanding, including the ability to display the heart, or parts of it, in various perspectives and slices. In addition, it should enable us to obtain precise volumetric measurements with no or only minimal geometric assumptions.

Both the technological and the clinical developments of transesophageal echocardiography have been truly international endeavors, with major contributions from numerous countries on at least three continents. The growing list of TEE applications has resulted in its increased use across a variety of clinical specialties, including cardiology, anesthesiology, and cardiac surgery. Given the versatility and cost-effectiveness of this imaging technique, there is little doubt that its future looks very bright and that we can anticipate continued growth and development.

This book is dedicated to the fascinating technique of TEE and attempts to summarize its current state, as well as point toward new developments. It is my hope that this book will provide a useful reference source to physicians, sonographers, and nurses interested in the use of transesophageal echocardiography.

References

1. Side CD, Gosling RG: Non-surgical assessment of cardiac function. *Nature* 232:335, 1971.
2. Duck FA, Hodson CJ, Tomlin PJ: An esophageal Doppler probe for aortic flow velocity monitoring. *Ultrasound Med Biol* 1:223, 1972.
3. Olson RM, Shelton DK: A nondestructive technique to measure wall displacement in the thoracic aorta. *J Appl Physiol* 32:147, 1972.
4. Frazin L, Talano JV, Stephanides L, et al: Esophageal echocardiography. *Circulation* 54:102, 1976.
5. Matsumoto M, Oka Y, Strom J, et al: Application of transesophageal echocardiography to continuous intraoperative monitoring of left ventricular performance. *Am J Cardiol* 46:95, 1980.
6. Matsumoto M, Hanrath P, Kremer P, et al: Evaluation of left ventricular performance during supine exercise by transoesophageal m-mode echocardiography in normal subjects. *Br Heart J* 48:61, 1982.
7. Hisanaga K, Hisanaga A, Hibi N, et al: High speed rotating scanner for transoesophageal cross-sectional echocardiography. *Am J Cardiol* 46: 837, 1980.
8. Schlüter M, Langenstein BA, Polster J, et al: Transoesophageal cross-sectional echocardiography with a phased array transducer system: Technique and initial clinical results. *Br Heart J* 48:67, 1982.
9. Hisanaga K, Hisanaga A, Ichie Y: Tranoesophageal pulsed Doppler echocardiography. *Lancet* 1:53, 1979.
10. Schlüter M, Langenstein BA, Hanrach P, et al: Assessment of transesophageal pulsed Doppler echocardiography in the detection of mitral regurgitation. *Circulation* 66:784, 1982.
11. Kyo S, Takamoto S, Matsumura M, et al: Immediate and early postoperative evaluation of cardiac surgery by transesophageal two-dimensional Doppler echocardiography. *Circulation* 76 (suppl V): 113, 1987.
12. Omoto R, Kyo S, Matsumura M, et al: Recent technological progress in transeosphageal color Doppler flow imaging with special reference to newly developed biplane and pediatric probes, in Erbel R, Khanderia BK, Brennecke, et al (eds): *Transesophageal Echocardiography*, Heidelberg, Springer-Verlag, 1989, p 21.
13. Omoto R, Kyo S, Matsumura M, et al: New direction of biplane transesophageal echocardiography with special emphasis on real-time biplane imaging and matrix phased-array biplane transducer. *Echocardiography* 7:691, 1990.
14. Flachskampf FA, Hoffmann R, Verlande M, et al: Initial experience with a multiplane transesophageal transducer: Assessment of diagnostic potential. *Eur Heart J* 13: 1201, 1992.

15. Roelandt JRTC, Thomson IR, Vletter WB, et al: Multiplane transesophageal echocardiography: Latest evolution in an imaging revolution. *J Am Soc Echocardiogr* 5:361, 1992.

16. Seward JB, Khanderia BK, Freeman WK, et al: Multiplane transesophageal echocardiography: Image orientation, examination technique, anatomic correlations, and clinical applications. *Mayo Clin Proc* 68:523, 1993.

17. Seward JB, Khanderia BK, Tajik AJ: Widefield transesophageal echocardiographic tomography: Feasibility study. *Mayo Clin Proc* 65:39, 1990.

18. Hsu TL, Weintraub AR, Ritter SB, et al: Panoramic transesophageal echocardiography. *Echocardiography* 8:677, 1991.

19. Pandian NG, Nanda NC, Schwartz SL, et al: Three-dimensional and four-dimensional transesophageal echocardiographic imaging of the heart and aorta in humans using a computed tomographic imaging probe. *Echocardiography* 9:677, 1992.

2

Transesophageal Echocardiography: Current Instrumentation and Future Prospects

Jean-Claude Tardif
Tsui-Lieh Hsu
Steven L. Schwartz
Natesa G. Pandian

Transesophageal echocardiography (TEE) was first used on an experimental basis in the late 1970s.[1] Since then, rapid technologic advances such as transducer size reduction, the development of phased-array systems housed in flexible endoscopes, and incorporation of spectral and color Doppler capabilities have greatly changed the practice of TEE examination and have led to its widespread clinical use.[2–9] While single-plane TEE examination has become an important part of cardiovascular imaging, recent developments such as bi- and multiplane devices provide incremental information and enable a more comprehensive examination of the heart and related structures.[10–17] Furthermore, ongoing work with panoramic TEE, acoustic quantification, and three-dimensional reconstruction holds out great promise to further aid in the proper assessment of cardiovascular pathology and improve diagnostic capability.[18–23]

In this chapter, we first review the examination with established single, biplane, and pediatric probes, and then focus on the echo-anatomic correlations and clinical applications of multiplane and panoramic TEE. Clinical experience with acoustic quantification and three-dimensional reconstruction is also described.

Currently Available Instrumentation

Single-plane transesophageal endoscopes have a single set of 5-MHz phased-array transducer elements incorporated into the flexible probe tip (Fig. 2-1). The two wheels at the handle are used for flexion of the probe tip, with 90° of forward and backward mobility and 70° of lateral mobility. The diameters of the endoscope tip and shaft are 10 to 13 mm and 9 mm, respectively. The length of the probe varies from 60 to 110 cm. Using these transducers, images are acquired in a single transverse plane at different levels. A comprehensive examination entails transgastric short-axis views of the ventricles, transverse plane imaging from the lower esophagus (classic four-chamber view, imaging at the coronary sinus level, and at the left ventricular outflow tract and aortic valve level) and serial basal short-axis views of the great vessels and adjacent structures. Examination is completed with the evaluation of the descending aorta and aortic arch.

Newer transesophageal probes that incorporate two transducers that image the heart in two orthogonal planes have been introduced to clinical practice. These biplane TEE probes operate at 5 to 7 MHz for two-dimensional imaging and 3.5 MHz for Doppler imaging. Within the tip of the scope, two sets of transducer elements perpendicular to each other are stacked, one above the other, 1.5 mm apart

(Fig. 2-1). The centers of the distal horizontal array and the proximal longitudinal array are separated by 1 cm. The dimensions and possible manipulations of single and biplane probes are similar; the endoscope tip can be advanced, withdrawn, rotated, and flexed in the anterior, posterior, left, and right directions. Longitudinal planes of section offered by biplane TEE examination provide additional morphologic information for the assessment of various abnormalities.

While improvised use of biplane devices can provide additional imaging planes, this requires extensive probe manipulation.[24] Furthermore, desired planes cannot always be obtained with such manipulations. Continuous visualization of the cardiac structures offered by multiplane TEE as the array is steered through the 180° arc provides a better understanding of the spatial relationship of the structures (Fig. 2-2). The multiplane TEE instrument (Omniplane, Hewlett-Packard) is composed of a 64-element phased-array transducer that has a dual-frequency feature allowing two-dimensional imaging at 5 and 3.7 MHz, and pulsed, continuous-wave, and color Doppler capabilities (Fig. 2-1). The transducer array encased within the tip of the endoscope can be rotated through a 180° arc by touching a button on the handle of the probe (Fig. 2-3). An icon in the form of a semicircle with a needlelike indicator points out the angle of the imaging plane as the transducer array is steered (Fig. 2-4). Two rotary knobs at the handle of the probe control the anteroposterior and lateral flexion of the

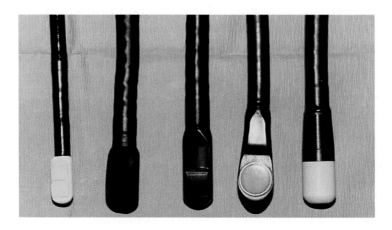

Figure 2-1
Photograph of different types of transesophageal probes. From left to right, pediatric, single-plane, biplane, multiplane, and panoramic probes are identified.

Figure 2-2
Schematic showing the two planes of section (transverse and longitudinal) offered by biplane TEE on the left and the multiple imaging planes provided by multiplane as the array is steered from 0 to 180° on the right.

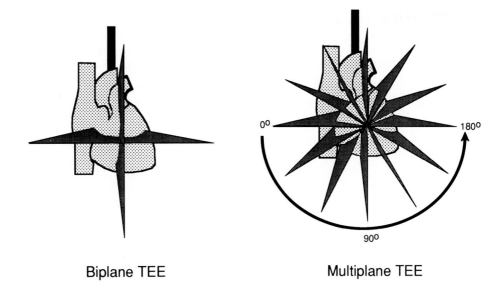

Biplane TEE

Multiplane TEE

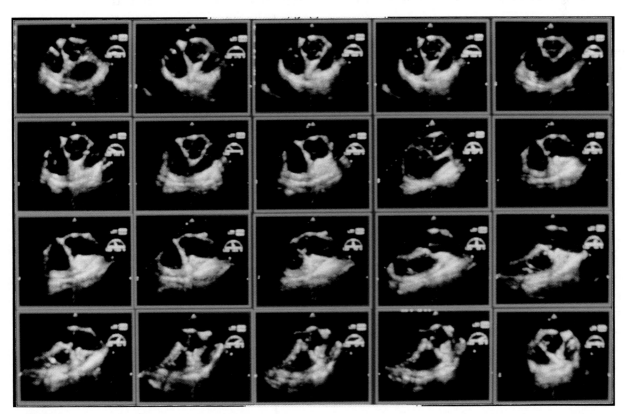

Figure 2-3
Vast assembly of images offered by multiplane TEE from a single location as the array is steered.

probe tip. The multiplane probe is interfaced to the ultrasound imaging console, and the operation on the console is similar to that of conventional echocardiography. In addition to

this commercially available probe, a number of prototype multiplane TEE probes are being evaluated and refined.

The advent of small pediatric-sized trans-

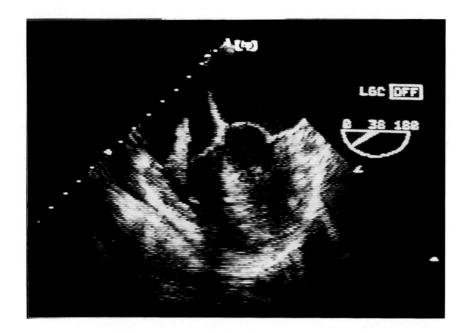

Figure 2-4
Multiplane TEE image from a patient with tricuspid valve vegetation. Four-chamber view from the esophagus depicts the left ventricle (at the bottom) and atrium on the viewer's right and the right ventricle and atrium on the viewer's left. This imaging plane was the most useful in this patient. An icon in the form of a semicircle with a needlelike indicator points out the angle of the imaging plane.

esophageal probes has dramatically changed the role of TEE in this population.[25,26] The device is 14 by 6.8 by 6.4 mm with a 26-element 5-MHz transducer and is mounted on a flexible 70-cm endoscope (Fig. 2-1). Further advances have already begun, including even smaller probes capable of being used in premature infants and biplane capability.

The panoramic TEE probe consists of an annular-array ultrasound transducer with a rotating crystal at the end of an endoscope. The transducer is cylindrical and is mounted in a 13-mm housing incorporated to the end of an endoscopic probe. The diameter of the probe shaft is 10 mm (Fig. 2-1). The probe tip can be steered to 90° anteroflexion, 45° retroflexion, and 60° lateral flexion. The transducer operates at 4 to 10 MHz for two-dimensional imaging and 3.3 MHz for spectral and color Doppler modalities. The widest angle of imaging field is 270°, but it can be reduced to the smallest sector angle of 15°. The frame rate is 20 per second at the maximum angle and 60 per second at lower angles. The field for color flow imaging can be varied from sectors with 10 to 180° angles. When desired, two-dimensional or color Doppler imaging can be performed with a small sector angle and the display can be magnified like other conventional echocardiographic instruments.

Clinical Applications of Single and Biplane TEE

The clinical indications for TEE examination have expanded, with technical improvements leading to its use in numerous cardiovascular disorders in a variety of clinical scenarios (Table 2-1). Poor transthoracic echocardiographic image quality in patients with obesity, chronic obstructive pulmonary disease, chest tubes, or bandages, or in those who are not movable because of mechanical ventilation, pain, recent catheterization, or surgery, and in whom questions of clinical significance cannot be answered adequately constitutes settings where TEE is useful. TEE is also indicated when the diagnostic sensitivity of transthoracic echocardiography is inadequate [27] to evaluate valvular insufficiency, vegetation, or thrombus in native or prosthetic valves,[28,29] to assess the presence of cardiogenic sources of emboli and specifically detect left atrial chamber and appendage thrombi and spontaneous echo contrast,[30–32] atheromatous plaques in the ascending aorta, interatrial septum abnormalities[33–35] such as patent foramen ovale or aneurysm, and tumors; TEE is also clearly superior to other imaging modalities in the detection of endocarditis[36–39] and aortic dissection.[40] Fur-

TABLE 2-1   TEE Technology

Strengths	Weaknesses	Future Directions
Single-plane TEE • Improved imaging of cardiac structures as compared to transthoracic approach in technically difficult patients • Increased diagnostic sensitivity and utility in almost all varieties of cardiovascular disorders	• Incomplete visualization of cardio-vascular structures	
Biplane TEE • Imaging in two orthogonal planes yields better morphologic information as compared to single-plane TEE	• Significant amount of flexion and rotation is necessary to derive imaging planes in between transverse and longitudinal planes • Suboptimal structure visualization	• Smaller-sized probes
Multiplane TEE • Better understanding of spatial relationship of the structures • Recognition of the most useful imaging planes • Less discomfort to patient compared to biplane TEE • Less flexion and rotation necessary • Shorter examination time		• Smaller-sized probes • Higher-frequency MPTEE • 3D reconstruction • Panoramic imaging field
Panoramic TEE • Better visual perspective of anatomy: aortic arch, entire left atrium, complex congenital heart disease • Better detection of paracardiac, pericardial, and extracardiac diseases	• Single-plane imaging	• Multiplane panoramic TEE • Improved resolution • 3D reconstruction
3D TEE • Better assessment of anatomy: ventricular geometry and function, MV, eccentric regurgitation, and mitral valve prolapse		• Improved resolution and data processing

thermore, better delineation of cardiovascular disorders or their complications can often be obtained with TEE, as with assessment of the severity of valvular disease by visualization of the valve (planimetry of stenosed aortic valve) and subvalvular apparatus (mitral valve), evaluation of regurgitant flow (particularly eccentric types), and hemodynamic consequence of the disorder (pulmonary venous blood flow, for instance). Similarly, better evaluation of pericardial and congenital heart diseases is possible with TEE. Finally, it is a very useful tool intraoperatively to monitor ventricular function and preload status and to evaluate surgical results.

Echo-Anatomic Correlations and Clinical Applications of Multiplane TEE

Continuous visualization of the cardiac structures as the ultrasound beam is steered through the arc allows a more reliable appraisal of any given abnormality (Fig. 2-5). Initial screening of cardiac anatomy allows recognition of the most useful imaging planes that would help in providing the maximum information (Figs. 2-6 and 2-7). There is thus greater diagnostic

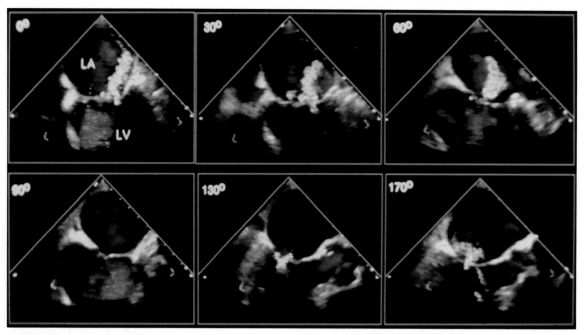

Figure 2-5
Enhanced delineation of mitral regurgitation provided by multiplane TEE as the array is steered. LA = left atrium; LV = left ventricle.

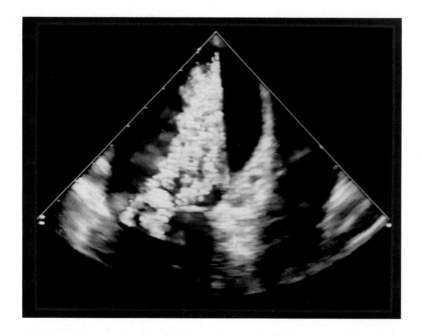

Figure 2-6
An off-axis view reveals two mitral regurgitation jets. One of these jets is associated with valvular fenestration. These abnormalities were more clearly delineated in this view than in the conventional transverse and longitudinal views in this particular patient.

assurance in the detection and delineation or exclusion of cardiac lesions. Moreover, considerably less flexion and rotation is necessary with multiplane than with biplane TEE, and the examination time is also shorter, leading to less discomfort to the patient. Although different array rotations can be suggested for visualizing various structures, optimal angles at which specific elements and their related disorders are best assessed vary between pa-

Figure 2-7
Multiplane TEE images from a patient with atrial septal defect. The defect is clearly depicted only in certain views. LA = left atrium; LV = left ventricle; RA = right atrium; RV = right ventricle.

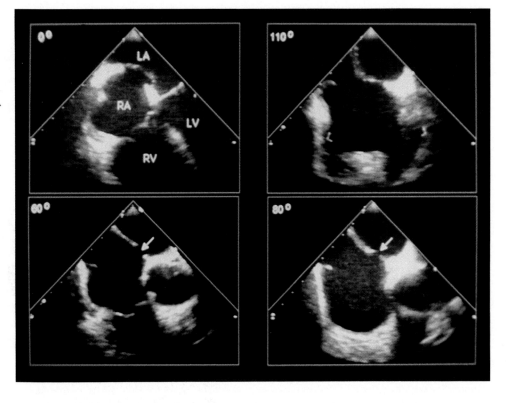

tients. Thus the most productive imaging planes for a given pathology in an individual patient must be used. A complete cardiac examination is accomplished by systematic acquisition of ultrasound images in various planes at different levels in the esophagus and gastric fundus. The sequence in which the different views are obtained varies with the clinical indication for TEE. Generally, the best approach is to start at the transesophageal level when valvular or aortic disease has to be evaluated and start with transgastric imaging for the assessment of left ventricular function. The planes of sections used to image the heart and thoracic aorta will be described.

Transgastric Imaging

Proximal Transgastric Views

Starting at 0°, variable amount of anteflexion and advancement of the probe will result in serial short-axis views of the ventricles, particularly at the mitral valve (MV) and papillary muscle (PM) levels (Fig. 2-8). The left ventricle (LV) is then displayed on the viewer's right, with the inferoposterior walls of both ventricles at the top of the monitor and the anterior walls at the bottom. As the ultrasound beam is steered to 40 to 60° while imaging the left heart, the basal lateral wall is visualized on the right and the distal interventricular septum on the left. A two-chamber view ensues at 90°, with the apex of the left ventricle on the viewer's left and left atrium on the right. The inferior wall, posteromedial papillary muscle, and posterior leaflet of the mitral valve are displayed on top and the anterior wall, anteromedial PM, and anterior MV leaflet at the bottom. Chordal structures are often also best evaluated in this view, and this is particularly useful in patients with rheumatic mitral valve disease, chordal rupture, or chordal vegetations. Furthermore, papillary muscle pathology can be more clearly delineated, as in patients with papillary muscle rupture or papillary muscle based masses. A long-axis image of the left ventricle is seen starting at about 120°, with the posterior wall noted on the upper part of the screen and the anterior septum, LV outflow tract, and aortic valve below. This long-axis view enables one to obtain the maximum aortic flow velocity. Orientation of 180° results in a

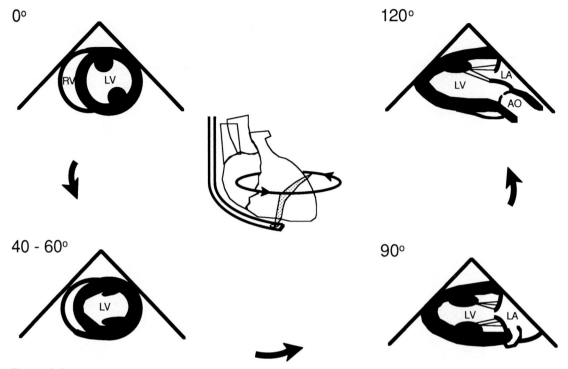

Figure 2-8
Schematic diagram showing representative sections of the left heart that can be obtained at the transgastric level by multiplane TEE as the array is steered. AO = aorta; LA = left atrium; LV = left ventricle; RV = right ventricle.

mirror image of the initial view, the left ventricle now being depicted on the viewer's left.

Serial planes of the right heart are obtained after initially centering the right ventricle (RV) in short axis while imaging at 0° (Fig. 2-9). All three leaflets of the tricuspid valve (TV) are visualized as the array is steered to 30°. The anterior leaflet is seen at the bottom, and a portion of the aorta adjoining the right atrium is brought into view as well. Further steering of the beam to about 80° yields the RV inflow view, displaying the right ventricle on the viewer's left and right atrium on the opposite side. The RV outflow region is visualized on the viewer's left in addition to the RV inflow at about 110°, as well as the superior vena cavae, which is seen on the viewer's right. As the array is steered beyond this orientation, the right ventricular apex is brought into view.

Distal Transgastric Views
Further advancement of the probe tip while maintaining anteflexion first results in a short-

axis view of the LV apex at 0°. Serial oblique sections of the apex are then obtained as the array is steered. This is very useful for delineating regional contraction abnormalities of the left ventricular apex and apical thrombi. Passage of the transducer tip farther into the stomach using maximum anteflexion yields the deep transgastric view, which is in fact similar to a transthoracic apical five-chamber view with the apex displayed on top, the atria at the bottom, and the left ventricle on the viewer's right. While the LV inflow and outflow regions can be evaluated in this plane of section, the left ventricle is commonly foreshortened.

Imaging from the Gastroesophageal Junction
Probe withdrawal to the gastroesophageal junction with clockwise rotation and ultrasound beam at 0° allows imaging of the right heart, coronary sinus, and its junction with the right atrium (Fig. 2-10). The anterior and septal leaflets of the tricuspid valve are seen, respec-

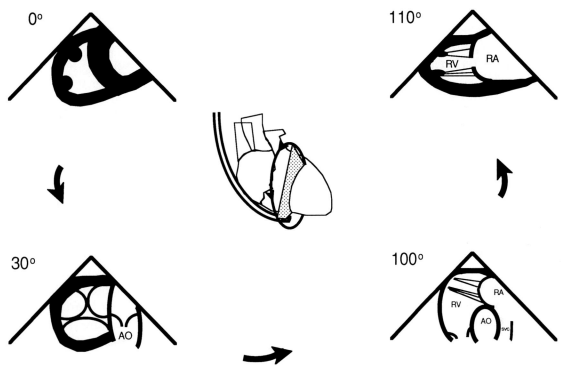

Figure 2-9
Schematic diagram showing representative sections of the right heart that can be obtained at the transgastric level by multiplane TEE. AO = aorta; RA = right atrium; RV = right ventricle; SVC = superior vena cava.

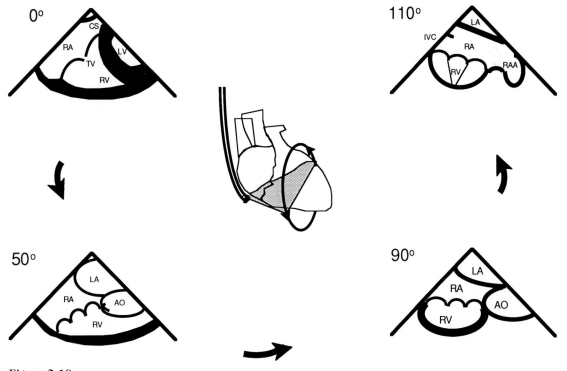

Figure 2-10
Schematic diagram showing some representative sections of the heart that can be obtained at the gastroesophageal junction or lower esophageal level. AO = aorta; CS = coronary sinus; IVC = inferior vena cava; LA = left atrium; LV = left ventricle; RA = right atrium; RAA = right atrial appendage; RV = right ventricle; TV = tricuspid valve.

tively, at the bottom left and top right of the image in this view. As the array is steered to 50 to 60°, the lower portion of the interatrial septum and posterior and septal leaflets of the tricuspid valve can be evaluated. At 90° orientation, the predominant portion of the tricuspid valve noted is the anterior leaflet. Further steering of the beam to 110° allows imaging of the right atrial appendage with superior vena cavae above it on the viewer's right and the inferior vena cavae and eustachian valve on the opposite side. Thus right heart anatomy is uniquely demonstrated by multiplane TEE, and this is useful in the assessment of various abnormalities such as tricuspid valve vegetations and masses, right atrial tumors and thrombi, tricuspid regurgitation, and right ventricular global or regional dysfunction.

Imaging from the Lower Esophagus

Imaging at this level with the transducer array at 0° yields a four-chamber view, with the left heart on the viewer's right, apex at the bottom, and atria on top (Fig. 2-11). Retroflexion is often required in this view to avoid foreshortening of the left ventricle. The midportion of the interventricular septum is seen between the LV and RV lateral walls which are respectively noted on the viewer's right and left. The anterior leaflet of the mitral valve is adjacent to the septum and the posterior leaflet is seen laterally. Likewise, anterior and septal leaflets of the tricuspid valve are respectively noted laterally and medially (Fig. 2-4). Clockwise rotation of the probe results in better visualization of the interatrial septum, which can be scanned by slowly advancing and withdrawing the probe and by steering the ultrasound beam. Abnormalities such as tumors (e.g., myxoma) and atrial septal defects (Fig. 2-7) are more precisely assessed as the ultrasound beam is steered with multiplane TEE. The right and left lower pulmonary veins are brought into view respectively by clockwise and counterclockwise rotation of the probe; color flow imaging can help in correctly identifying these

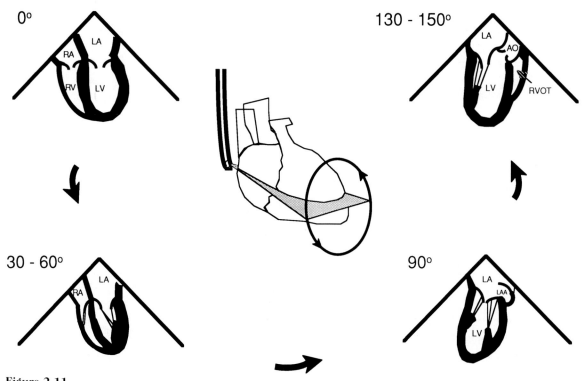

Figure 2-11
Schematic diagram showing some representative sections of the heart that can be obtained from the esophagus by multiplane TEE. AO = aorta; LA = left atrium; LAA = left atrial appendage; LV = left ventricle; RA = right atrium; RV = right ventricle; RVOT = right ventricular outflow tract.

veins. Reversal of the normal systolic pulmonary venous flow is found in patients with severe mitral regurgitation, but blunting of this component is also encountered in patients with mitral stenosis or left ventricular dysfunction. At approximately 35 to 45° (Fig. 2-11), more of the anterior mitral leaflet is seen on the viewer's left and the anterolateral scallop of the posterior leaflet is seen on the right. As the array is steered to 30 to 60°, the LV anterolateral wall, inferior septum, and posterior RV free wall are observed. Further steering of the ultrasound beam to 90° results in a two-chamber view, with the anterior wall of the left ventricle on the viewer's right and the inferior wall on the opposite side. With the array at 90 to 110° orientation, different planes of the mitral valve can be displayed by using various movements of the probe tip, which can result in visualization of either two distinct leaflets or only the posterior leaflet with its scalloped appearance (anterolateral and posteromedial scallops, respectively, on the viewer's right and left, with middle scallop in the center). Numerous views of the mitral valve can also be obtained as the array is steered. The left atrial appendage can commonly be seen at 90° orientation adjoining the base of the anterior wall, with the left upper pulmonary vein above and to the right. These two structures are separated by a muscular ridge. Counterclockwise rotation of the probe tip at this level allows visualization of the upper and lower left pulmonary veins draining into the left atrium, respectively, from the right and left of the screen. Clockwise rotation of the probe at 90° orientation will result in successive views already described with biplane TEE longitudinal imaging, which are the RV inflow-outflow view, ascending aorta–interatrial septum view, and vena cavae–interatrial septum view. Further clockwise rotation allows visualization of the right upper and lower pulmonary veins on the viewer's right and left. After initially centering the left heart in the sector, the long-axis view is displayed at 120 to 150° orientation. The anterior septum, LV outflow region, aortic valve, and RV free wall are seen on the right of the screen while LV posterior wall is noted on the viewer's left. This imaging plane is

particularly useful to delineate specific abnormalities such as aortic regurgitation, subaortic obstruction, or a posterobasal aneurysm.

Forward flexion of the probe tip or slight withdrawal of the probe yields a five-chamber view with the aortic valve cut in a tangential manner (Fig. 2-12). Steering the ultrasound beam to 30 to 60° yields a short-axis view of the aortic valve without requiring significant lateral flexion. Reliable determination of the aortic valve area by planimetry is possible at this orientation (Fig. 2-13).[41] Other abnormalities such as aortic regurgitation or vegetation can also be further assessed. The right coronary cusp is seen at the bottom, the left coronary cusp above and to the viewer's right, and the noncoronary cusp above and to the viewer's left. The RV inflow and outflow regions as well as the tricuspid and pulmonic valves are noted and can be evaluated as the array is steered to 60 to 100° orientation. Further steering of the array beyond this orientation results in a long-axis view of the ascending aorta arising from the aortic valve. Better delineation of lesions of these structures is possible as the array is steered.

Imaging from the Upper Esophagus

Serial transverse images of the base of the heart are seen with withdrawal and anteflexion of the probe tip (Fig. 2-14). At 0° orientation, the aortic valve is seen in a tangential presentation with the RV outflow region noted below. Adequate short-axis view of the aortic valve can be obtained with right lateral flexion of the probe tip but is more easily obtained by steering the array to 30°. Slight probe withdrawal at 0° orientation displays the ascending aorta in short axis above the pulmonic valve cut in an oblique manner. Fine adjustments of the localization of the probe tip along with steering of the beam allow visualization of variable portions of the left main coronary artery and its bifurcation into the circumflex artery posteriorly and the left anterior descending artery anteriorly. The left atrium is seen behind the aorta, the SVC and right atrial appendage on the viewer's left. Further withdrawal of the probe tip or forward flexion brings into view the left atrial appendage and left

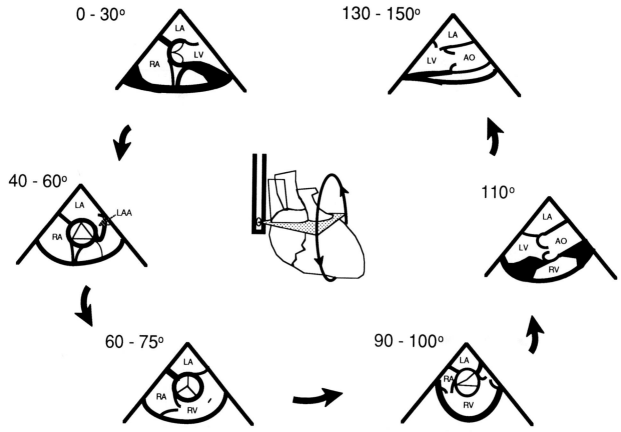

Figure 2-12
Schematic diagram showing some representative sections of the aortic valve and right ventricular outflow region that can be obtained from the esophagus by multiplane TEE. AO = aorta; LA = left atrium; LAA = left atrial appendage; LV = left ventricle; RA = right atrium; RV = right ventricle.

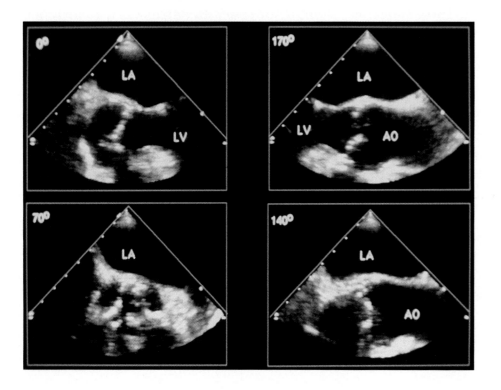

Figure 2-13
Multiplane TEE images from a patient with thickened, stenotic aortic valve. Steering of the array provides views of the aortic valve in short- and long-axis orientations. AO = aorta; LA = left atrium; LV = left ventricle.

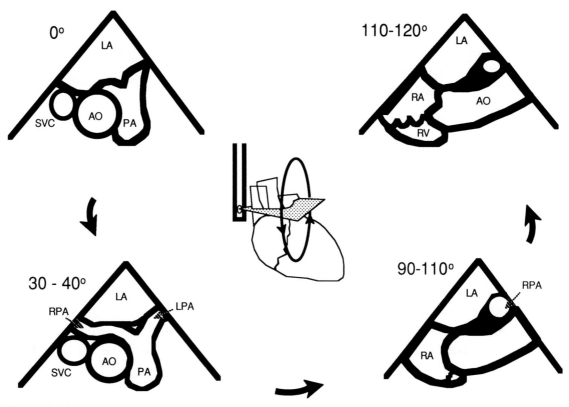

Figure 2-14
Schematic diagram showing some representative sections of the aorta and pulmonary artery that can be obtained from the upper esophagus by multiplane TEE. AO = aorta; LA = left atrium; LPA = left pulmonary artery; PA = pulmonary artery; RA = right atrium; RPA = right pulmonary artery; RV = right ventricle; SVC = superior vena cava.

upper pulmonary vein above it on the viewer's right. A multitude of imaging planes of the left atrial chamber and appendage are available as the array is steered from 0 to 180°, and this is especially useful in the detection and delineation or exclusion of thrombi and tumors. The right upper pulmonary vein is noted after clockwise rotation on the viewer's left just above the SVC. The right lower pulmonary vein can sometimes be seen in this orientation at the top left of the screen. As the probe is withdrawn further, the main pulmonary artery (PA) and its bifurcation into the right pulmonary artery, which is seen coursing behind the aorta, and the left pulmonary artery are displayed. Only a short section of the left pulmonary artery, coursing to the viewer's right, is seen until the view is obscured by the left main stem bronchus. Multiplane TEE provides enhanced assessment of PA abnormalities (e.g., tumors) by offering multiple imaging

planes as the array is steered. Oblique planes of section of the ascending aorta are displayed as the array is steered, until a true long-axis view is demonstrated at 110° orientation with the right pulmonary artery in short axis seen above it and proximal right coronary artery below. Steering of the ultrasound beam improves delineation of aortic dissection and atherosclerotic plaque.

Imaging of the Descending Aorta and Aortic Arch

The examination is completed with evaluation of the descending aorta and arch. Counterclockwise rotation and gradual withdrawal of the probe allows imaging of the descending aorta from the upper abdomen to the level of the aortic arch. Circular transverse images of the descending aorta are displayed at 0° orientation, followed by oblique images as the array is steered and then longitudinal planes of section at 90° orientation. Further withdrawal of the probe brings the aortic arch and its major branches into view. The ascending arch is displayed on the viewer's left at 0° orientation. Multiple orientations of images of the arch can be acquired as the ultrasound beam is steered. Multiplane TEE clearly enhances the definition of aortic lesions, particularly at the arch level.

Thus multiplane transesophageal echocardiography offers continuous visualization of the cardiovascular structures as the ultrasound beam is steered through the 180° arc, yielding numerous imaging planes. This provides the flexibility to choose the desired imaging planes that yield the maximum information (Fig. 2-15). Multiplane TEE has proved to be valuable in virtually all types of cardiac disorders by providing incremental information and by enhancing delineation of abnormalities (Table 2-1). This versatility, coupled to the ease of obtaining these imaging planes without undue probe manipulation, makes multiplane TEE

extremely useful. Addition of acoustic quantification and the potential of multiplane TEE for three-dimensional reconstruction could further increase its interest.

Panoramic TEE

The concept of visualizing structures in a wider angle than the conventional probes allow has been explored in the past. The feasibility and usefulness of single-plane panoramic TEE in various clinical settings have been recently established (Fig. 2-16).[17,18] After initially performing two-dimensional imaging at a 270° angle, the width of the field is reduced to improve the frame rate and examine regions of interest at various magnifications. A 180° color Doppler display is then superimposed on the widest two-dimensional sector and similarly reduced to examine in greater detail

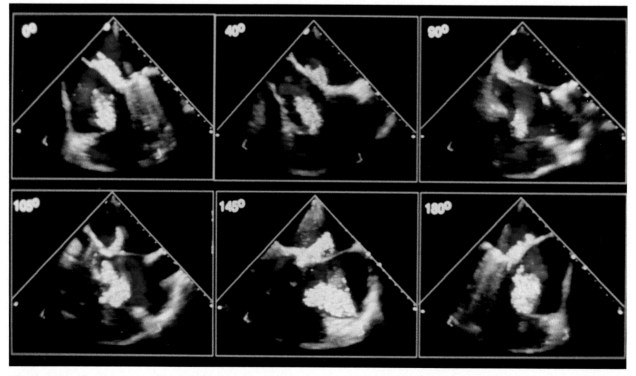

Figure 2-15
Multiplane TEE images from a patient with a mechanical prosthetic mitral valve. Enhanced delineation of the regurgitant jets from the mitral valve prosthesis and the tricuspid valve is possible as the array is steered.

Figure 2-16
Panoramic transesopha-geal two-dimensional and color Doppler im-ages showing the cardiac chambers and the de-scending thoracic aorta. AO = aorta; LA = left atrium; LV = left ventri-cle; RA = right atrium; RV = right ventricle.

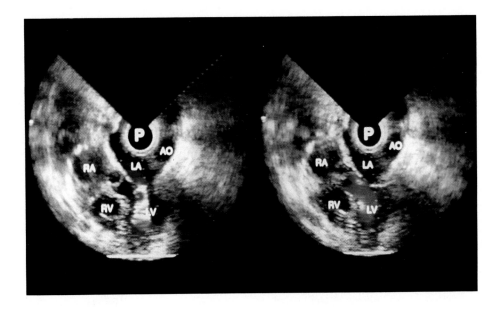

specific flow abnormalities. Spectral Doppler imaging is subsequently used.

Panoramic TEE results in better visual per-spective of cardiovascular anatomy (Table 2-1). Better evaluation of aortic disorders such as dissection and aneurysms, particularly by visu-alization of the whole arch in its transverse plane, ability to image the left atrium in its entirety, better recognition of spatial relation-ships in complex congenital diseases, and bet-ter assessment of pericardial and paracardiac abnormalities constitute some of the particular strengths of this technology. Furthermore, de-tection of extracardiac abnormalities such as mediastinal lymph nodes and masses, pleural effusions, collapsed lungs, and arteriovenous malformations is enhanced with wide-angle TEE. While a slower frame rate when using a wide sector represents a drawback, initial experience with panoramic TEE is encouraging and suggests clinical potential.

3D Reconstruction, Acoustic Quantification, and TEE

Until recently, three-dimensional (3D) evalua-tion required mental reconstruction of multiple two-dimensional images. Proper assessment of cardiovascular anatomy and pathology would be simplified if a method would provide objec-tive 3D reconstruction.[19–22] Diagnostic capabil-ity is further enhanced by visualization of the dynamic motion [four-dimensional (4D) imaging] of these three-dimensional images. Adequate temporal and spatial registrations of the images are crucial to achieve 3D and 4D reconstruction of images. Respiration and ECG-gated images contribute to temporal regis-tration. Different approaches have been devel-oped for appropriate spatial registration while using TEE. Fanlike scanning at predetermined angles and rotational scanning with multiplane TEE are promising avenues for 3D recon-struction.

Another method is to perform equidistant parallel slicing of the heart by pull-back scan-ning. A 5-MHz, 64-element, phased-array sin-gle-plane TEE probe that integrates 2D imaging and 3D reconstruction capabilities has recently been developed (Fig. 2-17). This probe is inter-faced to a computed tomographic ultrasound system capable of 3D and 4D data acquisition and processing. After intial diagnostic imaging, the distal portion of the probe, which consists of multiple semicircular segments lined on two cables, is straightened to form a rigid tube. The transducer is then pulled back within the carriage in 1-mm increments by means of a

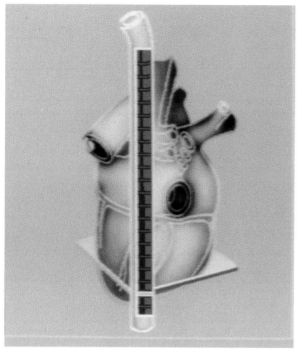

Figure 2-17
Single-plane TEE probe that integrates 2D imaging and 3D reconstruction capabilities. The distal portion of the probe can be straightened and the transducer then pulled back within the carriage.

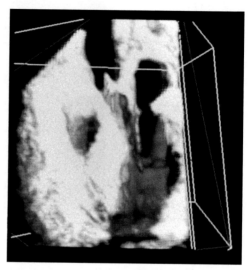

Figure 2-18
Three-dimensional display of the left heart.

computer-controlled motor. Images are recorded at each level during a complete cardiac cycle and then processed to yield 3D and 4D reconstruction as well as visualization of the heart in any desired dynamic plane of section (Fig. 2-18). Data acquisition is limited to a few minutes. Three-dimensional reconstruction will likely be of value for better assessment of ventricular geometry and function, and better evaluation of complex structures like the mitral valve or abnormalities such as eccentric regurgitation or mitral valve prolapse. Thus recent advances suggest that three- and four-dimensional imaging will be useful adjuncts to TEE.

Acoustic quantification (AQ) consists of automated border extraction based on integrated backscatter analysis, in which unprocessed acoustic signals are analyzed to detect interfaces between tissue and blood along every scan line of every frame in real time.[23] This enables calculation of total blood area, fractional area change, and time rate of area change within a user-defined region of interest in real-

time imaging. Work currently in progress will help to demonstrate whether this technology can provide reliable on-line derivations of left ventricular volume and ejection fraction using the multiple-disk method in patients. The feasibility of quantitative volumetric evaluation of regional abnormalities such as LV aneurysms is also being investigated. While major errors can result with inappropriate use of technical controls such as TGC and imaging planes, they can easily be corrected and optimized with care in the use of AQ. This new technology is a major step in quantitative echocardiography to study abnormal ventricles and to recognize changes over time.

Other Emerging Advances

Intravascular ultrasound (IVUS) and intracardiac echocardiography (ICE) are evolving catheter-based methods that use miniaturized ultrasound crystals interfaced to an ultrasound console to image vessels and cardiac structures.[42-45] Because low-frequency catheters have greater depths of field for imaging but less resolution, 10- to 20-MHz transducers carried by 6 to 10 French catheters are used for ICE and 20 to 35-MHz transducers with 3.5 to 9 F catheters are employed for IVUS imaging. These devices use either mechanical or phased-array systems. One of the several types of mechanical systems has a small ultrasound element affixed to the tip of a drive shaft and encased within a catheter. A motor rotates the drive shaft and transducer at 900 rpm. The processed signals are displayed as circular images at 15 frames per second on a monitor. Other designs of mechanical systems use a deflecting mirror, which can be either rotating with a fixed ultrasound element or fixed when the transducer is rotated by a motor. A phased-array instrument uses up to 64 elements activated electronically in sequence and carried by 3.5 to 7.8 F catheters. Because no rotating component is required with this multielement system, the central lumen of the catheter can be used for guidewires or for fluid injection. Instruments that combine ultrasound and other capabilities such as balloon angioplasty catheter, atherectomy device, or fiberoptic angioscopy are being developed to aid in the performance of interventional procedures.

Intravascular Ultrasound

Coronary and Peripheral Arteries

While TEE allows limited evaluation of coronary arteries, IVUS yields detailed images of coronary artery anatomy by providing circular, high-resolution cross sections in real time. Using IVUS imaging, reliable quantitation of arterial luminal area, wall thickness, plaque thickness, and arterial stenosis can be performed, and composition of the plaque can be identified (fatty, fibrous, or calcific). Complex lesions can be identified and intimal flaps, dissection, and intraarterial clots can be demonstrated. This technique is also a useful tool to identify atherosclerosis in angiographically normal arterial segments and to unmask left main coronary stenosis. Evolving applications of intravascular ultrasound include the study of regression of atherosclerosis, assessment of vasomotor function, and better evaluation of various catheter-based interventions. IVUS will

likely become the gold standard in the assessment of coronary and peripheral arterial pathology.

Aorta and pulmonary arteries

Intravascular imaging has been found to be useful in evaluation of aortic disease such as atheromatous disease, dissection, and coarctation. Atherosclerotic disease of the aorta and its major branches presents a similar spectrum of abnormalities on IVUS images as seen in other vessels. Detection and delineation of the extent of aortic dissection is possible with IVUS, and the contents of the true and false lumen and branch involvement can be identified as well. Nevertheless, IVUS cannot be considered more useful than TEE as a clinical tool to evaluate aortic dissection. In patients with aortic coarctation, IVUS imaging helps in evaluation of its severity and in the assessment of balloon dilatation results.

IVUS catheters can be safely introduced into the pulmonary arteries to image proximal and distal segments. Structural and functional changes in the pulmonary vasculature associated with pulmonary hypertension can be evaluated with IVUS imaging. Validation of IVUS images with histology and anatomic measurements is currently in progress, in terms of intimal proliferation and fibrosis, medial hypertrophy, muscularization of nonmuscularized arteries, and plexiform and thrombotic lesions. Thus this approach could aid in assessing the state of reversibility of pulmonary hypertension, study vasomotor function, and ultimately provide a fundamental basis for possible clinical studies of its pathogenesis, evolution, and treatment. Promising results also suggest a role for intravascular ultrasound in depicting pulmonary embolism and assessing peripheral pulmonary artery stenosis.

Intracardiac Echocardiography

ICE catheters can be used in different cardiac chambers to visualize cardiac structures in real time. Several cardiac diseases have been identified with these catheters, such as interatrial septum abnormalities, pericardial effusion, and pulmonic stenosis. While catheters with 20-MHz transducers yield high-resolution

22

images of chamber walls, interatrial septum, ostium of the coronary sinus, and portions of the valves, the depth of the imaging field is too restricted to allow adequate visualization of cardiac chambers or valves. Catheters bearing low-frequency (10- and 12.5-MHz) elements have recently been developed and appear capable of providing images similar to TEE. Retrograde catheterization is currently required for better imaging of the left side of the heart. Although the present clinical use of ICE is limited, early experience indicates that low-frequency catheters can provide high-resolution images of cardiac chambers and valves and could help to delineate valvular, myocardial, and pericardial disorders when conventional imaging methods are difficult or inadequate. Potential applications of intracardiac echocardiography include monitoring of ventricular function during coronary interventions or bypass surgery, guidance during interventions such as transseptal catheterization, valvuloplasty, occluder placements for atrial or ventricular septal defects, or ablation procedures for arrhythmias, and assessment of efficacy and complications of surgery.

Future Directions

Many major advances have made TEE a powerful diagnostic tool. Incorporation of color and spectral Doppler modalities and development of biplane, multiplane, and panoramic imaging have increased the versatility of this technique. Three-dimensional and four-dimensional reconstructions of the ventricles and valves, using rotational and fanlike scanning with multiplane TEE, a computed tomographic imaging probe, panoramic TEE, or intracardiac echocardiography, hold out great promise to provide clinically applicable information. Faster 3D image acquisition and reconstruction would strengthen its clinical potential. Further validation of acoustic quantification in relation to ventricular area, volume, and ejection fraction is in progress. Development of a panoramic multiplane TEE can also be contemplated. Use of stress TEE could be of valuable help to the

clinician as well. Development of even smaller probes capable of being used in premature infants and of pediatric-sized multiplane and panoramic TEE will offer additional information. Miniaturization of intravascular imaging devices, refinement of combination devices, development of forward-looking instruments, and on-line three-dimensional vascular imaging will also be highly useful. Low-frequency devices are also necessary for whole heart imaging from the venous side. Three-dimensional reconstruction and acoustic quantification of intracardiac images, and ICE assessment of myocardial perfusion, constitute some of the concepts for future developments of intracardiac echocardiography. Further research work and refinements will play an important role in expanding the horizons of echocardiography.

References

1. Frazin L, Talano JV, Stephanides L, et al: Esophageal echocardiography. *Circulation* 54:102, 1976.
2. Hisanaga K, Hisanaga A, Nagata K, et al: A new transesophageal real-time two-dimensional echocardiographic system using a flexible tube and its clinical application. *Proc Jpn Soc Ultrason Med* 32:43, 1977.
3. Hisanaga K, Hisanaga A, Hibi N, et al: High speed rotating scanner for transesophageal cross-sectional echocardiography. *Am J Cardiol* 46:837, 1980.
4. Hanrath P, Kremer P, Langestein BA, et al: Transosophageale Echokardiographie: Ein neues Verfahren zur dynamischen Ventrikelfunktions-analyse. *Dtsch Med Wochenschr* 106:523, 1981.
5. Matsumoto M, Oka Y, Strom J, et al: Application of transesophageal echocardiography to continuous intraoperative monitoring of left ventricular performance. *Am J Cardiol* 46:95, 1980.
6. Souquet J, Hanrath P, Zitelli L, et al: Transesophageal phased array for imaging the heart. *IEEE Trans Biomed Eng* 29:707, 1982.
7. Schluter M, Hinrichs A, Thier W, et al: Transesophageal two-dimensional echocardiography: Comparison of ultrasonic and anatomic sections. *Am J Cardiol* 53:1173, 1984.
8. Matsuzaki M, Ikee Y, Yorozu T: Clinical appli-

cation of esophageal echocardiography to the mitral valve prolapse syndrome. *Proc Jpn J Med Ultrason* 31:89, 1977.

9. Thier W, Schluter M, Kremer P, et al: Transesophageal 2-dimensional echocardiography: Better demonstration of intra-atrial structures. *Dtsch Med Wochenschr* 108:1903, 1983.

10. Seward JB, Khanderia BK, Edwards WD, et al: Biplanar transesophageal echocardiography: Anatomic correlations, image orientation, and clinical applications. *Mayo Clin Proc* 65:1193, 1990.

11. Richardson SG, Weintraub AR, Schwartz SL, et al: Biplane transesophageal echocardiography utilizing transverse and sagittal imaging planes. *Echocardiography* 8:293, 1991.

12. Omoto R, Kyo S, Matsumura M, et al: New direction of biplane transesophageal echocardiography with special emphasis on real-time biplane imaging and matrix phased-array biplane transducer. *Echocardiography* 7:691, 1990.

13. Nanda NC, Pinheiro L, Sanyal RS, et al: Transesophageal biplane echocardiographic imaging: Technique, planes and clinical usefulness. *Echocardiography* 7:771, 1990.

14. Bansal RC, Shakudo M, Shah PM, et al: Biplane transesophageal echocardiography: Technique, image orientation and preliminary experience in 131 patients. *J Am Soc Echocardiogr* 3:348, 1990.

15. Flachskampf FA, Hoffmann R, Verlande M, et al: Initial experience with a multiplane transesophageal transducer: Assessment of diagnostic potential. *Eur Heart J* 13:1201, 1992.

16. Pandian NG, Hsu TL, Schwartz SL, et al: Multiplane transesophageal echocardiography. Imaging planes, echocardiographic anatomy, and clinical experience with a prototype phased array omniplane probe. *Echocardiography* 9:649, 1992.

17. Roelandt JRTC, Thomson IR, Vletter WB, et al: Multiplane transesophageal echocardiography: Latest evolution in an imaging revolution. *J Am Soc Echocardiogr* 5:361, 1992.

18. Hsu TL, Weintraub AR, Ritter SB, et al: Panoramic transesophageal echocardiography. *Echocardiography* 8:677, 1991.

19. Wollschlager H, Zeiher AM, Klein HP: Transesophageal echo computer tomography: A new method for dynamic 3D imaging of the heart (abstract). *Circulation* 80:II-569, 1989.

20. Pandian NG, Nanda NC, Schwartz SL, et al: Three-dimensional and four-dimensional transesophageal echocardiographic imaging of the heart and aorta in humans using a computed tomographic imaging probe. *Echocardiography* 9:677, 1992.

21. Azevedo J, Chapman J, Angelsen B, et al: 3-dimensional reconstruction of the left ventricular cavity from transthoracic and multiplane transesophageal echocardiograms within minutes after echo examination. *Circulation* 86: I-529, 1992.

22. Fulton D, Pandian NG, Wollschlager H, et al: Dynamic three-dimensional echocardiographic imaging of congenital heart defects in infants and children by computer-controlled tomographic parallel slicing using a single integrated ultrasound instrument. *Circulation* 86:I-498, 1992.

23. Cao QL, Azevedo J, Hsu TL, et al: Realtime automated border detection and acoustic quantification in biplane and multiplane transesophageal echocardiography and factor influencing its accuracy. *Circulation* 86:I-263, 1992.

24. Weintraub A, Richardson G, Hsu TL, et al: Multiplane transesophageal echocardiography with improvised manipulation of a biplane transesophageal echocardiography probe: Newer imaging planes, echo-anatomic correlations and clinical applications. *J Am Soc Echocardiogr* 4:277, 1991.

25. Ritter SB, Thys D: Pediatric transesophageal color flow imaging: Smaller probes for smaller hearts. *Echocardiography* 6:431, 1989.

26. Stumper OFW, Elzenga NJ, Hess J, et al: Transesophageal echocardiography in children with congenital heart disease: An initial experience. *J Am Coll Cardiol* 16:433, 1990.

27. Matsuzaki M, Toma Y, Kusukawa R: Clinical applications of transesophageal echocardiography. *Circulation* 82:709, 1990.

28. Nellessen U, Schnittger I, Appleton CP, et al: Transesophageal two-dimensional echocardiography and color Doppler flow velocity mapping in the evaluation of cardiac valve prostheses. *Circulation* 78:848, 1988.

29. Taams MA, Gussenhoven EJ, Calahan MK, et al: Transesophageal Doppler color flow imaging in the detection of native and Björk-Shiley mitral valve regurgitation. *J Am Coll Cardiol* 13:95, 1989.

30. Aschenberg W, Schluter M, Kremer P, et al: Transesophageal two-dimensional echocardiography for the detection of left atrial thrombus. *J Am Coll Cardiol* 7:163, 1986.

31. Daniel WG, Nellessen U, Schröder E, et al: Left atrial spontaneous echo contrast in mitral valve disease: An indicator for an increased thromboembolic risk. *J Am Coll Cardiol* 11:1204, 1988.

32. Taams MA, Gussenhoven EJ, Lancée CT: Left atrial vascularized thrombus diagnosed by transesophageal cross-sectional echocardiography. *Br Heart J* 58:669, 1987.

33. Hanrath P, Schluter M, Langenstein BA, et al: Detection of ostium secundum atrial septal defects by transesophageal cross-sectional echocardiography. *Br Heart J* 49:350, 1983.

34. Mügge A, Daniel WG, Klopper JW, et al: Visualization of patent foramen ovale by transesophageal color-coded Doppler echocardiography. *Am J Cardiol* 62:837, 1988.

35. Yoshida K, Yoshikawa J, Akasaka T, et al: Assessment of left-to-right atrial shunting after precutaneous mitral valvuloplasty by transesophageal color Doppler flow-mapping. *Circulation* 80:1521, 1989.

36. Geibel A, Hofmann T, Berhoz A, et al: Echocardiographic diagnosis of infective endocarditis—Additional information by transesophageal echocardiography. *Circulation* 76:IV-38, 1987.

37. Daniel WG, Schroder E, Mugge A, et al: Transesophageal echocardiography in infective endocarditis. *Am J Cardiac Imag* 2:78, 1988.

38. Erbel R, Rohmann S, Drexler M, et al: Improved diagnostic value of echocardiography in patients with infective endocarditis by transesophageal approach: A prospective study. *Eur Heart J* 9:43, 1988.

39. Daniel WG, Mugge A, Martin RP, et al: Improvement in the diagnosis of abscesses associated with endocarditis by transesophageal echocardiography. *N Engl J Med* 324:795, 1991.

40. Erbel R, Engberding R, Daniel W: Echocardiography in diagnosis of aortic dissection. *Lancet* 1:457, 1989.

41. Hoffman R, Flaschkampf FA, Hanrath P: Planimetry of stenotic aortic valve area using multiplane transesophageal echocardiography. *Circulation* 84:II-129, 1991.

42. Pandian NG: Intravascular and intracardiac ultrasound imaging. An old concept, now on the road to reality. *Circulation* 80:1091, 1989.

43. Pandian NG, Hsu TL: Intravascular ultrasound and intracardiac echocardiography: Concepts for the future. *Am J Cardiol* 69:6H, 1992.

44. Pandian NG, Kumar R, Katz SE, et al: Real-time, intracardiac, two-dimensional echocardiography. Enhanced depth of field with a low-frequency ultrasound catheter. *Echocardiography* 8:407, 1991.

45. Schwartz SL, Gillam LD, Weintraub AR, et al: Intracardiac echocardiography in humans using a small-sized, low-frequency (12.5 MHz) ultrasound catheter. *J Am Coll Cardiol* 21:189, 1993.

3

Intubation of the Upper Gastrointestinal Tract: Methodological, Anatomical, and Safety Considerations

Gerald Maurer
Edward Share

Safety Record— Gastrointestinal and TEE Experience

During recent years, transesophageal echocardiography (TEE) has become firmly established as a valuable diagnostic tool that is widely used by cardiologists throughout the world.[1,2] While TEE appears to be very safe,[3,4] it is nevertheless an invasive procedure with potential risks and with some discomfort to the patient. Because of its similarity to upper gastrointestinal endoscopy in terms of both instrumentation and probe manipulation, its risks and complications can be expected to be quite similar.

Flexible upper gastrointestinal fiberoptic, and subsequently videoendoscopy, have been performed since approximately 1970 and have been tolerated well, with only relatively few complications.[5] The largest study that evaluated these complications is a survey conducted by the American Society for Gastrointestinal

Endoscopy in 1974.[6] A total of 211,410 upper gastrointestinal endoscopic examinations were anonymously reported by 404 endoscopists. There were 70 perforations (0.03 percent), with 3 deaths (0.001 percent) from perforation. The majority of perforations occurred in the cervical esophagus, with fewer in the distal esophagus and stomach. There were 129 cardiopulmonary complications (0.06 percent). Considering the improvements in instrumentation and in technique since 1974, one might assume current complication rates to be even lower.

Compared to gastrointestinal endoscopy, TEE studies were initially thought to conceivably carry a higher risk, since they are performed by cardiologists with limited experience in endoscopic techniques, since they are often done in patients with severe cardiac diseases, and since the probe lacks the direct optical control. In an effort to assess the safety of TEE, a survey of 15 European centers performing TEE studies for at least 1 year was undertaken.[7]

25

TABLE 3-1   Reasons for TEE Study Interruption Before Completion [90 of 10,218 Examinations (0.88 Percent) with Successful TEE Probe Insertion]

	Patients (n)
Intolerance of TEE probe	65
Pulmonary complications	
Bronchospasm	6
Hypoxia	2
Cardiac complications	
Nonsustained ventricular tachycardia	3
Transient atrial fibrillation	3
Third-degree atrioventricular block	1
Severe angina pectoris	1
Bleeding complications	
Minor pharyngeal bleeding	1
Severe hematemesis due to malignant tumor; death on same day	1
Others	
Vomiting	5
TEE probe defect	2

Reproduced with permission. Daniel W, Erbel R, Kasper W, et al: Safety of transesophageal echocardiography: A multicenter survey of 10,419 examinations. *Circulation* 83:817, 1991. Copyright 1991, American Heart Association.

At the time of the survey, 10,419 studies had been performed by these institutions. There was only 1 death from bleeding complications resulting from a malignant lung tumor with esophageal infiltration. Thus, in this large series, the mortality rate for TEE was only 0.0098 percent. In 201 cases (1.9 percent), attempted insertion of the TEE probe was unsuccessful, because of poor patient cooperation or lack of operator experience (98.5 percent) or because of anatomical reasons (1.5 percent). The vast majority of these patients did not receive intravenous sedation, as is customary in the United States. With such sedation the success rate of probe insertion would have been even higher, although one may conceivably have faced an increase of complications related to the medications themselves. In 90 patients (0.88 percent) with successful probe insertion the examination had to be interrupted (Table 3-1) because of the patient's intolerance to the echoscope, because of pulmonary, cardiac, or bleeding complications, or for other reasons. In the United States, a review of 3827 TEE studies performed at the Mayo Clinic showed

the overall rate of minor and major complications to be 2.9 percent.[8] Major complications occurred in only 0.2 percent, and there was only 1 death (mortality rate 0.026 percent). Thus these surveys document similar low complication rates for upper gastrointestinal endoscopy and for TEE and demonstrate the safety of these procedures.

Training Requirements and Credentialing for TEE

Transesophageal echocardiography is a highly specialized procedure that should only be performed by physicians. Furthermore, these physicians should have undergone special training (Table 3-2), as recommended by the American Society of Echocardiography,[9] since considerable skills are needed to perform this procedure (Table 3-3). A sound knowledge of conventional echocardiography should be attained prior to training in TEE. The level of expertise should be at least equivalent to level II training in general echocardiography.[10] This training level requires the performance and primary interpretation (with proper supervision) of at least 300 general echocardiographic studies over a period of approximately 6 months or the achievement of an equivalent level of experience. Subsequently, probe passage and manipulation should be learned under the supervision of a cardiologist who is fully trained in TEE procedures, or of a trained gastrointestinal endoscopist, following accepted standards of practice in the community for TEE or upper endoscopic procedures. The American Society of Echocardiography recommends that the average trainee perform approximately 25 esophageal-gastric intubations under appropriate supervision, in order to develop the basic skills needed to begin performing TEE probe passage and manipulation independently.

Proper performance of a TEE procedure requires ongoing interpretation of data while performing the examination and is an interactive process that requires considerable knowledge of normal and abnormal cardiac

TABLE 3-2   Recommended Training Components for Developing and Maintaining Skills in TEE

Component	Objective	Duration	No. of Cases (approx.)
General echocardiography, level II	Background needed for performance and interpretation	6 months or equivalent	300
Esophageal intubation	TEE probe introduction	Variable	25
TEE examination	Skills in TEE performance and interpretation	Variable	50
Ongoing education	Maintenance of competence	Annual	50–75

By permission of the American Society of Echocardiography. From Pearlman A, Gardin J, Martin R, et al: Guidelines for physician training in transesophageal echocardiography: Recommendations of the American Society of Echocardiography committee for physician training in echocardiography. *J Am Soc Echocardiogr* 5:187, 1992.

TABLE 3-3   Skills Needed to Perform TEE

Cognitive skills

Knowledge of appropriate indications, contraindications, and risks of TEE

Understanding of differential diagnostic considerations in each clinical case

Knowledge of physical principles of echocardiographic image formation and blood flow velocity measurement

Familiarity with the operation of the ultrasonographic instrument, including the function of all controls affecting the quality of the data displayed

Knowledge of normal cardiovascular anatomy, as visualized tomographically

Knowledge of alterations in cardiovascular anatomy resulting from acquired and congenital heart diseases

Knowledge of normal cardiovascular hemodynamics and fluid dynamics

Knowledge of alterations in cardiovascular hemodynamics and blood flow resulting from acquired and congenital heart diseases

Understanding of component techniques for general echocardiography and TEE, including when to use these methods to investigate specific clinic questions

Ability to distinguish adequate from inadequate echocardiographic data, and to distinguish an adequate from an inadequate TEE examination

Knowledge of other cardiovascular diagnostic methods for correlation with TEE findings

Ability to communicate examination results to patient, other health care professionals, and medical record

Technical skills

Proficiency in performing a complete standard echocardiographic examination, using all echocardiographic modalities relevant to the case

Proficiency in safely passing the TEE transducer into the esophagus and stomach, and in adjusting probe position to obtain the necessary tomographic images and Doppler data

Proficiency in operating correctly the ultrasonographic instrument, including all controls affecting the quality of the data displayed

Proficiency in recognizing abnormalities of cardiac structure and function as detected from the transesophageal and transgastric windows, in distinguishing normal from abnormal findings, and in recognizing artifacts

Proficiency in performing qualitative and quantitative analysis of the echocardiographic data

Proficiency in producing a cogent written report of the echocardiographic findings and their clinical implications

By permission of the American Society of Echocardiography. From Pearlman A, Gardin J, Martin R, et al: Guidelines for physician training in transesophageal echocardiography: Recommendations of the American Society of Echocardiography committee for physician training in echocardiography. *J Am Soc Echocardiogr* 5:187, 1992.

anatomy and physiology. While some basis for such expertise can and should be acquired through reading, reviewing teaching material and case studies, the actual skill can only be attained by doing procedures "hands on." It is therefore recommended that a minimum of 50 studies should be performed under supervision of an experienced (level III) echocardiographer who is also an expert at TEE procedures.

The credentialing requirements for physicians who are not in a cardiology training program represent a particular problem. Physicians who wish to attain proficiency at TEE should undergo training that is comparable to that which would be obtained during TEE training in a cardiology fellowship program. Cardiologists in practice should also first have attained level II training in general echocardiography, either during or subsequent to their fellowship. They then need to undergo supervised training on probe insertion and manipulation and actual performance of TEE studies, as outlined above. Attending a short postgraduate course on TEE does not of itself constitute adequate training in TEE, although it may be a useful adjunct.

Physicians without formal cardiology training are recommended to undergo a period of intensive training (approximately 6 months) in an active echocardiography program, in order to develop the necessary skills. Attendance at occasional interpretation sessions and review of selected videotapes clearly is not sufficient training to perform TEE independently. The noncardiologist who performs TEE as a primary operator (for example, for intraoperative monitoring during anesthesia) needs to develop a close working relationship with an experienced echocardiographer who can provide consultation and assist in the event of unsuspected and confusing findings.

Maintenance of competence in TEE requires the regular performance of TEE examinations, and it is recommended that at least 50 to 75 studies per year should be done. As with most procedures, infrequent performance of TEE studies may result in an increase in complications, missed diagnoses, and misinterpretation of the observed findings.

TABLE 3-4   Potential Complications of TEE

Trauma to oropharynx, esophagus, or stomach
Esophageal or gastric perforation
Ventricular and atrial arrhythmias
Hypo- or hypertension
Transient hypoxemia
Myocardial ischemia (in patients with coronary artery disease)
Complications related to used medications:
    Respiratory depression
    Hypotension
    Allergic reactions

Potential Complications

Some of the more significant potential complications of transesophageal echocardiography are outlined in Table 3-4. In addition to trauma or perforation of the upper gastrointestinal tract, atrial and ventricular arrhythmias can occur. These can be related to increase in sympathetic or vagal tone, to myocardial ischemia, medications, or hypoxemia. The changes in oxygen saturation during upper gastrointestinal endoscopy have been investigated, and a decrease from a mean of 95 to 92 percent has been observed.[11] The reported incidence of desaturation below 90 percent has varied from 7 to 24 percent. No definite correlation between hypoxemia and age, sex, or type or dose of medication has been documented. There are conflicting data regarding the correlation between hypoxemia and the length of the procedure, the use of intravenous sedation, and whether preprocedure pulmonary function testing was beneficial. Correlation between the occurrence of hypoxemia and endoscope diameter,[12] the additive effect of a narcotic when used in combination with a benzodiazepine,[13] and the presence of obstructive pulmonary disease[14] has been reported. Hypoxemia can be particularly problematic in patients with severe cardiac or pulmonary disease. While damage to the esophagus is uncommon,[15,16] Mallory-Weiss tears have been reported as rare complications of TEE,[17] as previously described with gastrointestinal endoscopy.[18,19] While patients undergoing intraoperative TEE were not found to have an increased incidence of dysphagia,[20] transient vocal cord paralysis has been reported in two patients after lengthy neurosurgical procedures performed in the upright position.[21] Other potential complications that need to be considered include the occurrence of myocardial ischemia in patients with coronary artery disease,[22] changes in blood pressure (both hypo- and hypertension), as well as adverse reactions caused by the used medications.

Contraindications

The contraindications to transesophageal echocardiography are outlined in Table 3-5. Most of them should be viewed as relative rather than absolute contraindications, where the actual risk must be assessed individually for each patient.

Uncooperative patients may injure themselves, the examiner, or the instrument. Sedation or general anesthesia with or without paralytic agents may make the procedure possible in these patients. Perforation may result from passage of the TEE probe in presence of all forms of esophageal obstruction, whether due to cancer, a web, a distal ring, or a stricture. Obviously, TEE should not be performed in the presence of upper gastrointestinal bleeding or of a perforated viscus. In patients who have esophageal varices without active bleeding, TEE should only be performed after having obtained clearance from a gastroenterologist. While there is little evidence that passage of an endoscope causes variceal bleeding, one should nevertheless advance the instrument carefully and make sure that it does not impact against the esophageal wall. An esophageal diverticulum (Fig. 3-1) may be easily perforated by the instrument, and thus puts the patient at high risk. Large cervical osteophytes (Fig. 3-2) can also result in perforation, since the

TABLE 3-5   Contraindications to TEE

Uncooperative patient
Esophageal obstruction (cancer, web, stricture, ring)
Active upper gastrointestinal bleed
Perforated viscus
Esophageal diverticulum
Large cervical osteophytes
Esophageal varices
Severe cervical arthritis
Profound oropharyngeal distortion
Past oropharyngeal surgery
History of neck irradiation

May require endotracheal intubation or anesthesiology standby:

Severe pulmonary disease or congestive heart failure
Impaired ability to handle secretions (impaired gag reflex)

posterior wall of the esophagus can be eroded between the instrument and the protruding osteophyte. One can apply neck flexion and gentle pressure, but if resistance is encountered, force should not be used. In patients with cervical arthritis neck flexion may be contraindicated, but a cervical collar can be used and the procedure attempted without neck flexion. Profound oropharyngeal distortion, such as seen after surgery in this region, can also make passage of the instrument difficult, and necessitates great care and gentle handling. Patients who have had oropharyngeal surgery and/or radiation may have a stiff, noncompliant, or narrowed pharynx. The tissues may be thin and the pharyngeal muscles atrophic, so the endoscopist must take great care not to cause any damage. Patients with severe pulmonary disease or with congestive heart failure, who are at danger of developing hypoxia during the procedure, or those whose impaired ability to handle secretions (for example, after a stroke) puts them at an increased risk for aspiration, may require short-term endotracheal intubation or at least standby of a qualified anesthesiologist in order for TEE to be performed.

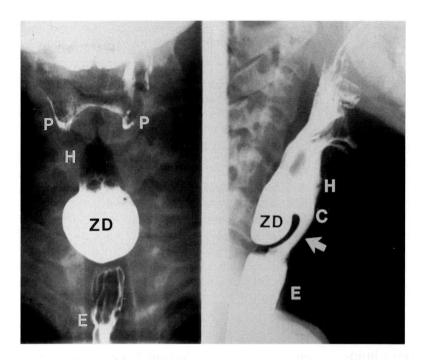

Figure 3-1
Radiograph with barium contrast of a posterior pharyngeal (Zenker's) diverticulum in anteroposterior (left panel) and lateral projection (right panel). The diverticulum may fill with food and secretions and push the posterior esophageal wall anteriorly, which results in narrowing of the lumen (arrow). A TEE probe can be passed inadvertently into the diverticulum and may cause perforation. C = cricopharyngeus; E = esophagus; H = hypopharynx; P = piriform sinus; ZD = Zenker's diverticulum.

Safety Considerations

Ancillary Equipment
Transesophageal echocardiography is being performed in a variety of settings and locations, such as dedicated laboratories, at bedside, in intensive care units, in operating rooms, and in emergency departments. In all these settings it is important to maintain safety standards that include the presence or the immediate availability of ancillary equipment (Table 3-6) that is needed to perform TEE with the utmost

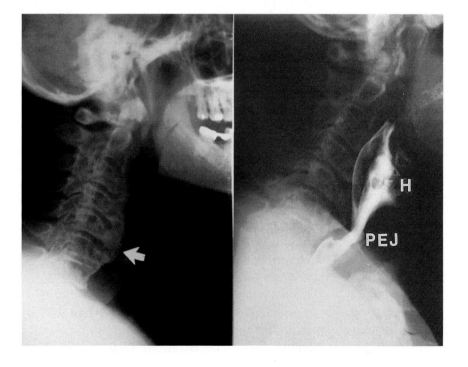

Figure 3-2
Protruding cervical osteophytes (arrow) push the posterior wall of the esophagus anteriorly, narrowing the lumen at the level of the pharyngoesophageal junction. Passage of a TEE probe may be difficult or even impossible in this setting. Forceful pressure may result in pharyngeal perforation. H = hypopharynx; PEJ = pharyngoesophageal junction.

TABLE 3-6   Ancillary Equipment for TEE

Crash cart
Suction
Pulse oximeter
EKG monitor
Blood pressure monitor
Oxygen
Bite block

safety. The presence of a "crash cart," which contains a defibrillator and other equipment and medication needed for cardiopulmonary resuscitation, is absolutely essential. A suction device should be available to remove oropharyngeal secretions or vomited material. Noninvasive pulse oximetry should also be available for monitoring the level of blood oxygen saturation. Oxygen should also be available for administration as needed. An automatic blood pressure measuring device that can be set to obtain measurements at predetermined intervals offers the convenience of hands-off measurements; however, the use of an ordinary blood pressure cuff is also acceptable. A dedicated EKG monitor is optional, since the patient's cardiac rhythm can also be observed using the EKG display on the echocardiography machine. Other items that should be readily available include bite blocks, gloves, and the various medications needed for the procedure. Of particular importance is the availability of medications that can rapidly reverse the action of agents used for sedation, as in cases where sedation causes significant respiratory depression or hypotension or when it results in a paradoxical response with agitation and confusion. The medications that should be available include flumazenil (Mazicon), which is an antagonist to benzodiazepines, as well as naloxone (Narcan), which is a narcotic antagonist.

Cleaning and Disinfection of TEE Probes

Standards for the cleaning and disinfection of gastrointestinal endoscopes have changed over the last decade, in the wake of the AIDS epidemic. Cases of bacterial[23–25] and hepatitis B viral[26,27] cross infection between patients have been documented with endoscopy. Even though

transmission of HIV by endoscopy has not yet been reported, it has to be assumed possible.[28]

Contamination, as well as effectiveness of washing and disinfection of endoscopes, has been assessed in a number of studies. In one such study, 20 endoscopes that were used in AIDS patients were cultured before washing, after washing, and after disinfection.[29] Seven of the 20 unwashed endoscopes were positive for human immunodeficiency virus and 6 were positive for *Candida albicans, Staphylococcus aureus,* and *Pseudomonas aeruginosa.* Washing alone removed all detectable organisms in all but two endoscopes, which were positive for *Neisseria* species. Disinfection with a 2 percent glutaraldehyde solution removed the remaining organisms. Another study was designed to assess whether heavier than usual HIV contamination might be more resistant to cleaning and disinfection.[30] Five endoscopes were contaminated by aspiration of high-titer HIV into the suction and biopsy channels. Contamination was measured before and after manual cleaning in a detergent solution. Four of the five instruments were negative for HIV after cleaning only, and the fifth was negative after 2 min in glutaraldehyde. Similar results have been found using the more hydrophilic polio virus. Cleaning is thus an extremely important and effective part of the disinfection process, as it removes organic materials and allows for unimpaired action of subsequently applied chemical disinfectants.

TEE probes should be inherently even easier to disinfect than gastrointestinal endoscopes, since they do not have the long and narrow channels used for suction and biopsy. These channels are difficult to clean and have been believed to contribute to the higher positive culture rates of gastrointestinal endoscopes, as compared to other types of endoscopic instrumentation.[31]

Standards for dealing with TEE probes should be based on the larger experience with gastrointestinal endoscopy. The American Society for Gastrointestinal Endoscopy[32] and a Working Party of the British Society of Gastroenterology[33] have published guidelines for the cleaning and disinfection of gastrointestinal endoscopes. The essential features that are

32

relevant to the TEE probes include the following:

1. Initial mechanical cleaning with a detergent to remove blood, mucus, and organic material is essential.

2. Disinfection by soaking for a minimum of 20 min is necessary to kill common bacteria, viruses (including HIV and hepatitis B), fungi, and mycobacteria. Glutaraldehyde-based formulations (such as 2 percent activated glutaraldehyde) are the first-line agents and are most frequently used.

3. Rinsing for at least 30 s is needed to remove a disinfectant from the equipment. A 70 percent alcohol solution is commonly used to rinse the equipment prior to storage.

4. Cleaning and disinfection of endoscopic equipment is a specialized procedure and should be carried out by staff that is properly trained. This includes procedures done on an emergency basis.

5. All endoscopic equipment must be cleaned between patient examinations and at the end of the day.

6. Automated washing machines are commonly used in gastrointestinal laboratories and have advantages, such as standardized cleaning cycles and keeping assistants away from potentially toxic disinfectants and contaminated equipment, but are not necessarily more effective than washing by hand. It should be remembered that mechanical cleaning must be done prior to placing the equipment in the washing machine.

7. Universal precautions should be followed in all patients, and all patients should be considered as "potentially at risk." A separate policy for the cleaning and disinfection of equipment for use in patients infected with HIV is not necessary.

Protection of TEE Personnel

Physicians and assistants participating in TEE have to be aware of the potential dangers of handling contaminated equipment and of interacting with infected patients. Since the patients' infective state may not be known at the time of TEE, it is advisable to follow precautions in all procedures. These include the wearing of gloves when coming in contact with potentially contaminated probes, secretions, or blood. The use of gowns, masks, and eye coverings should also be considered when anticipating an unusual amount of splattering or contact with blood or secretions.[34] Hand washing should be done before and after every procedure, even if gloves were worn. Needles should be safely discarded without recapping. After the procedure, exposed surfaces should be thoroughly cleaned and disinfected. In order to minimize the danger of being bitten, bite blocks should be used routinely. While the danger of being infected with hepatitis B is very small, TEE personnel should nevertheless consider immunization.[35]

Electrical and Thermal Safety

Damage to the outer skin of the transducer can potentially result in current leaks and may represent an electrical hazard. Because of the high safety standards required in designing and building these devices, this has, however, not proved to be a significant problem. It is nevertheless important to check the integrity of the probe before and after every examination, in order to avoid this potential complication.

Another theoretical concern is the possibility of thermal injury to the esophagus. The esophagus is an organ that is very resilient to thermal injury, which does not even seem to occur with the intake of very hot food and liquids. Although ultrasound transducers generate a certain amount of heat, the temperature elevation is usually not high enough to pose a hazard. There has been particular concern about intraoperative monitoring, where prolonged TEE examinations may occur in hypothermic patients. In this setting a thermal gradient between the transducer and the hypothermic esophagus has been felt to possibly increase the potential for thermal injury. So far this concern has not been substantiated, but it is nevertheless advisable to periodically shut down the equipment in such a setting, in order to allow for cooling of the transducer. Most manufacturers now incorporate thermistors into TEE probes. Some of them provide the examiner with a continuous digital temperature readout on the screen and most of the probes automatically shut down at a preset temperature. This feature can result in difficulties with examining febrile patients and has proved to be more of a hindrance than a useful safety feature.

Procedure

Informed Consent

Because of the potential risks associated with TEE, it is mandatory to obtain legally adequate informed consent prior to performing the procedure. No guidelines on informed consent specific for TEE have been made available to date; however, the American Society of Gastrointestinal Endoscopy has published a statement on informed consent for gastrointestinal endoscopy.[36] It states that the following information needs to be disclosed to the patient: (1) the nature of the proposed procedure; (2) the underlying reason why the procedure is necessary and its goals; (3) the risks and complications of the procedure, including their relative incidence; (4) reasonable alternatives to the proposed procedure. The endoscopist must be mindful of the fact that informed consent is a process of disclosure and deliberation, not merely the signing of a form. The only exceptions when the duty of obtaining informed consent may not apply are: (1) the emergency exception (in the case of life-threatening emergencies or to relieve pain and suffering); (2) incompetency (in this setting, consent should be obtained from the patient's legal guardian); (3) therapeutic privilege (assumption by the physician that the patient may be harmed by the disclosure, which should be applied most cautiously); and (4) waiver by the patient to obtain disclosure.

History

It is very important to obtain a thorough history prior to the procedure. In addition to general questions about the overall health status, it is essential to focus on any potential swallowing problems. Careful questioning can generally help exclude a Zenker's diverticulum, large cervical osteophytes, esophageal strictures, rings, or webs with a high degree of likelihood.[37] Specifically, one should ask the patient if there is any difficulty swallowing solids or liquids, or if coughing occurs with or soon after meals. Solid food dysphagia suggests a mechanical narrowing, such as a ring, web, or stricture. Dysphagia that is worse for liquids than for solids suggests a pharyngeal neuromuscular problem, such as from a stroke. Dysphagia for both solids and liquids suggests an esophageal motility problem or a Zenker's diverticulum, the latter especially if there is regurgitation of food. Difficulty with neck flexion may indicate cervical arthritis. A history of oropharyngeal neoplasm, surgery, or radiation therapy may make swallowing of the instrument difficult or impossible.

It is also important to find out whether the patient is on anticoagulant therapy, or whether there is any history of a coagulopathy, in order to assess whether there is an increased risk of bleeding. In addition one should investigate whether there is a history of drug allergies or of drug intolerance, particularly to the medications that might be administered in conjunction with the procedure.

Medications

The use of medications for TEE (Tables 3-7 and 3-8) varies from country to country, from institution to institution, and from patient to patient. Medications are usually given for four purposes: for topical anesthesia, for sedation, as drying agents, and for antibiotic prophylaxis.

Topical Anesthesia

Most physicians prefer to spray the oropharynx with a local anesthetic agent, in order to diminish the gag reflex; in some institutions TEE and upper gastrointestinal endoscopy are done without sedation, using only topical anesthesia.[38] The most commonly used agents are benzocaine (Hurricaine), lidocaine (Xylocaine), or a blend of benzocaine and tetracaine

TABLE 3-7   Sedation and Premedication for TEE

"Verbal sedation"

Topical anesthesia
Local anesthetic spray to oropharynx
Viscous lidocaine lubricant

Intravenous sedation
Midazolam (Versed) IV (0.5–5 mg in increments)
    alone or in combination with
Meperidine (Demerol) IV (25–75 mg in increments) or
Fentanyl IV (25–100 µg in increments)

Drying agents
Glycopyrrolate (Robinul) 0.2 mg IV
(Atropine)

TABLE 3-8   Antibiotic Prophylaxis for TEE

Standard regimen
• Ampicillin 2.0 g IV or IM
• Gentamicin 1.5 mg/kg IV or IM (not to exceed 80 mg)
• Amoxicillin 1.5 g by mouth 6 h after the initial dose
• Alternatively, the parenteral regimen may be repeated once 8 h after the initial dose

Regimen for penicillin-allergic patients
• Vancomycin 1.0 g IV *over 1 h*
• Gentamicin 1.5 mg/kg IV or IM (not to exceed 80 mg)
• May be repeated once 8 h after the initial dose

(Cetacaine). Patients frequently complain about the unpleasant taste and the initial irritation and discomfort caused by all of these agents. It is important to instruct patients not to breathe during spraying, in order to avoid inhaling the aerosolized material. Some laboratories prefer not to use topical anesthetics if the patient is also sedated, since potentially there may be an increased risk of aspiration due to suppression of the gag reflex. For this reason, patients who received topical anesthetics should also be instructed not to eat for at least half an hour after the procedure, or for as long as the throat feels numb.

Sedation

While sedation is not used in all laboratories, it increases patient tolerance of the procedure, increases patient willingness to undergo repeat TEE, if necessary, and usually allows for better imaging, since there is less gagging and less patient motion. With proper administration of sedation, the increase in risk is only minimal. The main drawbacks of sedation are that it prolongs the preparatory phase of the procedure, since these medications have to be given slowly, and that it requires longer monitoring after the study until the patient can be discharged.

Today the most commonly used sedative agent in TEE and endoscopy is probably midazolam (Versed), which has largely displaced the use of diazepam (Valium) for this purpose.

Like diazepam, midazolam is also a benzodiazepine, but it has the advantage of shorter half-life. Midazolam is also 3 to 4 times more potent per milligram than diazepam. The onset of action can be as short as 2 to 3 min after intravenous injection. Its effect has usually largely worn off 2 to 6 h after administration. Midazolam also has an amnestic effect, so that the majority of patients have no or only limited recollection of the procedure. Its most serious side effects are respiratory depression and hypotension; however, these complications have mainly occurred when larger doses (several milligrams) of the drug were injected rapidly. When the drug is administered in small increments and the dosage is titrated to patient response, these complications are far less common. We usually start with a 1-mg injection and administer additional doses in 1-mg increments until the patient is adequately sedated. In small, elderly, or debilitated patients it may be preferable to use 0.5-mg increments. Responses to midazolam are difficult to predict and dosages at which sedation is achieved vary from patient to patient. Most patients do not require more than a total of 5 mg of the drug, but we occasionally use up to 8 mg. Flumazenil (Mazicon), a specific benzodiazepine antagonist that quickly reverses the action of midazolam, has recently become available and adds to the safety of using midazolam.

Many physicians who perform TEE use a narcotic in addition to midazolam, most commonly meperidine (Demerol). Meperidine is usually given intravenously prior to midazolam.

The usual dosage ranges from 25 to 75 mg, given in 25 mg increments. Naloxone (Narcan) is a narcotic antagonist that reverses the action of meperidine if needed.

Fentanyl, a shorter-acting and more potent narcotic is used increasingly by some laboratories and will probably replace the use of meperidine as a narcotic for TEE and for endoscopy, just as midazolam has replaced diazepam. Fentanyl has an almost immediate onset of action and a shorter duration of action than meperidine. The usual dosage is 25 to 100 μg, given intravenously in 25 μg increments.

Just as one needs to learn the proper technique for probe insertion, it is also important to learn how to administer these sedative and narcotic medications, how to minimize the incidence of complications, and how to deal with potential side effects.

Drying Agents

Anticholinergic agents, which decrease salivation and gastrointestinal motiliy, are used in some centers. The agent of choice for this application may be glycopyrrolate (Robinul), which is better tolerated than atropine and which has less effect on heart rate. Anticholinergic drugs are contraindicated in patients with glaucoma, urinary retention, or asthma. At our laboratory, these agents are almost never used, since secretions can usually be effectively removed by suctioning.

Antibiotic Prophylaxis

Some controversy exists about the need to administer antibiotic prophylaxis prior to TEE. A temporal and possibly causal relationship between TEE and endocarditis has been reported.[39] Some studies have claimed that probe insertion might cause bacteremia;[40] however, other investigators have disputed those findings and blamed them on contaminants.[41–43] In these studies the rate of transient bacteremia was indeed similar to the contaminant rate seen in microbiologic laboratories. Thus there is little evidence to clearly support the need for antibiotic prophylaxis with TEE. Indeed, higher rates of bacteremia have been said to occur with brushing teeth and defecation.[44] Because endocarditis can be a catastrophic event, and because there are only very limited data on the actual incidence of its occurrence in high-risk patients who did not receive prophylaxis, most laboratories nevertheless do administer antibiotics prior to TEE in selected cases. The recommendations of the American Heart Association on prevention of bacterial endocarditis state that antibiotic prophylaxis is not routinely recommended for endoscopy with or without gastrointestinal biopsy.[45] They do, however, also state that in patients who have prosthetic heart valves, a previous history of endocarditis, or surgically constructed systemic-pulmonary shunts or conduits, physicians may choose to administer prophylactic antibiotics even for low-risk procedures that involve the lower respiratory, genitourinary, or gastrointestinal tracts. The recommended drug regimens are shown in Table 3-8. Thus the standard regimen consists of a combination of parenteral ampicillin and gentamicin, given 30 min before the procedure, followed by oral amoxicillin, given 6 h after the initial dose. In penicillin-allergic patients, vancomycin and gentamicin are given 1 h before the procedure. It is important to infuse vancomycin over a 1-h period, in order to avoid unpleasant and potentially dangerous reactions.

Anatomy of the Oral Cavity, Pharynx, Esophagus, and Stomach

The anatomy of these structures is depicted in Figs. 3-3 and 3-4. The oral cavity extends from the lips to the tonsillar pillars, the superior border being the palate, the lateral borders the buccal mucosa. The pharynx can be divided into three compartments:[46] the nasopharynx, the oropharynx, and the hypopharynx.

The nasopharynx extends from the base of the skull to the top of the soft palate, the velum, and is part of the respiratory tract rather than of the alimentary tract. The oropharynx is bordered by the soft palate superiorly, the base of the tongue inferiorly, and the pharyngeal constrictor muscles at the lateral and posterior walls. The vallecula is the space between the epiglottis and the base of the tongue and serves to protect the larynx from entry of swallowed material.

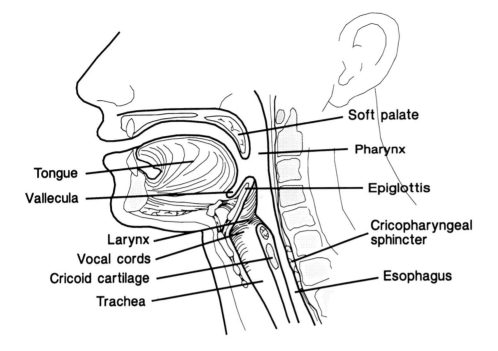

Figure 3-3
Diagram of the upper alimentary tract and airway.

The hypopharynx extends inferiorly from the base of the tongue to the cricopharyngeus muscle. The base of the hypopharynx is formed by the larynx anteriorly and the esophageal inlet posteriorly. There are two channels (one on each side of the larynx) called the piriform sinuses, which direct swallowed material into the esophageal inlet. At the posterior aspect of the larynx is an area called the posterior commissure. This is a rigid structure formed in part by an intact ring of cartilage called the cricoid cartilage. The joints of the vocal cords,

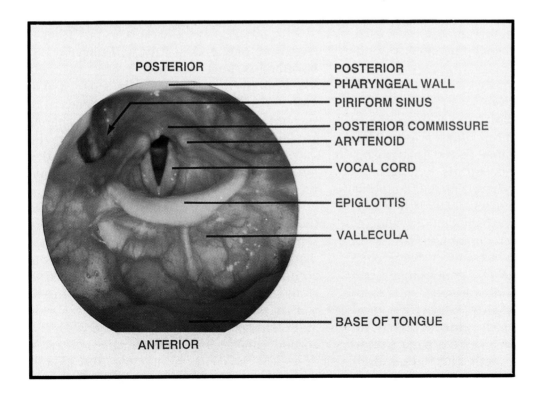

Figure 3-4
Normal hypopharynx and larynx, imaged by laryngoscopy.

the arytenoids, sit at the lateral ends of the posterior commissure. The space directly behind the posterior commissure is rigidly narrow, lying between the anterior vertebral bodies and the cricoid cartilage.

The esophagus starts just below the cricopharyngeus, courses through the posterior mediastinum, and passes through the esophageal hiatus of the diaphragm into the stomach.

Technique of Probe Insertion

It is important to explain the procedure to the patient, in order to reduce anxiety and to ensure patient cooperation ("verbal sedation"). A number of safety precautions should be followed, as outlined in Table 3-9. As described above, a careful history and informed consent have to be obtained. The patient should not have had any intake of food or drink for at least 4 to 6 h. Dentures or other forms of oral prostheses should be removed. We routinely place an intravenous line in all patients prior to the procedure. The patient should be placed in the left lateral decubitus position. This position helps diminish the danger of aspiration and facilitates the suctioning of secretions. After topical anesthetics and sedation are administered, a bite block is introduced between the teeth to protect the instrument and the examiner's finger. The neck is then flexed to facilitate passage into the esophagus, which is located posteriorly. The probe is gently passed into the oral cavity over the tongue and guided into the pharynx.[47] The probe should be guided posteriorly, against the posterior pharyngeal wall, in order to pass it behind the epiglottis and into the hypopharynx and in order to avoid getting trapped in the vallecula. When the instrument is below the epiglottis and above the larynx, the patient should be asked to swallow. This closes the vocal cords, brings the larynx up and forward under the posterior aspect of the tongue, and opens the cricopharyngeus muscle. At that time the probe is gently introduced into the esophagus. The instrument is then slowly and gently advanced while the echocardiographic screen is watched to ensure that the esophageal wall is moving by, in order to exclude impaction of the instrument in the esophagus or stomach.

TABLE 3-9   Safety Precautions for TEE

Obtain history:
   Upper gastrointestinal pathology
   Swallowing disorders
   Drug allergies
   Coagulopathies or anticoagulation
Obtain informed consent
NPO 4–6 h before, 1/2 h after
Remove dentures
IV access
Monitoring of vital signs
Observation after procedure
Predischarge instructions

Pitfalls and Tricks

When passed into the oral cavity, the probe must be kept in the midline, in order to prevent impaction against the tonsillar folds. In some patients this may require a finger to be passed alongside the instrument in order to guide it. When inserting the finger into the mouth, this should be done outside the bite block, which should stay in place for protection of the examiner's finger and the instrument.

The probe may get trapped in the vallecula, the space between the epiglottis and the back of the tongue. If this happens, the probe should be straightened and pushed gently against the posterior pharyngeal wall. If needed, a finger can be used to pull the epiglottis slightly forward, allowing the probe to pass into the hypopharynx. The TEE probe will pass through either the left or the right piriform sinus, down to and through the cricopharyngeus. It usually does not pass through the midline directly behind the posterior commissure, a narrow space bordered by the rigid cricoid ring and the anterior wall of the vertebral body.

If the instrument will not pass through the cricopharyngeus, or if the patient cannot swallow as requested, one may place 1 to 2 ml of water gently down the pharynx with a 5-ml syringe. This may stimulate swallowing with subsequent pharyngeal and esophageal peristalsis, carrying the instrument down the esophagus.

If resistance to passage occurs, the probe should not be advanced forcefully. If the resistance is at the level of the hypopharynx, the possibility of large cervical osteophytes, Zenker's diverticulum, or spasm of the pharyngeal muscles or of the cricopharyngeus should be considered. If cervical osteophytes are suspected to be the problem, one may flex the neck more forward to open the hypopharynx as much as possible. If there is spasm of the musculature, further sedation and renewed attempt to pass the probe several minutes later may be helpful. At times it is helpful to change the position of patients, having them sit upright for passage of the probe. With the support of an assistant, this can be done even with sedated patients.

If the probe is successfully passed into the esophagus but resistance is encountered on further passage, the patient should be asked to swallow to induce esophageal peristalsis. If these methods are unsuccessful, the procedure should be aborted. Obtaining a lateral x-ray study of the neck can help evaluate the cervical vertebrae. A barium swallow can help assess the presence of anatomical abnormalities such as webs, rings, strictures, or diverticula.

Passage of the TEE probe into the esophagus in a patient who has an endotracheal tube in place can sometimes be difficult. Patients are usually placed in the supine position, although one may use the left lateral position. If insertion is difficult, the endotracheal tube can be pushed to one side of the oral cavity and the neck can be flexed. At times it may be necessary to briefly deflate the endotracheal balloon during passage. Although nasogastric tubes generally do not pose a significant problem, they can occasionally interfere with TEE studies. If need be, the nasogastric tube can be either totally removed for the duration of the TEE procedure if it makes probe insertion difficult, or partially withdrawn if it interferes with imaging.

Monitoring During and After the Procedure

Guidelines for monitoring the patient receiving conscious sedation for upper gastrointestinal endoscopy have been published by the Standards of Practice Committee of the American Society for Gastrointestinal Endoscopy.[48] A well-trained assistant who works closely with the endoscopist (preferably a nurse), who helps the examiner with continuous and conscientious clinical assessment, is the most important part of the monitoring process. This clinical assessment should include the determination of heart rate and rhythm, blood pressure, as well as respiratory rate. If a pulse oximeter is used, it is also important to observe the patient's oxygen saturation levels. In addition, the need for suction should be assessed continuously.

After termination of the procedure, the patient should remain under observation until the effects of sedation have worn off. If a local anesthetic spray has been administered to the oropharynx, the patient should avoid eating or drinking until its effects have worn off. The patient should not be allowed to drive for several hours after the procedure and ideally should not leave alone, but together with a family member or another accompanying person.

References

1. Seward J, Khanderia B, Oh J, et al: Transesophageal echocardiography: Technique, anatomic correlations, implementation, and clinical applications. *Mayo Clin Proc* 63:649, 1988.

2. Schiller N, Maurer G, Ritter S, et al: Transesophageal echocardiography (position paper of the American Society of Echocardiography). *J Am Soc Echocardiogr* 2:354, 1989.

3. Geibel A, Kasper W, Behroz A, et al: Risk of transesophageal echocardiography in awake patients with cardiac diseases. *Am J Cardiol* 62:337, 1988.

4. Pearson A, Castello R, Labovitz A: Safety and utility of transesophageal echocardiography in the critically ill patient. *Am Heart J* 119:1083, 1990.

5. Shahmir M, Schuman B: Complications of fiberoptic endoscopy. *Gastrointest Endosc* 26:86, 1980.

6. Silvis S, Nebel O, Rogers G, et al: Endoscopic complications: Results of the 1974 American Society for Gastrointestinal Endoscopy survey. *JAMA* 235:928, 1976.

7. Daniel W, Erbel R, Kasper W, et al: Safety of transesophageal echocardiography: A multicenter survey of 10,419 examinations. *Circulation* 83:817, 1991.

8. Seward J, Khanderia B, Oh J, et al: Critical appraisal of transesophageal echocardiography: Limitations, pitfalls and complications. *J Am Soc Echocardiogr* 5:288–305, 1992.

9. Pearlman A, Gardin J, Martin R, et al: Guidelines for physician training in transesophageal echocardiography: Recommendations of the American Society of Echocardiography committee for physician training in echocardiography. *J Am Soc Echocardiogr* 5:187, 1992.

10. Pearlman A, Gardin J, Martin R, et al: Guidelines for optimal physician training in echocardiography: Recommendations of the American Society of Echocardiography committee for physician training in echocardiography. *Am J Cardiol* 60:158, 1987.

11. Bell G, Reeve P, Moshiri M, et al: Intravenous midazolam: A study of the degree of oxygen desaturation during UGI endoscopy. *Br J Clin Pharmacol* 23:703, 1987.

12. Lieberman D, Wuerker C, Katon R: Cardiopulmonary risk of EGD: Role of endoscope diameter and systemic sedation. *Gastroenterology* 88:468, 1985.

13. Rozen P, Fireman Z, Gilat T: The causes of hypoxemia in elderly patients. *Gastrointest Endosc* 28:243, 1982.

14. Rostykes P, McDonald G, Albert R: Upper intestinal endoscopy induces hypoxemia in patients with obstructive pulmonary disease. *Gastroenterology* 78:488, 1988.

15. O'Shea J, Southern J, D'Ambra N, et al: Effects of prolonged transesophageal manipulation on the esophagus—An echocardiographic pathologic study. *J Am Coll Cardiol* 17:1426, 1991.

16. Urbanowicz J, Kernoff R, Oppenheim G, et al: Transesophageal echocardiography and its potential for esophageal damage. *Anesthesiology* 72:40, 1990.

17. Dewhirst W, Stragand J, Fleming B: Mallory-Weiss tear complicating intraoperative transesophageal echocardiography in a patient undergoing aortic valve replacement. *Anesthesiology* 73:777, 1990.

18. Knauer C: Mallory-Weiss syndrome. A characterization of 75 Mallory-Weiss lacerations in 528 patients with upper gastrointestinal hemorrhage. *Gastroenterology* 71:5, 1976.

19. Watts HD: Mallory-Weiss syndrome occurring as a complication of endoscopy. *Gastrointest Endosc* 22:171, 1976.

20. Messina A, Paranicas M, Fiamengo S, et al: Risk of dysphagia after transesophageal echocardiography. *Am J Cardiol* 67:313, 1991.

21. Cucchiara R, Nugent M, Seward J, et al: Air embolism in upright neurosurgical patients. Detection and localization by two-dimensional transesophageal echocardiography. *Anesthesiology* 60:353, 1984.

22. Matsuzaki M, Toma Y, Kusukawa R: Clinical applications of transesophageal echocardiography. *Circulation* 82:709, 1990.

23. O'Connor H, Axon A: Gastrointestinal endoscopy: Infection and disinfection. *Gut* 24:1067, 1983.

24. Webb S, Vall-Espinosa A: Outbreak of Serratia marrescens associated with a flexible fiberbronchoscope. *Chest* 68:703, 1975.

25. Dean A: Transmission of Salmonella typhi by fiberoptic endoscopy (letter). *Lancet* 2:134, 1977.

26. Bond W, Moncada R: Viral hepatitis B infection risk in flexible fiberoptic endoscopy. *Gastrointest Endosc* 24:225, 1978.

27. Birnie G, Quigley E, Clements G, et al: Case report: Endoscopic transmission of hepatitis B virus. *Gut* 24:171, 1983.

28. Hanson P, Jeffries D, Collins J: Viral transmission and fiberoptic bronchoscopy. *J Hosp Infect* 18(suppl A): 136, 1991.

29. Hanson P, Clarke J, Nicholson G, et al: Contamination of endoscopes used in AIDS patients. *Lancet* 86, 1989.

30. Hanson P, Gor D, Jeffries D, et al: Elimination of high titer HIV from fiberoptic endoscopes. *Gut* 31:657, 1990.

31. Kaczmarek R, Moore R, McCrohan J, et al: Multistate investigation of the actual disinfection/sterilization of endoscopes in health care facilities. *Am J Med* 92:257, 1992.

32. Infection control during gastrointestinal endoscopy: Guidelines for clinical application. *Gastrointest Endosc* 34:37S, 1988.

33. Cleaning and disinfection of equipment for gastrointestinal flexible endoscopy: Interim recommendations of a working party of the British Society of Gastroenterology. *Gut* 29:1134, 1988.

34. Recommendations for prevention of HIV transmission in health care settings. Morbidity and Mortality Weekly Report. U.S. Department of Health and Human Services/Public Health

Service, Centers for Disease Control. Supplement 36:25, 1987.

35. Koretz R, Chin K, Gitnick G: The endoscopists' risks from endoscopic transmission of hepatitis. *Gastroenterology* 88:1454, 1985.

36. Informed consent for gastrointestinal endoscopy. *Gastrointest Endosc* 34:26S, 1988.

37. Pope C: Heartburn, dysphagia, and other esophageal symptoms. In Sleisenger M, Fordtran (eds): *Gastrointestinal Disease*, 4th ed. Philadelphia, Saunders, 1989, chap 10, p 200.

38. Ross W: Premedication for upper gastrointestinal endoscopy. *Gastrointest Endosc* 2:120, 1989.

39. Foster E, Kusumoto F, Sobol S, et al: Streptococcal endocarditis temporarily related to transesophageal echocardiography. *J Am Soc Echocardiogr* 3:424, 1990.

40. Görge G, Erbel R, Heinrichs J, et al: Positive blood cultures during transesophageal echocardiography. *Am J Cardiol* 65:1404, 1990.

41. Steckelberg J, Khanderia B, Anhalt J, et al: Prospective evaluation of the risk of bacteremia associated with transesophageal echocardiography. *Circulation* 84:177, 1991.

42. Melendez L, Chan K, Cheung P, et al: Incidence of bacteremia in transesophageal echocardiography. A prospective study of 140 consecutive patients. *J Am Coll Cardiol* 18:1650, 1991.

43. Nikutta P, Mantey-Stiers F, Becht I, et al: Risk of bacteremia induced by transesophageal echocardiography: Analysis of 100 consecutive procedures. *J Am Soc Echocardiogr* 5:168, 1992.

44. Khanderia B: Prophylaxis or no prophylaxis before transesophageal echocardiography? *J Am Soc Echocardiogr* 5:285, 1992.

45. Dajani A, Bisno A, Chung K, et al: Prevention of bacterial endocarditis—recommendations of the American Heart Association. *JAMA* 264:2919, 1990.

46. Jones B, Gayler B, Donner M: Pharynx and cervical esophagus, in Levine M (ed): *Radiology of the Esophagus*. Philadelphia, Saunders, 1989, p 311.

47. Fleischer D, Goldstein S: Transesophageal echocardiography: What the gastroenterologist thinks the cardiologist should know about endoscopy. *J Am Soc Echocardiogr* 3:428, 1990.

48. Fleischer D: Monitoring the patient receiving conscious sedation for gastrointestinal endoscopy: Issues and guidelines. *Gastrointest Endosc* 35:262, 1989.

4

Transesophageal Biplane Echocardiographic Imaging: Technique and Image Planes

Navin C. Nanda
Luiz Pinheiro
Rajat S. Sanyal
Octavia Storey
Gerald Maurer

In spite of its popularity and great clinical utility, transesophageal echocardiography has some limitations in its ability to obtain tomographic images of the heart, since the probe has only limited side-to-side maneuverability in the narrow confines of the esophagus. This limitation has been particularly obvious in conventional single-plane probes, which can only obtain transverse image planes of the heart and the great vessels. These planes can only be varied by moving the transducer up and down the esophagus, by angling the probe, and by rotating it from side to side. This

limitation has stimulated a continuous quest toward technological developments intended to offer the clinician an improved ability to obtain additional image planes. Currently the most widespread newer technology is biplane TEE,[1-3] with matrix phased-array,[4] multiplane probes[5,6] (see Chap. 2) and even three-dimensional transesophageal imaging[7] on the horizon. The biplane TEE probe provides a second transducer, which is located adjacent and proximally to the conventional transverse transducer utilized in single-plane probes. The channels of the additional transducer are oriented perpendicularly to those of the conventional distal transducer, making it possible to obtain longitudinal planes through the heart and the great vessels. This results in the capability of generating transverse and longitudinal planes that can be displayed in a sequential manner.

Reproduced with modifications and permission from Nanda NC et al: Transesophageal biplane echocardiographic imaging: Technique, planes, and clinical usefulness. *Echocardiography* 7: 771–788, 1990.

Even though the two transducers are located at different sites at the probe tip, it does not represent a significant disadvantage since the orthogonal relationship of the images obtained with both planes is maintained. Each transducer contains up to 64 elements; the distance between the centers of the two transducers is approximately 1 cm (Figs. 4-1 and 4-2). The incorporation of the second transducer has not resulted in any significant increase in probe width, so that patient comfort and tolerance have not been adversely affected. The addition of the second transducer for obtaining longitudinal planes has significantly expanded the diagnostic capability of transesophageal echocardiography and has led to an increased ability to obtain understanding of three-dimensional structural relationships in individual patients.

This chapter describes the various transverse and longitudinal planes that are generated using the biplane approach and how to obtain them. The sequence in which these planes are presented is from cranial to caudal, beginning

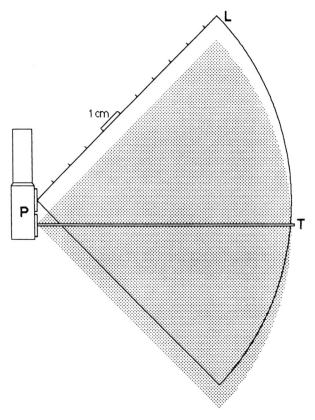

Figure 4-2
Schematic drawing of the biplane probe tip (P) illustrating the effect of the distance between the two transducers. Observe that the transverse plane (T) intersects the longitudinal plane (L) approximately 1 cm from the probe, resulting in a lack of overlay in the proximal field. The shaded area represents the hypothetical situation of the longitudinal plane originating from the same transducer as the transverse plane. It is generally not necessary to advance the probe tip minimally to obtain exact correspondence between the two planes unless one is examining proximal structures such as the descending thoracic aorta.

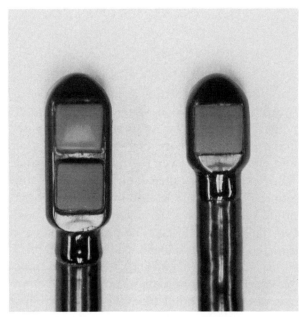

Figure 4-1
Biplane transesophageal probe. The tip of the Aloka biplane probe (left) has two transducers. The distal transducer is used to obtain transverse planes while the proximal one generates longitudinal planes. On the other hand, the conventional single-plane probe (right) has only one transducer that obtains transverse planes.

at the level of the great vessels and ending with the transgastric views and examination of the descending thoracic aorta. In this chapter, the image orientation for the transverse planes follows the recommendations of the American Society of Echocardiography.[8] According to them, the four-chamber view should appear with the cardiac apex down (sector apex up) and the left ventricle to the viewer's right, as seen in Fig. 4-8B. All other views are displayed as they arise from the transducer element or crystal orientation and firing sequence required to generate this four-chamber view. No official recommendations exist yet for the newer longitudinal views. We display our images so that a longitudinal view of the ascending aorta will be shown with superior structures on the right side of the screen, and with inferior structures to the left (Fig. 4-4D and E). All other longitudinal views are displayed as derived from this orientation.

Figure 4-3 is a diagrammatic representation of the various longitudinal planes passing through the heart, as obtained by the transesophageal probe positioned in the esophagus at the level of the pulmonary artery bifurcation. This corresponds approximately to a transverse section of the chest at the level of the sixth vertebral body. Plane 1 passes through the right pulmonary artery and the superior vena cava, plane 2 traverses the right pulmonary artery and the aortic root, plane 3 passes through the main pulmonary artery, pulmonary valve, and the right ventricular outflow tract, while plane 4 is directed posteriorly through the descending thoracic aorta. Figure 4-4 demonstrates conventional transverse imaging of the aortic root, and displays all three

leaflets of the aortic valve in short axis (A, B, and C) while the longitudinal plane at the same level (A, D, and E) demonstrates the aortic valve and the proximal ascending aorta in long axis (corresponding to plane 2 in Fig. 4-3). In the subsequent images, examples are demonstrated of an aortic regurgitation jet (Fig. 4-4F), aortic valve vegetation with aortic regurgitation (Fig. 4-4G), and aortic dissection with communication between the perfusing and the nonperfusing lumens (Fig. 4-4H and I) using the biplane transducer. The transverse plane in Fig. 4-4F is taken at a somewhat lower level and hence demonstrates the five-chamber view. Slight leftward rotation of the transducer in the long-axis plane results in the visualization of a large segment of the dissection flap as well as its relation to the aortic valve (Fig. 4-4H).

By withdrawing the transducer slightly from the level of the aortic valve (Fig. 4-4J), a transverse plane can be obtained, which demonstrates the ascending aorta and superior vena cava in short axis and the main pulmonary artery in long axis; the right pulmonary artery, also imaged in long axis, is seen posteriorly. The longitudinal plane at this level demonstrates, as

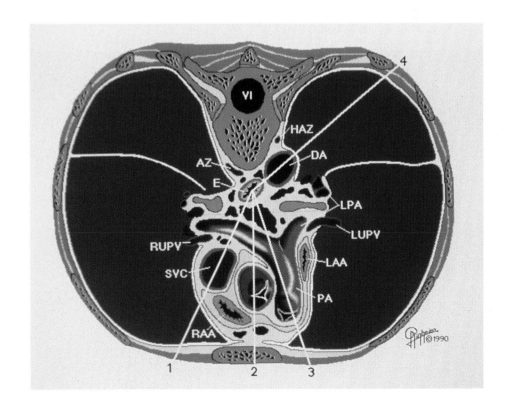

Figure 4-3
Schema at the level of the sixth vertebral body showing various longitudinal planes that can be obtained by the transesophageal probe positioned at this level. AZ = azygos vein; DA = descending thoracic aorta; E = esophagus; HAZ = hemiazygos vein; LAA = left atrial appendage; LPA = left pulmonary artery; LUPV = left upper (superior) pulmonary vein; PA = pulmonary artery; RAA = right atrial appendage; RUPV = right upper pulmonary vein; SVC = superior vena cava.

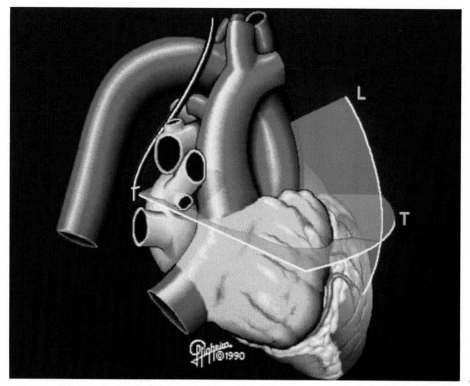

A.

Figure 4-4
A. Schematic of the heart in right lateral view showing the transverse plane (T) passing through the heart at the level of the aortic root. The corresponding longitudinal plane (L) passes through the ascending aorta.

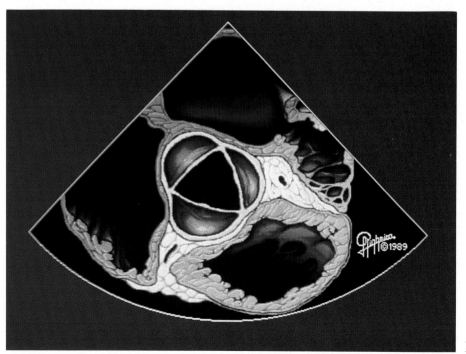

B.

Figure 4-4
B, C. Anatomical representation (*B*) and transesophageal image (*C*) obtained with the transverse plane at the level of the aortic root. All three cusps of the aortic valve are clearly seen. LA = left atrium; LCC = left coronary cusp; NCC = noncoronary cusp; PV = pulmonary valve; RA = right atrium; RCC = right coronary cusp; RVOT = right ventricular outflow tract.

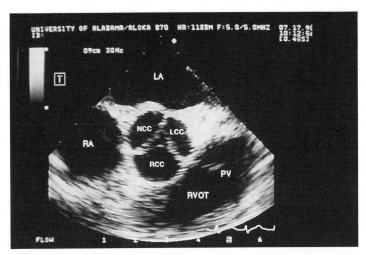

C.

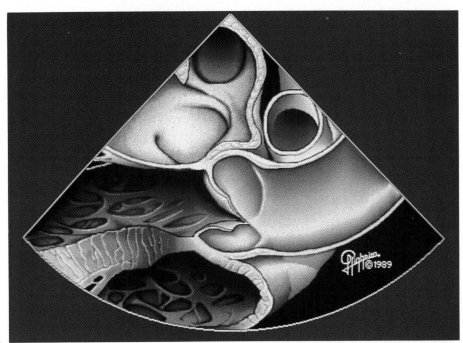

D.

Figure 4-4
D, E. Anatomical representation (*D*) and transesophageal image (*E*) obtained with the longitudinal plane showing the ascending aorta in long axis. AMVL = anterior mitral valve leaflet; AO = aorta; AV = aortic valve; LVOT = left ventricular outflow tract; RPA = right pulmonary artery; RV = right ventricle.

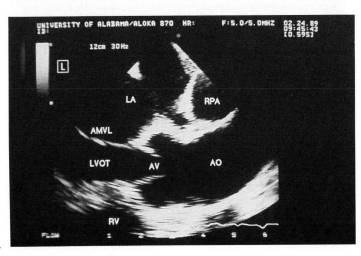

E.

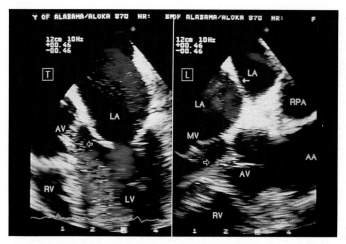

F.

Figure 4-4
F. Aortic regurgitation jet (arrows) imaged in five-chamber (transverse plane) and aortic long-axis (longitudinal plane) views. AA = ascending aorta; LV = left ventricle; MV = mitral valve.

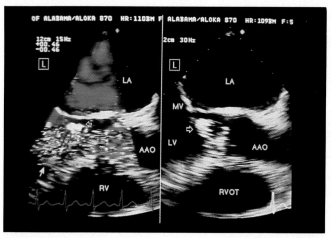

G.

Figure 4-4
G. Aortic valve vegetations (open arrow) and aortic regurgitation (solid arrow) imaged in aortic long-axis view (longitudinal plane). AAO = ascending aorta.

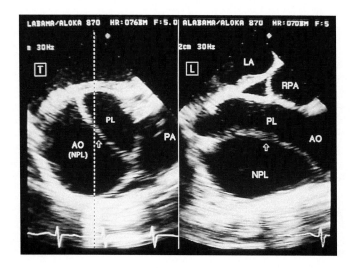

H-a.

Figure 4-4
H, I. Biplane imaging in a patient with aortic dissection showing a prominent flap (arrow in *H*) and flow signals (blue) moving from the perfusing lumen (PL) into the nonperfusing lumen (NPL) through a communication (arrows in *I*) to the superior vena cava.

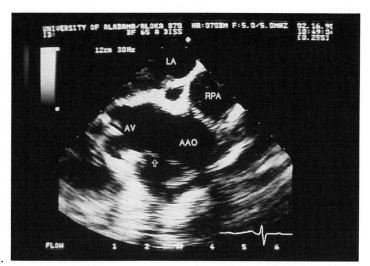

H-b.

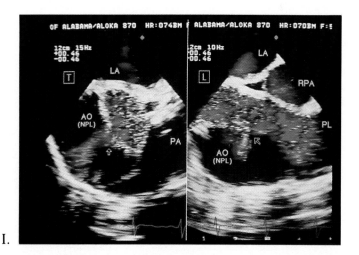

I.

Figure 4-4

J. Ascending aorta at the level of pulmonary artery bifurcation examined using transverse and longitudinal planes. The arrow points to a catheter in the superior vena cava (SVC). The dotted line in the transverse plane image shows the level at which the longitudinal plane was obtained.

J.

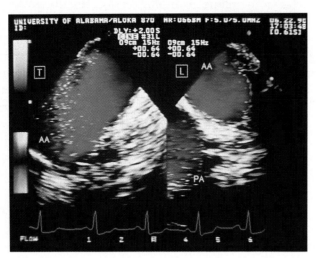

Figure 4-4
K. Distal ascending aorta (AOO) and aortic arch (AA) examined using transverse and longitudinal planes.

K.

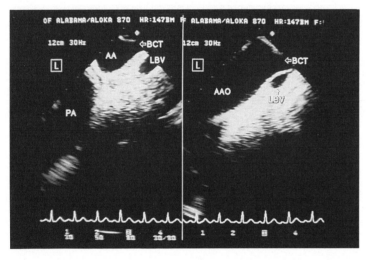

Figure 4-4
L, M. Biplane examination of the proximal aortic arch. The brachiocephalic trunk (BCT, innominate artery) is imaged in the longitudinal plane. LBV = left brachiocephalic vein (left innominate vein).

L.

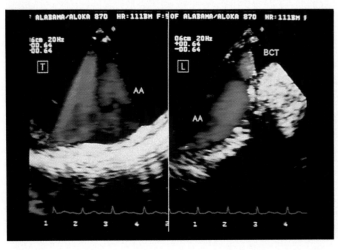

M.

would be expected, the right pulmonary artery in short-axis and the ascending aorta in long-axis view. Further withdrawal of the transducer from this position often results in imaging of the distal ascending aorta and the proximal aortic arch in an oblique long-axis view, when using the transverse plane (Fig. 4-4K). At this level, slight transducer manipulation, which minimally displaces the longitudinal plane, frequently demonstrates the brachiocephalic trunk (innominate artery) at its origin from the proximal aortic arch. The left brachiocephalic (innominate) vein and the main pulmonary artery may also be imaged (Fig. 4-4L and M). Because of the proximity of the esophagus to the aorta, TEE is an ideal tool for imaging aortic structures. However, it is important for the clinician to be aware that the air-filled trachea and left mainstem bronchus can obstruct visualization of a small portion of the distal ascending aorta.[9] This problem has been somewhat alleviated but not completely resolved by the introduction of biplane TEE. By rotating the probe clockwise and displacing the ultrasonic beam to the right (corresponding to plane 1 in Fig. 4-3), the longitudinal plane passes through the right atrium and superior vena cava, which are displayed in long axis (Fig. 4-5A, B, C, and D). Minimal leftward tilting of the probe from this position demonstrates the right upper pulmonary vein in long axis (Fig. 4-5E). Advancing the transducer slightly may also demonstrate the entrance of the inferior vena cava into the right atrium (Fig. 4-5F). Figure 4-5G represents a transverse section demonstrating the ascending aorta and the superior vena cava in short axis, the right upper pulmonary vein in oblique axis, and the right pulmonary artery in long axis more posteriorly. The corresponding long-axis section at this level demonstrates the superior vena cava in long axis and the right pulmonary artery in short axis. Figure 4-5H was taken after an intravenous injection of indocyanine green and initially demonstrates opacification of the superior vena cava, followed by opacification of the right pulmonary artery, both viewed in the longitudinal plane. Figure 4-5I and J demonstrates two different patients with ostium secundum atrial septal defects. In both

Figure 4-5
A, B, and C. Schema showing a longitudinal plane passing through the superior vena cava, right atrium, interatrial septum, and the left atrium.

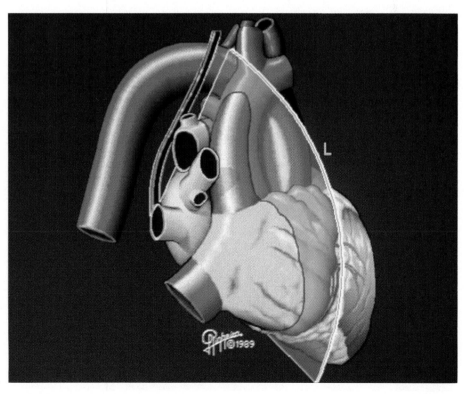

A.

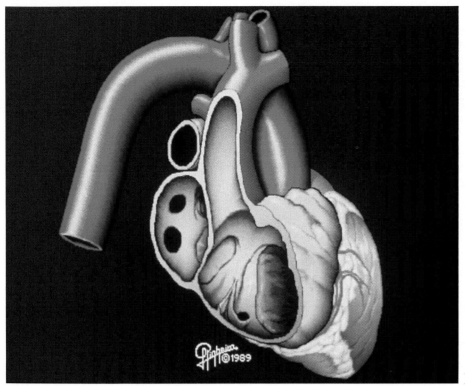

B.

Figure 4-4
(continued)

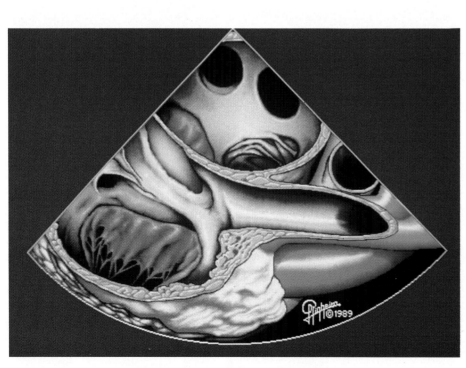

C.

Figure 4-5
D. The corresponding transesophageal image. The arrow points to the crista terminalis. IAS = interatrial septum.

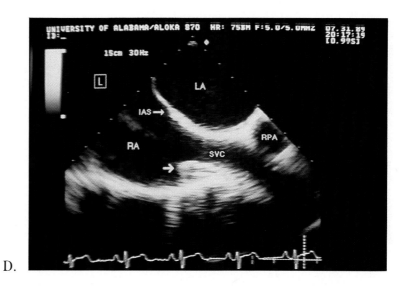

D.

Figure 4-5
E. Demonstrates the relationship of the right upper pulmonary vein (RUPV) to the superior vena cava.

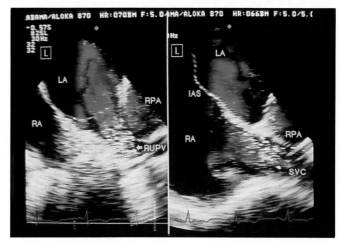

E.

Figure 4-5
F. Demonstrates both superior and inferior vena cava and a portion of the right atrial appendage (RAA). EV = eustachian valve.

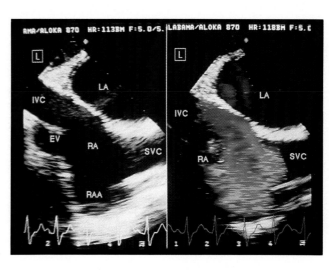

F.

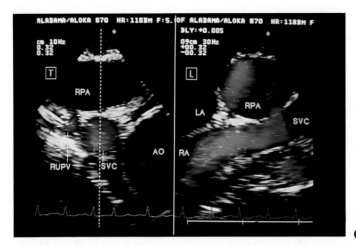

G.

Figure 4-5
G. Shows the relationship of the superior vena cava to the right pulmonary artery (which is dilated) using transverse and longitudinal planes.

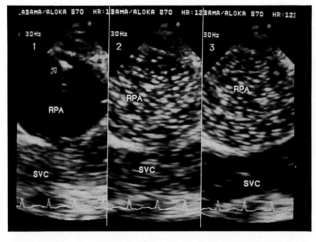

H.

Figure 4-5
H. Intravenous contrast injection using indocyanine green demonstrates opacification of the superior vena cava (left) followed by opacification of the right pulmonary artery (middle and right). A Swan-Ganz catheter (arrow) is seen in the right pulmonary artery.

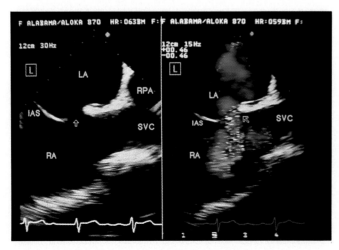

I.

Figure 4-5
I. Demonstrates the relationship of a large ostium secundum atrial septal defect (arrows) to the superior vena cava in an adult using the longitudinal plane.

Figure 4-5
J. Large ostium secundum atrial septal defect (arrows) in another adult patient viewed using both transverse and longitudinal planes.

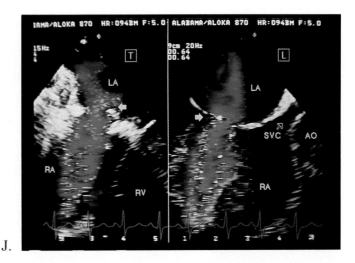

J.

intact interatrial septal tissue can be seen separating the defect from the superior vena cava. The combined use of transverse and longitudinal planes permits viewing of the atrial septum in two orthogonal planes, which allows for improved characterization and accurate sizing of atrial septal defects.

By rotating the probe counterclockwise and displacing the ultrasonic beam toward the left,

the right ventricular outflow tract, pulmonic valve, and main pulmonary artery can be displayed in long axis using the biplane transducer (Fig. 4-6*A*, *B*, *C*, *D*, and *E*). Angulation of the transducer tip using the probe's lateral control knob also demonstrates the aortic valve in true short axis using the longitudinal imaging plane (Fig. 4-6*F*). As shown in Fig. 4-6*F*, the conventional transverse plane demonstrates the aortic

Figure 4-6
A, B, and *C.* Schema showing a longitudinal plane passing through the long axis of the main pulmonary artery and the right ventricular outflow tract.

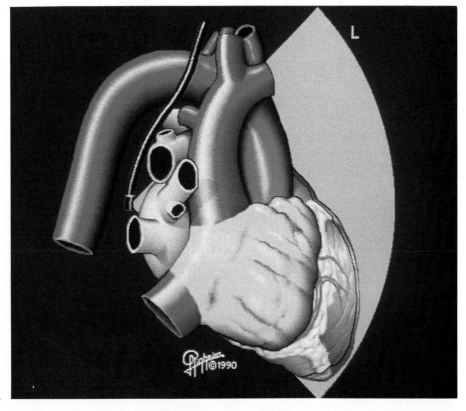

A.

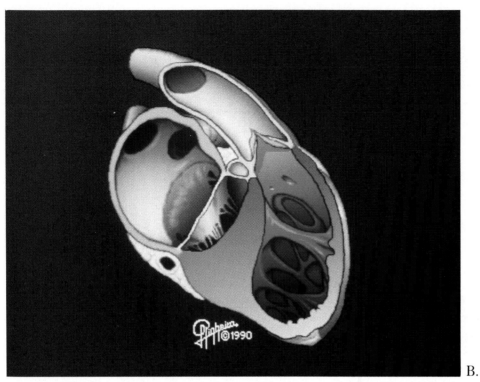

B.

Figure 4-6

(continued)

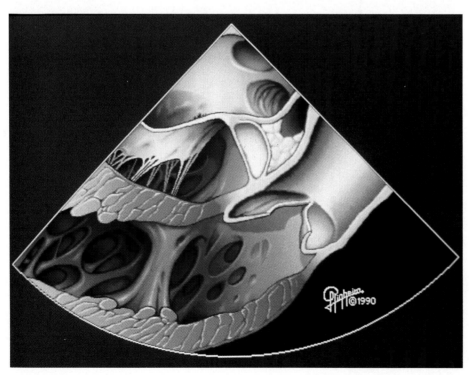

C.

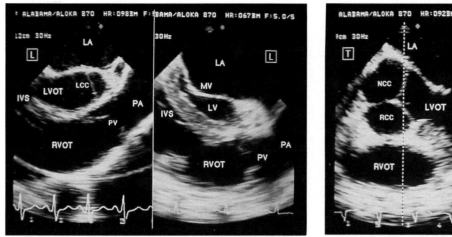

D.

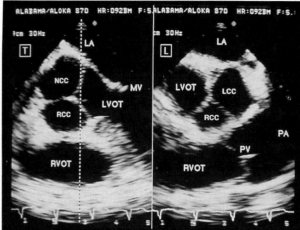

E.

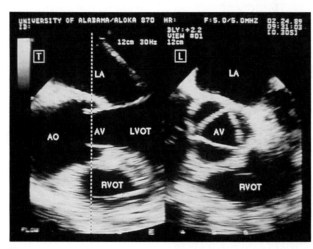

F.

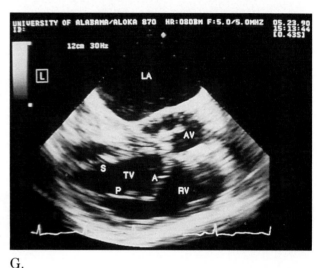

G.

Figure 4-6

D, E, F, and *G* represent the corresponding transesophageal images. *F* shows the aortic valve in true short axis using the longitudinal plane. This was obtained in a patient with a dilated aortic root and ascending aorta. The dotted lines in *E* and *F* represent the level in the transverse plane image at which the longitudinal plane was taken. In *G,* all three leaflets of the tricuspid valve are viewed in the longitudinal plane. This was accomplished by rotating the probe to the right. A = anterior tricuspid leaflet; AV = aortic valve; IVS = interventricular septum; LCC = left coronary cusp; LVOT = left ventricular outflow tract; MV = mitral valve; NCC = noncoronary cusp; P = posterior tricuspid leaflet; PA = main pulmonary artery; RCC = right coronary cusp; RVOT = right ventricular outflow tract; S = septal tricuspid leaflet; TV = tricuspid valve.

leaflets in the enlarged ascending aorta in long axis, while the longitudinal plane shows the aortic root and valve in true short axis. With further rotation of the probe to the right, all three leaflets of the tricuspid valve may be demonstrated in the longitudinal plane (Fig. 4-6*G*).

Figure 4-7 represents a schematic drawing that shows the longitudinal planes passing through the heart and the descending aorta at the level where a transesophageal four-chamber view can be obtained (which generally corresponds to the level of the eighth vertebral body). Plane 1 passes through the left and right atria and the right ventricle, plane 2 is shown passing through the left atrium and the left ventricle, and plane 3 traverses the descending thoracic aorta. Figure 4-8*A* represents a diagram showing orthogonal planes commonly used to examine the atrioventricular valves

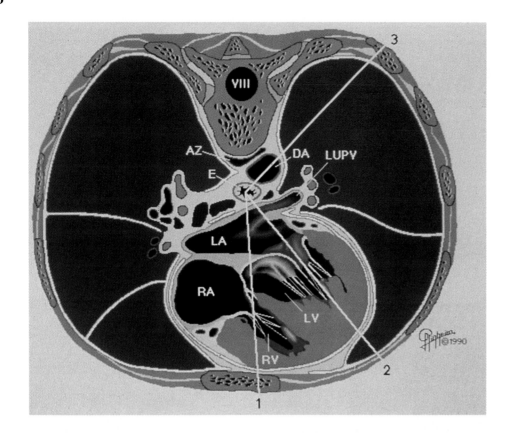

Figure 4-7
Schematic at the level of the eighth vertebral body showing various longitudinal planes that can be obtained by positioning the transesophageal probe at this level. AZ = azygos vein; DA = descending thoracic aorta; E = esophagus; LUPV = left upper pulmonary vein.

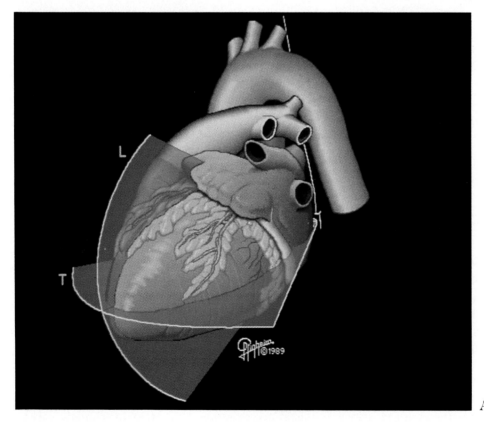

A.

Figure 4-8
A, B, and C. Schematics showing the four-chamber view obtained from the transverse plane (T) and the two-chamber view acquired utilizing the longitudinal plane (L).

Figure 4-8

(continued)

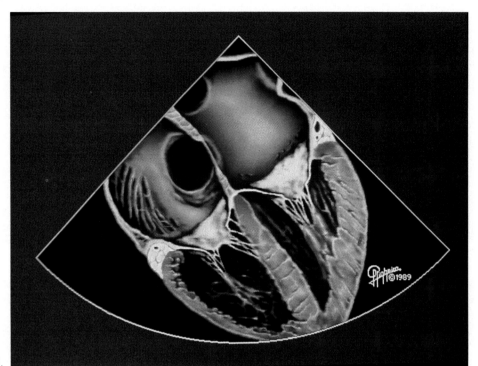

B.

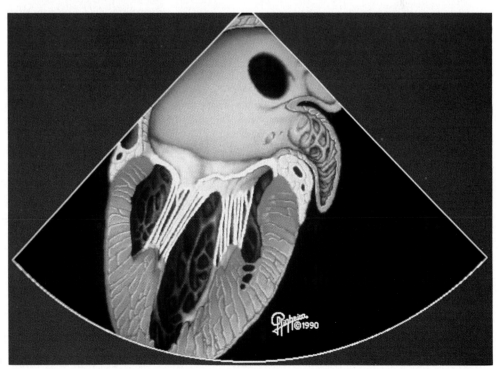

C.

Chapter 4

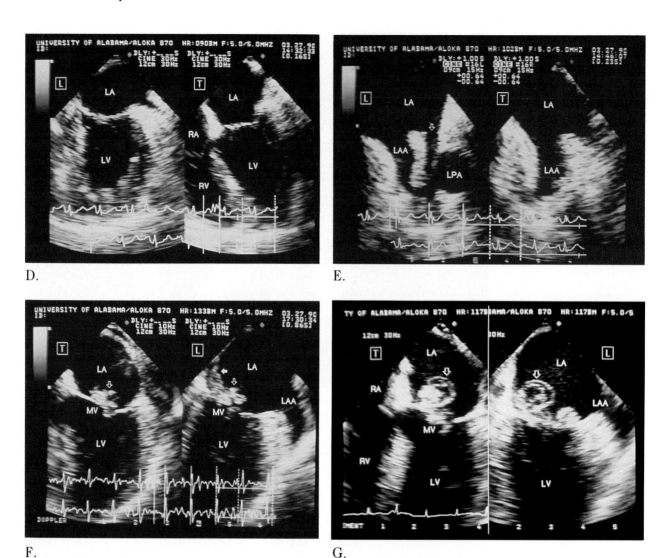

D.

E.

F.

G.

Figure 4-8

D. Demonstrates the corresponding transesophageal images. *E.* Shows examination of the left atrial appendage (LAA) using both longitudinal and transverse planes. The arrow points to the left upper pulmonary vein. LPA = left pulmonary artery. *F, G.* Biplane images in a patient with a large staphylococcal mitral valve vegetation (open arrows). Extension of the vegetation to involve the left atrial free wall (closed arrow) was noted only in the longitudinal plane. A large rounded abscess cavity (arrows) was noted in this patient a few days later (G).

and the ventricular cavities, particularly the left ventricle. The transverse plane demonstrates a typical four-chamber view showing the ventricular septum as well as the left ventricular posterolateral wall (Fig. 4-8B). The longitudinal plane, on the other hand, demonstrates the anterolateral and the inferior walls of the left ventricle and a portion of the left atrium, including the left atrial appendage. The appendage is seen adjacent to the basal anterior wall of the left ventricle. Both the anterolateral and

the posteromedial papillary muscles may also be visualized in this plane (Fig. 4-8C, corresponds to plane 2 in Fig. 4-7). Figure 4-8D shows an adult patient in whom the left atrium and the left ventricle are interrogated using both transverse and longitudinal planes. Figure 48E depicts the left atrial appendage viewed using both the transverse and longitudinal planes. In the longitudinal plane, the left superior pulmonary vein and the left pulmonary artery are seen adjacent to the left atrial ap-

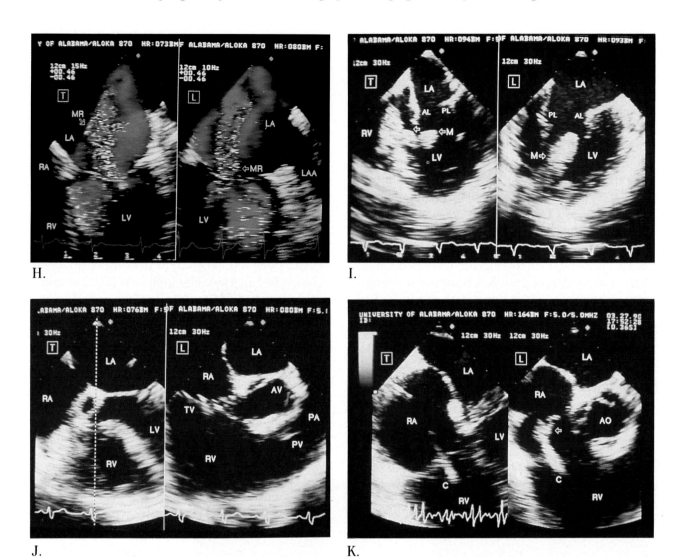

H.

I.

J.

K.

Figure 4-8

H. Color Doppler interrogation of mitral regurgitation (MR) using orthogonal planes. *I.* Left ventricular myxoma examined using four-chamber (transverse plane) and two-chamber (longitudinal plane) views. Although the two heads (arrows) of the tumor mass (M) were well visualized in the transverse plane, the apical attachment of the tumor was identified only when the longitudinal plane was utilized. AL = anterior mitral valve leaflet; PL = posterior mitral valve leaflet. *J.* Demonstrates the inflow and the outflow tracts of the right ventricle utilizing the longitudinal plane. A catheter is seen passing through the tricuspid valve. The corresponding transverse plane shows the inflow and outflow tracts of the left ventricle (five-chamber view). *K.* Minimal advancement of the transesophageal probe results in the detection of a vegetation (arrow) involving the right heart catheter (C) seen in *J*. The vegetation was best visualized in the longitudinal plane.

pendage, while in the transverse plane the left pulmonary artery is not visualized. Figure 4-8*F* demonstrates a large staphylococcal vegetation involving the mitral valve, as viewed in both transverse and longitudinal planes. Extension of the vegetation to involve the left atrial free wall is shown in the longitudinal plane; this finding could not be diagnosed using the standard transverse imaging plane. Figure 4-8*G*,

taken a few days later, shows the development of a large circular abscess cavity in the same patient. The use of biplane imaging for Doppler color flow mapping is also effective for demonstrating mitral regurgitation in two orthogonal planes (Fig. 4-8*H*). The additional planes provided by biplane imaging offer a more comprehensive examination of the mitral regurgitation, which can be very valuable for more reliable assessment of regurgitant severity, particularly when dealing with eccentric jets. Biplane examination in a patient with a left ventricular myxoma demonstrated the two heads of the tumor in the four-chamber view and its point of attachment in the apex in the two-chamber plane (Fig. 4-8*I*). Figure 4-8*J* demonstrates a standard five-chamber view using the transverse plane; the corresponding long-axis plane taken at this level shows aortic, pulmonic, and tricuspid valves, as well as the inflow and outflow tracts of the right ventricle (corresponds to plane 1 in Fig. 4-7). A catheter is also observed traversing the tricuspid valve. Figure 4-8*K* demonstrates a prominent vegetation involving a right heart catheter noted in the longitudinal plane; the vegetation was not well visualized in the corresponding four-chamber view obtained by the transverse plane. Figure 4-9*A*, *B*, *C*, and *D* shows the standard transverse transgastric plane viewing the left ventricle in short axis and the corresponding longitudinal plane viewing it in long axis. The dotted line in Fig. 4-9*D* shows the level at which the longitudinal plane was obtained. By slightly withdrawing and adjusting the probe, the left atrial appendage, the left pulmonary artery, the left upper pulmonary vein, the left circumflex coronary artery, and the coronary sinus may be brought into view utilizing the longitudinal plane; in this patient, a thrombus is seen in the left atrial appendage (Fig. 4-9*E*). Figure 4-9*F* shows the transgastric transverse and longitudinal planes taken at the level of the papillary muscles in a patient with left ventricular hypertrophy. Figure 4-9*G* shows transgastric transverse and longitudinal images of the same left ventricular myxoma previously shown in Fig. 4-8*I*. The long-axis plane is taken at the level of mitral valve leaflets and chordae, as shown by the dotted line in the short-axis view, and demonstrates the head of the tumor between the two papillary muscles. Note absence of any attachment of the myxoma to the papillary muscles in this patient.

Figure 4-10*A* illustrates the transverse and longitudinal planes passing through the descending thoracic aorta in the course of biplane

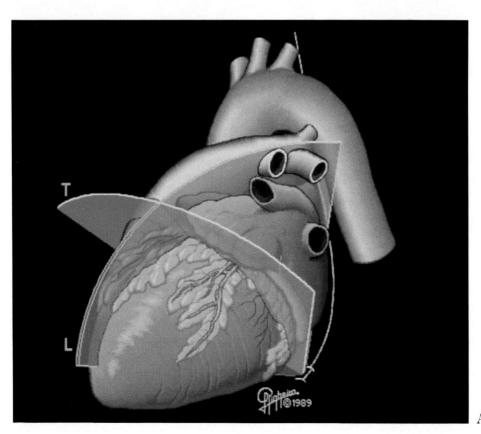

Figure 4-9

A, *B*, and *C*. Schematic representation of transgastric orthogonal planes demonstrating the left ventricle in short-axis (transverse plane) and two-chamber (longitudinal plane) views.

A.

Figure 4-9

(continued)

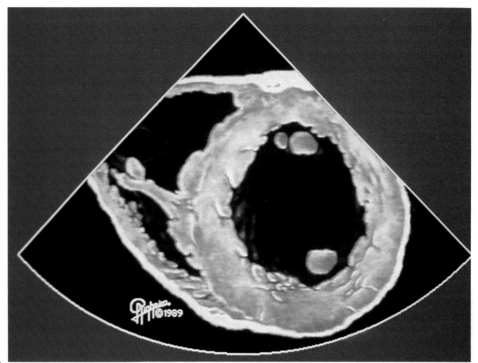

B.

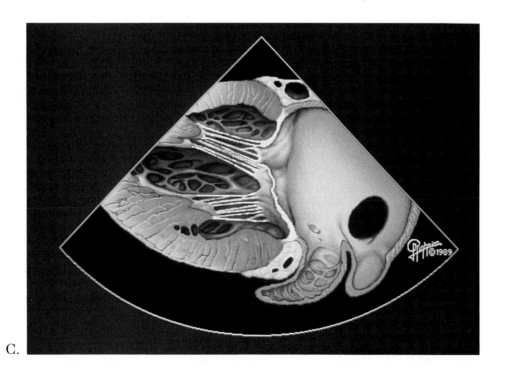

C.

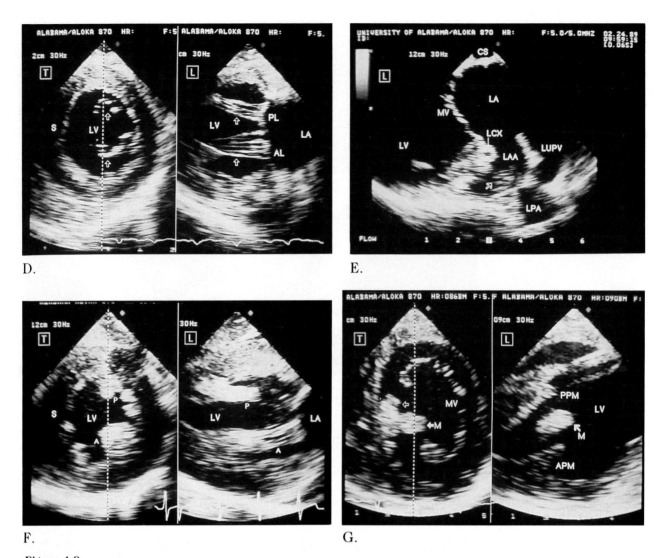

D.

E.

F.

G.

Figure 4-9

D. Demonstrates the corresponding transgastric images. The dotted line on the short-axis image shows the level at which the longitudinal plane was obtained. The arrows point to the mitral valve chordae. AL = anterior mitral valve leaflet; PL = posterior mitral valve leaflet. *E.* Represents a transgastric left heart two-chamber view showing the coronary sinus (CS), the left circumflex coronary artery (LCX), and the left pulmonary artery (LPA) in short axis. Note the presence of a clot (arrow) in the left atrial appendage (LAA) which is imaged next to the left upper pulmonary vein (LUPV). *F.* Transgastric examination in a patient with left ventricular hypertrophy demonstrates hypertrophied walls and papillary muscles in both transverse and longitudinal planes. A = anterolateral papillary muscle; P = posteromedial papillary muscle. *G.* Transgastric examination in the patient with a left ventricular myxoma (see Fig. 4-8*I*) demonstrates absence of any attachment of the tumor mass (M) to the anterior (APM) or posterior (PPM) papillary muscles in the longitudinal plane. Note that the dotted line on the transverse plane image representing the level at which the longitudinal plane was obtained passes through a head of the tumor.

interrogation. The corresponding images are shown in Fig. 4-10*B*. The vertebral bodies are imaged as echolucent spaces due to the inability of the ultrasonic beam to penetrate through bone. Intervertebral disks, on the other hand, can be penetrated by ultrasound and are visualized as linear echoes interposed between the vertebral bodies. The relationship of the esophagus to the descending thoracic aorta varies depending upon the vertebral level at which it is examined (Fig. 4-10*C*). The large echo-free space surrounding the descending

Figure 4-10
A. Schema representing transverse and longitudinal planes passing through the descending thoracic aorta.

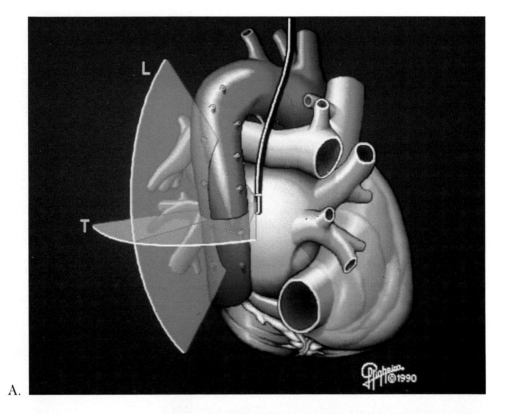

A.

Figure 4-10
B. Shows the corresponding transesophageal images. Since these images were obtained in the distal descending thoracic aorta, the aorta is imaged between the probe and the vertebral bodies (VB). The arrow points to a posterior intercostal vein. D = intervertebral disks.

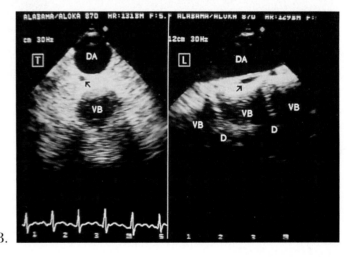

B.

aorta in Fig. 4-10D represents a large pleural effusion viewed in orthogonal planes. Figure 4-10E shows prominent atherosclerotic plaques in the descending thoracic aorta imaged utilizing the transverse and longitudinal transesophageal planes.

The ability of biplane TEE to image the heart and great vessels in multiple tomographic sections and to provide instantaneous information about morphology and blood flow has made it a valuable tool, which has found numerous and diverse clinical applications.[10–24]

A sound anatomical understanding of the obtainable biplane transesophageal echocardiographic views is the prerequisite for performing this procedure and will also serve as a solid basis for understanding the additional information provided by the new multiplane probes.

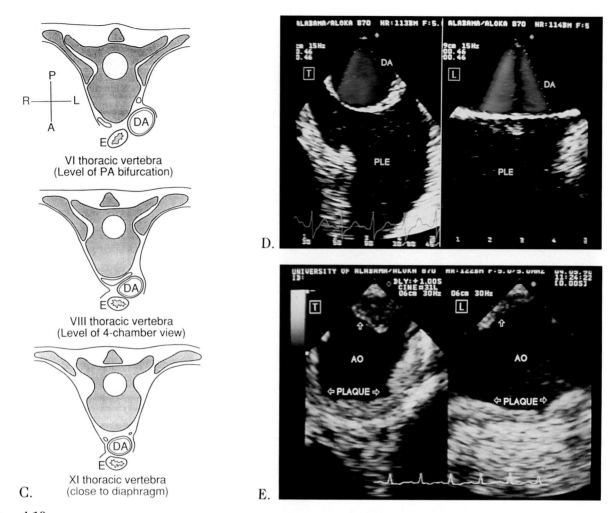

Figure 4-10

C. Schema showing the relationship of the esophagus (E) to the descending thoracic aorta (DA). The proximal portion of this vessel lies posteriorly and to the left of the esophagus but sebsequently it courses toward the midline and at the level of the 9th to 12th vertebral bodies positions itself directly posterior to the esophagus. *D.* Shows a large left pleural effusion (PLE) surrounding the descending thoracic aorta (DA) in both longitudinal and transverse planes. *E.* Prominent atherosclerotic plaques (arrows) in the descending thoracic aorta (AO) are imaged in both transverse and longitudinal planes.

References

1. Nanda N, Pinheiro L, Snayal R, et al: Transesophageal biplane echocardiographic imaging: Technique, planes, and clinical usefulness. *Echocardiography* 7:771, 1990.

2. Bansal R, Shakudo M, Shah P, et al: Biplane transesophageal echocardiography: Technique, image orientation, and preliminary experience in 131 patients. *J Am Soc Echocardiogr* 3:348, 1990.

3. Seward J, Khanderia B, Edwards W, et al: Biplanar transesophageal echocardiography: Anatomic correlations, image orientation, and clinical applications. *Mayo Clin Proc* 65:1193, 1990.

4. Omoto R, Kyo S, Matsumura M, et al: Biplane color Doppler transesophageal echocardiography: Its impact on cardiovascular surgery and further technological progress in the probe, a matrix phased-array biplane probe. *Echocardiography* 6:423, 1990.

5. Pandian N, Hsu TL, Schwartz S, et al: Multiplane transesophageal echocardiography: Imaging planes, echocardiographic anatomy, and clinical experience with a prototype phased array omniplane probe. *Echocardiography* 9:649, 1992.

6. Nanda N, Pinheiro L, Sanyal R, et al: Multiplane echocardiographic imaging and three-dimensional reconstruction: A preliminary study. *Echocardiography* 9:667, 1992.

7. Pandian N, Nanda N, Schwartz S, et al: Three-dimensional and four-dimensional transesophageal echocardiographic imaging of the heart and aorta in humans using a computed tomographic imaging probe. *Echocardiography* 9:677, 1992.

8. Schiller N, Maurer G, Ritter S, et al: Transesophageal echocardiography (position paper of the American Society of Echocardiography) *J Am Soc Echocardiogr* 2:354, 1989.

9. Seward J, Khanderia B, Oh J, et al: Transesophageal echocardiography: Technique, anatomic correlations, implementation, and clinical applications. *Mayo Clin Proc* 63:649, 1988.

10. Nellesen IJ, Schnittger I, Appleton CP, et al: Transesophageal two-dimensional echocardiography and color Doppler flow velocity mapping in the evaluation of cardiac valve prostheses. *Circulation* 78:848, 1989.

11. Taams MA, Gussenhoven EJ, Cahalan MK, et al: Transesophageal Doppler color flow imaging in the detection of native and Björk-Shiley mitral valve regurgitation. *J Am Coll Cardiol* 13:95, 1989.

12. Erbel R, Engberding R, Daniel W, et al: Echocardiography for diagnosis of aortic dissection. *Lancet* 1:457, 1989.

13. Ballal R, Nanda N, Gatewood R, et al: Usefulness of transesophageal echocardiography in assessment of aortic dissection. *Circulation* 84:1903, 1991.

14. Daniel W, Mügge A, Martin R, et al: Improvement in the diagnosis of abscesses associated with endocarditis by transesophageal echocardiography. *N Engl J Med* 324:795, 1991.

15. Mehta RH, Helmcke F, Nanda NC, et al: Transesophageal color Doppler echocardiographic assessment of atrial septal defect. *J Am Coll Cardiol* 16:1010, 1990.

16. Ritter SB, Thys D: Pediatric transesophageal color flow imaging: Smaller probes for smaller hearts. *Echocardiography* 6:431, 1990.

17. Smith JS: Intraoperative detection of myocardial ischemia in high-risk patients: Electrocardiography versus two-dimensional transesophageal echocardiography. *Circulation* 72:1015, 1985.

18. Kyo S, Takamoto S, Matsumura M, et al: Immediate and early postoperative evaluation of results of cardiac surgery by transesophageal two-dimensional Doppler echocardiography. *Circulation* 76(suppl V):113, 1987.

19. Maurer G, Siegel R, Czer L: The use of color flow mapping for intraoperative assessment of mitral valve repair. *Circulation* 84(suppl I):250, 1991.

20. Ballal R, Mahan EF III, Nanda NC, et al: Utility of transesophageal echocardiography in interatrial septal puncture during percutaneous mitral balloon valvuloplasty. *Am J Cardiol* 66:230, 1990.

21. Kay GN, Holman WL, Nanda NC: Combined use of TEE and endocardial mapping to localize the site of origin of ectopic atrial tachycardia. *Am J Cardiol* 65:1284, 1990.

22. Boogaerts J, Samdarshi TE, Nanda NC, et al: Anomalous separate origin of left circumflex coronary artery from a separate ostium in the left coronary sinus: Identification by transesophageal color Doppler echocardiography. *Echocardiography* 7:165, 1990.

23. Samdarshi TE, Chang LK, Gatewood R, et al: Usefulness and limitations of transesophageal color Doppler echocardiography in the assessment of proximal coronary artery stenosis. *J Am Coll Cardiol* 19:572, 1992.

24. Coy K, Maurer G, Goodman D, et al: Transesophageal echocardiographic detection of aortic atheromatosis may provide clues to occult renal dysfunction in the elderly. *Am Heart J* 123:1684, 1992.

5

Transesophageal Echocardiographic Evaluation of Valvular Heart Disease

Cheryl L. Reid
Shiro Yamachika
Julius M. Gardin

Introduction

Doppler two-dimensional echocardiography by the transthoracic approach has been a valuable noninvasive technique in the assessment of patients with known or suspected native valve disease.[1] Hemodynamic data, including transvalvular gradients, blood flows, valve area, intracardiac pressures, and ventricular function, can be estimated and the presence and severity of valvular regurgitation assessed by transthoracic echocardiography.[2–7] Transesophageal echocardiography has extended our imaging fields and provided unique information regarding native valvular morphology and function. The posterior location of the echocardiographic transducer within the esophagus permits detailed examination of intracardiac chambers and structures that may be obscured by transthoracic echocardiographic imaging (Table 5-1). The left atrium particularly is well visualized by transesophageal echocardiogra-

phy. The presence of left atrial thrombi or mitral regurgitation, which may be obscured by poor imaging or acoustic shadowing from calcification or prosthetic valves with transthoracic echocardiography, can be detected. Because of the proximity of the ultrasound transducer and the superior resolution of transesophageal echocardiography, abnormalities of valvular structure, such as flail leaflets and the presence of vegetations, are also better visualized. Finally, structures such as the pulmonary veins are more easily evaluated by transesophageal echocardiography and have proved useful in estimating the severity of mitral regurgitation. Recent advances in technology have made possible hemodynamic measurements, including valve areas, gradients, and intracardiac pressures, by transesophageal Doppler echocardiography. Thus clinically diagnostic information can be obtained in patients with valvular disease by the combined application of transthoracic and transesophageal echocardiography.

TABLE 5-1   Role of Transesophageal Echocardiography in the Evaluation of Left-Sided Native Valve Disease

Left and right ventricular size and function
Left and right atrial size and function
Left atrial pressure
Presence of atrial thrombi
Mitral valve morphology
   Stenosis: Valve thickening and calcification,
     commissural fusion and calcification, leaflet mobility,
     and subvalvular disease
   Regurgitation: Proplapse, flail leaflets, chordal rupture,
     systolic anterior motion, vegetations, and annular
     dilatation and calcification
Aortic valve morphology
   Stenosis: Thickening and calcification, congenital
     abnormalities
   Regurgitation: Prolapse, flail leaflets, perforation,
     vegetations, annular dilatation, aortic dissection
Hemodynamic severity
   Mitral: Valve area, gradient, presence and severity of
     regurgitation, pulmonary artery systolic pressure
   Aortic: Valve gradient, area, presence and severity of
     regurgitation

This chapter describes the contribution of transesophageal echocardiography in the assessment of native valve stenosis and regurgitation. The complementary roles of transthoracic and transesophageal Doppler echocardiography in the diagnosis of valvular abnormalities and the assessment of the hemodynamic consequences are emphasized.

Left-Sided Lesions

Imaging Views

Mitral Valve

The mitral valve and its supporting structures can be completely visualized by transesophageal echocardiographic imaging with the probe in the transgastric and midesophagus positions.[8-11] Midesophageal transverse imaging provides a four-chamber view in which the medial or lateral segments of the anterior mitral valve leaflet, middle or lateral segment of the posterior mitral valve leaflet, atria, and ventri-

cles can be assessed. Longitudinal views from the midesophagus include the two-chamber view in which the middle scallop of the posterior mitral leaflet, the lateral segment of the anterior mitral leaflet, left atrium, left atrial appendage, and left ventricle can be evaluated. In the midesophagus imaging planes, shadowing from a heavily calcified mitral valve or annulus may prevent optimal visualization of the subvalvular and left ventricular areas. Advancement of the probe into the fundus of the stomach with anteflexion of the tip yields a short-axis view of the mitral valve in the transverse plane. The mitral valve opening and both segments of the anterior leaflet and all three scallops of the posterior leaflet can be evaluated. The longitudinal plane results in a transgastric two-chamber view in which the medial scallop of the posterior leaflet and lateral segment of the anterior leaflet are imaged. In this view, the subvalvular papillary muscles and chordal attachments to the mitral valve leaflets can be fully visualized. By imaging in these multiple tomographic views, the various components of the mitral valve apparatus, including the segments of the anterior leaflet, the scallops of the posterior leaflets, commissures, chordae tendineae, and papillary muscles can be evaluated. The morphology of the mitral valve can be assessed for abnormalities that may result in valvular regurgitation or stenosis. Continuous-wave Doppler interrogation of the high-velocity mitral valve flows in patients with mitral stenosis can be recorded from the midesophagus transverse four-chamber view. Color flow imaging should be performed in each view to evaluate for the presence of abnormal flow patterns and valvular regurgitation.

Pulmonary Veins

Images of the pulmonary veins can be obtained in the basal views with the probe in the upper esophagus position.[8-11] The left upper pulmonary vein is the most easily identified and lies superior and to the right of the left atrial appendage in the transverse and longitudinal basal views. With slight withdrawal of the probe, the right upper pulmonary vein can be visualized in the basal longitudinal view. Color and pulsed-wave Doppler imaging can be performed to record the pulmonary venous velocity profiles.

Aortic Valve

The aortic valve can be visualized and assessed for abnormalities by imaging with the probe in the midesophagus and basal positions.[8–11] The aortic cusps and leaflets can be evaluated in the transverse and longitudinal basal short-axis views. The left ventricular outflow tract is evaluated by the combined use of the midesophagus transverse five-chamber and the longitudinal ascending aorta views. Normal blood flows of the left ventricular outflow tract and aortic valve can be interrogated with pulsed and color Doppler. The severity of aortic regurgitation can be assessed with color Doppler flow mapping. In patients with valvular aortic stenosis, the high-velocity jets across the aortic valve may be recorded using continuous-wave Doppler. It may be difficult, however, to assure that the Doppler beam is parallel to the stenotic jet—with the lack of a parallel beam resulting in underestimation of the maximal jet velocity.

Stenotic Lesions

Mitral

Mitral stenosis, in adults, is most commonly due to the late effects of acute rheumatic carditis. Stenosis results from calcification of the valve leaflets, commissural fusion, and fusion and calcification of the subvalvular apparatus.[12] In patients with mitral stenosis, the treatment is generally commissurotomy, with either percutaneous balloon commissurotomy or surgical commissurotomy. Several studies have shown that results of these treatments are influenced by the morphology of the mitral valve apparatus.[13–15] By transthoracic echocardiography, the mobility of the mitral valve leaflets, the presence and severity of subvalvular disease, and valvular thickening can be visualized. In patients in whom the transthoracic echocardiogram is inadequate, transesophageal echocardiography can provide the same detailed analysis of mitral valve morphology (Fig. 5-1A and B).[17] Similar scores for valve mobility and thickening are obtained by both transesophageal and transthoracic echocardiography. These two components of valve morphology have been shown to be the most important predictors of the results of balloon commissurotomy.[14,18] Subvalvular thickening and calcification may be underestimated by monoplane transesophageal echocardiography, probably due to masking of the subvalvular region from thickening and calcification in the mitral valve leaflets. Biplane transesophageal echocardiography improves imaging of the subvalvular region with the additional transgastric longitudinal imaging plane.

In addition to being used to assess morphologic abnormalities of the mitral valve in patients with mitral stenosis, transesophageal imaging is useful in evaluating associated valvular disease, left atrial and left ventricular function, and right heart function. Transesophageal echocardiography has been shown to be superior to transthoracic echocardiography in the imaging of the left atrial appendage and in the detection of left atrial thrombi.[19,20] The presence of a left atrial thrombus is considered to be a contraindication to the performance of mitral balloon commissurotomy.[21] Since the catheters must traverse the left atrium, dislodgment of a thrombus may occur with a resultant systemic embolus. In most patients, the mitral valve gradient and area can be measured by transthoracic continuous-wave Doppler. With the development of transesophageal imaging technology, including continuous-wave Doppler, these measurements can now be determined in the occasional patient in whom the transthoracic echocardiogram is inadequate, or for intraoperative monitoring (Fig. 5–2).[22] The mitral valve area can be determined by the pressure half-time method and valve gradient by the modified Bernoulli equation as applied in transthoracic Doppler echocardiography.[2,3]

The status of the mitral valve, whether it is stenotic or regurgitant, alters the normal pulmonary venous flow patterns. In patients with mild to moderate mitral stenosis in normal sinus rhythm, the diastolic phase is prolonged and significantly reduced with decreased systolic flow. The atrial phase shows marked retrograde flow.[23] In patients with severe mitral stenosis in normal sinus rhythm, diastolic flow

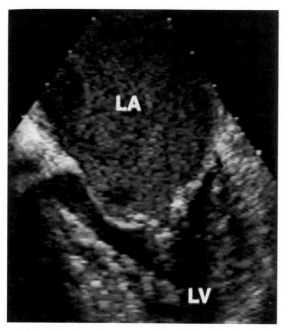

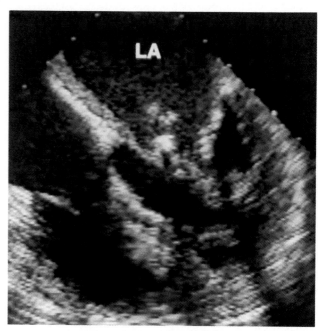

A.   B.

Figure 5-1

Midesophagus transverse four-chamber view of two patients with mitral stenosis. *A.* The mitral leaflets appear thin and pliable without calcification. No subvalvular disease is noted. Spontaneous contrast is visualized within the left atrium (LA). *B.* The mitral leaflets appear thickened with focal areas of calcification. The subvalvular apparatus shows thickened chordae tendineae without calcification. The increase in valve area with balloon or surgical commissurotomy would be expected to be less with this valve than that expected from the mitral valve shown in *A.* LV = left ventricle.

is absent or severely reduced and systole becomes the predominant filling phase of the left atrium from the pulmonary veins. Marked retrograde flow into the pulmonary veins occurs with atrial contraction. In contrast, in patients with severe mitral stenosis and atrial fibrillation, the major portion of left atrial filling occurs in the diastolic phase with a markedly reduced systolic phase. The pulmonary venous flow pattern observed in patients with mitral stenosis results from the prolonged atrioventricular pressure gradient during diastole between the left atrium and left ventricle. Because of the prolonged gradient, left atrial pressure remains elevated during diastole, resulting in decreased filling of the left atrium from the pulmonary veins. In the presence of atrial fibrillation, pulmonary systolic flow decreases because of the lack of atrial relaxation and volume change.

Aortic

Congenital abnormalities of the aortic valve, with visualization of the number of cusps, valve mobility, and leaflet thickening, can be easily evaluated by transesophageal echocardiography (Fig. 5-3). Direct measurement of the aortic valve orifice by transthoracic two-dimensional echocardiography in adult patients with aortic stenosis is difficult. The resolution of the images is a major limitation to the ability to completely define the entire aortic valve orifice. With transesophageal echocardiography this limitation can be overcome. Care must be given to define the smallest aortic orifice by scanning in the transverse short-axis view (Fig. 5-4*A* and *B*). The orifice can be measured at the maximal opening in systole in those patients in whom the entire circumference can be visualized without echo dropout. Aortic valve orifice area determined by transesophageal echocardiogra-

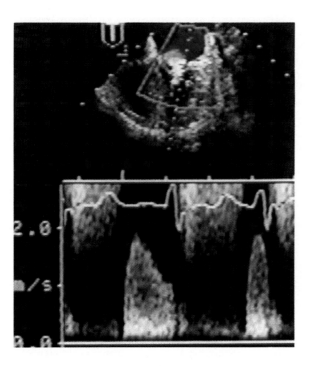

Figure 5-2
Continuous-wave Doppler ultrasound examination of a patient with rheumatic mitral stenosis and atrial fibrillation performed from the midesophagus transverse four-chamber view. The flow velocity tracing has been inverted and shows an increased velocity and prolonged pressure half-time typical of mitral stenosis.

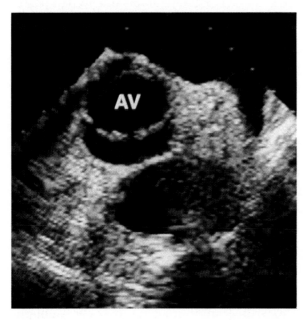

Figure 5-3
Basal short-axis transverse view of the aortic valve (AV) during systole. The orifice shows two leaflets of a bicuspid valve.

phy has been reported to be reliable, with a correlation value of $r = 0.92$ with cardiac catheterization determined aortic valve area.[24] The aortic valve orifice in one study would be directly measured in 83 percent of patients, while severe aortic stenosis (valve area <0.75 cm^2) could be predicted with a sensitivity of 100 percent and specificity of 73 percent. The presence of severe calcification of the valve leaflets or distortion of the leaflets in congenital abnormalities prevents imaging of the true orifice in one plane and may preclude direct measurement by both transthoracic and transesophageal imaging. This can lead to overestimation of the aortic valve area. In patients in whom the transthoracic study is inadequate for the assessment of aortic valve morphology and its hemodynamic consequences, transesophageal echocardiography may be a valuable alternative.

Regurgitation

Mitral

Anatomic Assessment Transesophageal echocardiography is superior to transthoracic echocardiography in the detection of the anatomic abnormalities responsible for mitral regurgitation. The precise definition of the structural defect is necessary to guide the selection of patients for mitral valve repair. Mitral valve abnormalities that can lead to severe regurgitation include myxomatous degeneration, rheumatic, annular calcification, papillary muscle rupture due to infarction, systolic anterior motion in patients with hypertrophic cardiomyopathy, flail chordae tendineae, and endocarditis with vegetations, perforations, and rupture. Transthoracic echocardiography is particularly limited in patients with severe lung disease, chest deformities or obesity, prosthetic mitral valves, and heavy calcification of the mitral leaflets or annulus. With transesophageal echocardiography, due to the proximity of the probe to the posterior cardiac structures, the left atrium, mitral valve, and its supporting structures can be visualized for assessment of the mechanism of the regurgitation.

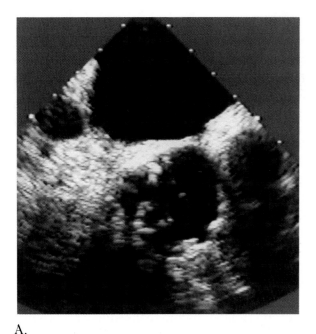

A.

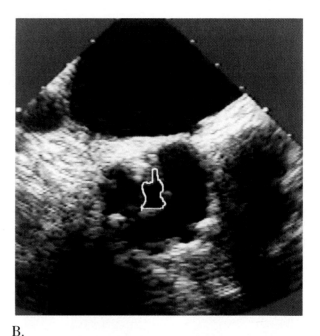

B.

Figure 5-4
Basal short-axis transverse view of a stenotic aortic valve. By careful scanning in this plane the smallest orifice of the aortic valve can be identified (*A*) and planimetered (*B*) to determine the valve area. The aortic

valve area by planimetry is 0.6 cm², which correlates well with the echocardiographic and Doppler determined aortic valve area of 0.7 cm² and cardiac catheterization determined area of 0.9 cm². (Courtesy of Dr. Harry Peled.)

Several studies have shown that transesophageal is more sensitive than transthoracic echocardiography for the detection of flail mitral leaflets due to ruptured chordae tendineae.[25–29] Hozumi et al. studied 17 patients with severe mitral regurgitation undergoing mitral valve repair and found that transesophageal was 100 percent sensitive and specific for the detection of ruptured chordae tendineae compared to 65 percent sensitivity and 100 percent specificity for transthoracic echocardiography.[26] Direct visualization of the ruptured chordae tendineae by transthoracic echocardiography was possible in only 35 percent of the patients. By transesophageal echocardiography, a ruptured chordae tendineae is seen as abnormal coaptation of the mitral leaflets or the presence of thin undulating echo structures within the left atrial cavity during systole. Flail mitral leaflets are also invariably associated with eccentric regurgitation jets (Fig. 5-5). The direction of the jet aids in identifying the abnormal mitral leaflet. Eccentric jets that are directed along the posterolateral wall of the

left atrium are associated with flail anterior mitral leaflets. Eccentric jets due to flail posterior mitral leaflets are directed along the interatrial septum (Fig. 5-6).[30] Regurgitant jets due to lack of leaflet coaptation, as in rheumatic disease or with a dilated annulus, are usually centrally directed (Fig. 5-7). The diagnostic criteria for mitral valve prolapse by transesophageal echocardiography have not been determined.

Rupture of a papillary muscle is a rare but life-threatening mechanical complication of acute myocardial infarction. A rapid diagnosis is necessary for improved survival with surgical intervention. Transthoracic echocardiography has been shown to be useful in the diagnosis of a ruptured papillary muscle; however, in the setting of critically ill patients who are often mechanically ventilated, transthoracic echocardiography imaging may be suboptimal.[31–33] Transesophageal echocardiography in these patients provides clear images in which the head of the ruptured papillary muscle and its chordae tendineae can be visualized within

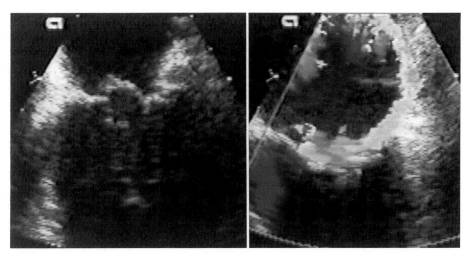

Figure 5-5
Midesophagus transverse four-chamber view of a patient who developed acute mitral regurgitation due to ruptured chordae tendineae. Left panel: The anterior mitral valve leaflet shows bulging into the left atrium with abnormal coaptation during real-time analysis. Right panel: Color Doppler flow mapping that shows a regurgitant jet directed along the lateral wall of the left atrium. (Courtesy of Dr. Harry Peled.)

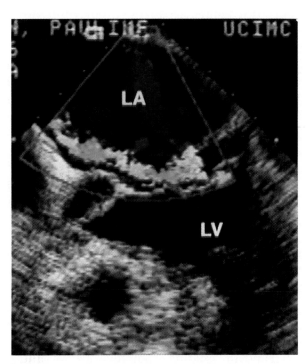

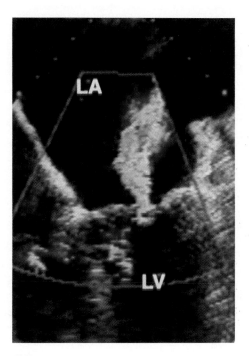

Figure 5-6
Transesophageal echocardiogram in the transverse midesophagus view of a patient with prolapse of the posterior leaflet of the mitral valve. Color Doppler flow mapping shows the regurgitant jet directed along the interatrial septum. LA = left atrium; LV = left ventricle.

Figure 5-7
Systolic frame from the midesophagus transesophageal four-chamber view. The regurgitant jet is centrally directed due to a dilated mitral annulus in this patient with an idiopathic cardiomyopathy. LA = left atrium; LV = left ventricle.

the body of the left atrium during systole (Fig. 5-8).

In addition to the evaluation of the mechanism of mitral regurgitation, the presence and severity of the regurgitation can be assessed by color and pulsed-wave Doppler ultrasound. Difficulty in assessing the presence and severity of the mitral regurgitation may occur with transthoracic echocardiography in patients with suboptimal images. The presence of mitral stenosis with heavy calcification or prosthetic mitral valves obstructs the transmission of the Doppler ultrasound to the left atrium with transthoracic imaging.[34] Transesophageal echocardiography eliminates these difficulties of lung and rib interference and "flow masking" from strong echo reflectors between the transducer and left atrium. The sensitivity of transesophageal echocardiography compared to left ventriculography in the assessment of the presence of mitral regurgitation has been reported to be 96 to 100 percent.[35, 36] Specificity ranges from 38 to 44 percent, with regurgitant jet areas of <1.5 cm² detected by transesophageal echocardiography in patients without regurgitation by left ventriculography. Small regurgitant jet areas have been reported in 62 percent of patients without mitral regurgitation by left ventriculography.[37]

Color Doppler Jet Size The assessment of the severity of mitral regurgitation by both transesophageal and transthoracic echocardiography is based upon the spatial distribution of the regurgitant jet. Semiquantitative grading of the severity of the mitral regurgitation has shown a good correlation with angiography when performed by transthoracic echocardiography.[38,39] However, the criteria for the assessment of the severity of the mitral regurgitation by color Doppler jet size differ between transthoracic echocardiography and transesophageal echocardiography. A variety of factors influence the spatial distribution of the regurgitant jet by both techniques. Instrument settings that affect the jet size include the color flow gain, transducer frequency, pulse-repetition frequency, and color flow map used.[40–42] It must be recognized that the size of the jet is more dependent upon the velocity of the regurgitant jet or driving pressure between the left ventricle and left atrium than upon the actual volume of the regurgitation.[43] Eccentric jets that impinge upon the atrial wall or interatrial septum may have their spatial distribution distorted by the Coanda effect (Fig. 5-9).[44] Finally, physiologic factors such as left atrial compliance and ventricular afterload have been shown to affect the size of the regurgitant jet.[45] All these factors must be considered when estimating the severity of the regurgitation by either transthoracic echocardiography or transesophageal echocardiography.

With the advent of transesophageal echocardiography, it was assumed that the same standards employed for transthoracic echocardiography in grading the severity of mitral regurgitation could be applied to the transesophageal echocardiographic images. However, the closer proximity of the transducer to the flow, the shallower depth setting, decreased attenuation of the Doppler signals, and higher

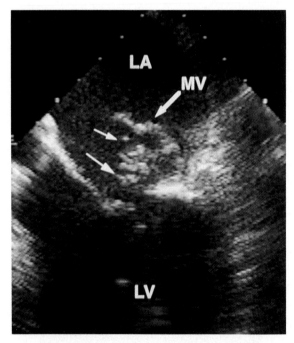

Figure 5-8
Flail posterior leaflet of the mitral valve (MV) due to myocardial infarction. The ruptured head of the papillary muscle (arrows) can be visualized within the left atrium (LA) in this midesophagus transverse five-chamber systolic frame. LV = left ventricle. (Courtesy of Dr. Harry Peled.)

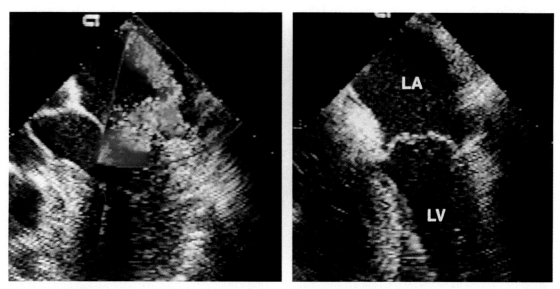

Figure 5-9
Left panel: Color Doppler flow mapping shows a mitral regurgitant jet that impinges upon the lateral wall of the left atrium (LA) in this midesophagus transverse five-chamber systolic frame. Right panel: The regurgitation was due to marked prolapse of both the anterior and posterior mitral valve leaflets. LV = left ventricle.

transducer frequency by transesophageal echocardiography alter the size of the color jet compared to that imaged by transthoracic echocardiography. Because of these technical factors, the size of the perceived color flow disturbance is larger with transesophageal echocardiography than when imaged by transthoracic echocardiography.[46] Thus there is a tendency to overestimate the severity of the regurgitation by transesophageal imaging when using the same criteria applied in transthoracic echocardiography.

Despite the list of variables known to influence jet size and the differences between imaging by transesophageal and transthoracic echocardiography, studies have shown that a semiquantitative assessment of the severity of mitral regurgitation can be made by Doppler color flow imaging. The maximal jet area visualized in any imaging plane should be utilized. Biplane transesophageal echocardiography improves the correlation of the assessment of regurgitation severity when compared to left ventricular angiography.[47] The best correlation with left ventriculography is obtained with the maximal regurgitant jet from either the transverse or longitudinal imaging planes (Fig.

5-10). Examination in multiple planes is particularly important in the evaluation of maximal area in eccentric jets. The optimal method for measurement of the area of disturbed flow is unclear. The most widely used clinical method is to include the central aliased velocities and the surrounding low-velocity laminar flow. A jet area greater than 7 cm^2 predicts severe regurgitation with a sensitivity of 83 percent and specificity of 100 percent.[47] A jet area less than 4 cm^2 predicts an angiographic grading of mild regurgitation with a sensitivity and specificity of 82 and 95 percent, respectively. Recent data, however, suggest that for transesophageal studies, the more central mosaic pattern provides the least variability and the best correlation with left ventricular angiography, whereas in transthoracic studies, both the central aliased area and surrounding laminar flow should be included.[48] If only the mosaic area is considered, a jet area less than 3 cm^2 predicts mild regurgitation with a sensitivity of 96 percent and specificity of 100 percent; in contrast, a jet area less than 6 cm^2 predicts severe mitral regurgitation with a sensitivity and specificity of 91 and 100 percent, respectively.[48]

TRANSVERSE

LONGITUDINAL

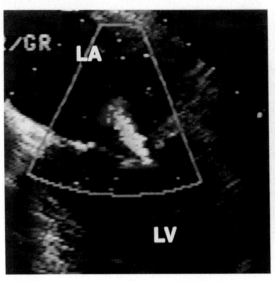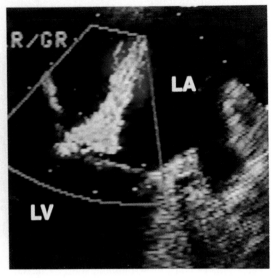

Figure 5-10
Biplane transesophageal imaging of a patient with mild mitral regurgitation. Left panel: In the midesophagus transverse four-chamber view, the jet is centrally directed and is minimal. The maximal jet area is 1.5 cm². Right panel: In the longitudinal midesophagus view, the regurgitant jet area appears much larger and measures 3.5 cm². LA = left atrium; LV = left ventricle.

Pulmonary Veins Pulmonary venous flow has recently been shown to reflect changes in left atrial pressure during the cardiac cycle.[49] The pulmonary veins act as a conduit between the lungs and left atrium in a pulsatile flow pattern that is influenced by left atrial pressure, mitral valve function, and left ventricular compliance. Abnormalities of pulmonary venous flow can be expected in a variety of cardiac diseases whose hemodynamic changes are determined by these factors. Pulsed-wave Doppler echocardiography from both the transthoracic and transesophageal approaches can be used to record the pulmonary venous flow patterns. By transthoracic echocardiography, the right or left upper pulmonary veins can be visualized from the apical window; however, because of the location of the pulmonary veins in the far field it is often difficult to place and maintain the pulsed Doppler sample volume distal to the pulmonary vein orifice. With the advent of transesophageal echocardiography, it is often possible to provide excellent images of all four pulmonary veins. Color Doppler echocardiography can be used with both transthoracic and

transesophageal echocardiography to identify the flow signals and optimize placement of the pulsed-wave sample volume. Because of the location of the pulmonary veins in the far field by transthoracic echocardiography, the quality of the flow velocity tracings is often poor, with spectral broadening that makes quantitative analysis difficult. Biphasic systolic flow is not usually visualized, and reversed flow due to atrial contraction in one study was visualized in only 37 percent of normal subjects, but in 100 percent of normal subjects by transesophageal echocardiography.[50] Thus the flow patterns and velocities detected will differ slightly between transthoracic and transesophageal echocardiography.

Normal pulmonary venous flow consists of three major phases: (1) forward systolic inflow that may consist of two components due to atrial relaxation and ventricular contraction with the downward motion of the mitral annulus, (2) diastolic flow following mitral valve opening, and (3) a variable negative signal due to atrial contraction. The pulmonary venous flow pattern is shown in Fig. 5-11. Normal

Figure 5-11
In the longitudinal midesophagus imaging plane the left upper pulmonary vein can be seen adjacent to the left atrial appendage. Color Doppler flow imaging of the red jet aids in the placement of the pulsed Doppler sample volume distal to the orifice of the pulmonary vein at maximal blood flow. In the lower portion of the picture, the pulsed Doppler spectral tracing illustrates the two forward flows in systole (S) and diastole (D) and the reversed flow that occurs with atrial (A) contraction. In this patient, the forward systolic flow is less than the diastolic forward flow due to the presence of moderate mitral regurgitation.

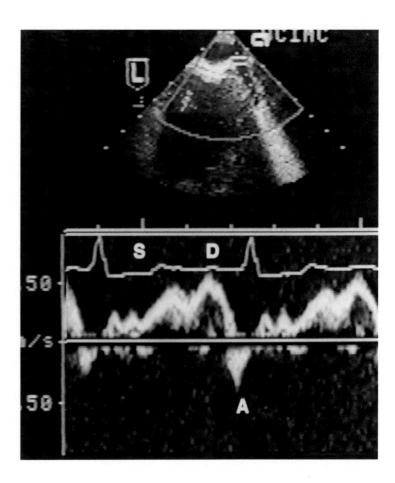

pulmonary venous flow velocities for transthoracic and transesophageal echocardiography are shown in Table 5-2. Pulmonary venous and mitral flow velocities have been shown to be influenced by a number of hemodynamic variables, including loading conditions and ventricular compliance in addition to abnormal disease states.[51–53] Factors that affect measurement of pulmonary venous flow are listed in Table 5-3.

TABLE 5-2   Pulmonary Venous Velocities by Transesophageal and Transthoracic Echocardiography in Normal Subjects

| | Transesophageal* | | Transthoracic* |
	LUPV	RUPV	RUPV
Systolic (early)	39 ± 11		
Peak systolic (cm/s)	60 ± 17	52 ± 15	50 ± 14
Peak diastolic (cm/s)	44 ± 9	44 ± 14	41 ± 6
S/D ratio	1.4 ± 0.3	1.3 ± 0.4	1.2 ± 0.3
Peak A reversal (cm/s)	24 ± 14	17 ± 10	21 ± 16
Systolic FVI	15 ± 3.1	12 ± 4.4	11 ± 1.5
Diastolic FVI	8 ± 3	7.8 ± 4	8.5 ± 3.1
A Wave FVI	2 ± 1.3	1.8 ± 0.6	2 ± 1

Source   Castello et al: *J Am Coll Cardiol* July 1991; reprinted with permission.

*Data are presented as mean ± standard deviation.

Abbreviations: A = atrial; FVI = flow velocity integral; LUPV = left upper pulmonary vein; RUPV = right upper pulmonary vein; S/D = systolic/diastolic.

TABLE 5-3   Factors Influencing Pulmonary Venous Flow

Systolic
    Left atrial pressure
    Cardiac output
    Atrial relaxation
    Left atrial area change and volume
    Left atrial compliance
    Left ventricular systolic function
    Mitral regurgitation
    Rhythm
Diastolic
    Left ventricular end-diastolic pressure
    Left atrial pressure
    Left ventricular compliance
    Left ventricular relaxation
    Viscoelastic myocardial forces
Atrial
    Rhythm
    Left atrial compliance
    Left ventricular compliance
    Left atrial contractility

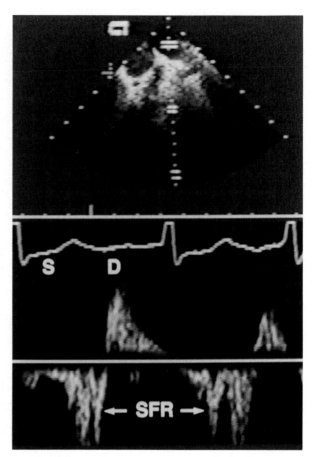

Figure 5-12
Pulsed Doppler examination of the left upper pulmonary vein is shown in the upper portion of the picture. In the lower portion of the picture, the spectral flow tracing shows systolic flow reversal (SFR) in a patient with severe mitral regurgitation due to infective endocarditis. D = diastole; S = systole.

Recently, pulmonary venous flow has been used to semiquantitatively estimate the severity of mitral regurgitation.[54–57] Systolic reflux of contrast dye during left ventriculography has been noted to be a sign of severe (4+) mitral regurgitation. The mechanism for the systolic reflux into the pulmonary veins reflects the increased left atrial pressure A and V waves due to the severe mitral regurgitation. This is similar to the mechanism for blunted systolic pulmonary venous flow, with predominant diastolic pulmonary venous flow, reported in patients with elevated left atrial pressure and no mitral regurgitation.[48] In a study by Klein et al. 26 of 28 (93 percent) patients with 4+ mitral regurgitation by color Doppler flow mapping with transesophageal echocardiography had reversed pulmonary systolic flow.[54] The sensitivity and specificity of reversed pulmonary systolic flow was 86 and 81 percent, respectively, when compared to 4+ mitral regurgitation by left ventriculography (Fig. 5-12). As the degree of mitral regurgitation increases, the peak systolic flow velocity integral decreases. In patients with 0 to 1+ mitral regurgitation, the peak systolic–peak diastolic flow ratio exceeds 1.0.[54,55] Blunted systolic flow reportedly has a sensitivity of only 61 percent, but a high specificity (97 percent) for detecting 3+ mitral regurgitation by transesophageal echocardiography color flow mapping (Fig. 5-13). The presence of atrial fibrillation, which is known to blunt systolic forward flow, did not alter the findings. Patients with atrial fibrillation and insignificant mitral regurgitation continued to show biphasic forward systolic and diastolic flow signals.[54]

It is important when assessing the severity of mitral regurgitation by pulmonary venous flow patterns that both the left and right upper pulmonary veins be interrogated. The sample volume should be placed from 0.5 to 1.0 cm

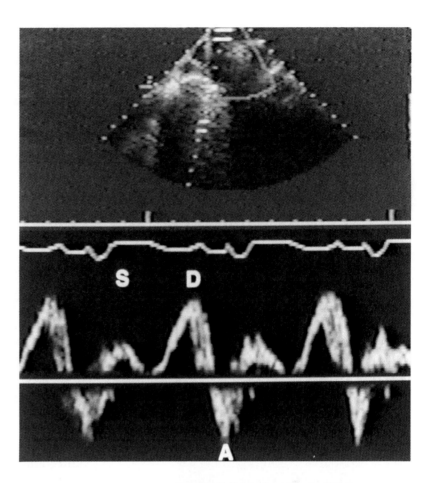

Figure 5-13
Blunted forward systolic (S) flow is seen in the pulsed Doppler spectral tracing of the pulmonary vein in a patient with moderate mitral regurgitation due to mitral valve prolapse. A = atrial contraction; D = diastole.

from the orifice into the left atrium.[55] In one study, 77 percent of patients had similar flow characteristics in both the left and right pulmonary veins. In patients with severe (4 +) mitral regurgitation, sampling of the left pulmonary vein alone may underestimate the severity of the mitral regurgitation.[54]

Flow Convergence Region Because of the technical and hemodynamic factors that influence the assessment of the severity of mitral regurgitation by color Doppler flow mapping, improved methods for assessing mitral regurgitation are needed. Recently, it has been recognized that color Doppler flow mapping can be used to identify a region of proximal flow convergence through a regurgitant or stenotic orifice.[58–61] As flow accelerates toward a regurgitant or stenotic orifice, a series of isovelocities occur until the flow reaches its maximal velocity. A blue-red aliasing radius can be visualized that can be used to calculate a proximal isovelocity surface area (PISA, Fig. 5-14). This flow

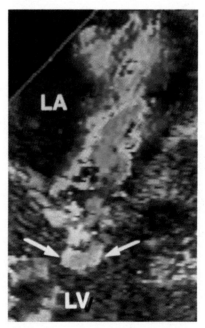

Figure 5-14
Proximal isovelocity surface area (arrows) is seen as a red-blue interface on the ventricular side of the mitral valve leaflets in this patient with moderate mitral regurgitation. LA = left atrium; LV = left ventricle.

convergence area can be made to be hemispherical in shape by shifting the color Doppler zero baseline to produce apparent aliasing velocities in the range of 10 to 20 cm/s.[62] Maximum volume flow rate can then be calculated as maximum PISA (in cm^2) isovelocity (in cm/s). The PISA method can be used to measure regurgitant flow rates, or in conjunction with continuous-wave Doppler to estimate regurgitant orifices based on the continuity equation. This method has some advantages over other color Doppler methods since the PISA appears to be independent of machine settings and orifice shape.[63] In vitro studies of pulsatile flow have yielded excellent correlations with varying flow rates.[59, 61] Initial clinical studies have shown that the regurgitant volume calculated by the PISA method correlates with the color Doppler regurgitant jet area in patients with moderate or severe mitral regurgitation.[64] In patients with mild mitral regurgitation, a region of flow convergence may not be visualized. Thus the appearance of a flow convergence region often suggests severe regurgitation.

Aortic

Transesophageal echocardiography is of greatest value in the identification of valvular pathology associated with aortic regurgitation. Transesophageal echocardiography has been shown to be superior to transthoracic echocardiography in the assessment of vegetations caused by infective endocarditis.[65, 66] Complications of aortic valve infective endocarditis, including paravalvular abscess formation, valve perforation, and rupture, are more easily identified by transesophageal echocardiography. Aortic dissection, which can be detected by transesophageal echocardiography (see Chap. 11), may cause aortic regurgitation due to disruption of the aortic valve annulus. A limitation, however, of transesophageal echocardiography in the evaluation of aortic valve disease is the acoustic shadowing of the left ventricular outflow tract from a calcified aortic or mitral valve. This limitation is reduced with the additional longitudinal planes available using biplane transesophageal echocardiography.

The severity of aortic regurgitation can be estimated semiquantitatively by both color Doppler transesophageal echocardiography and transthoracic echocardiography. In both approaches, semiquantitation is based on the ratio of the regurgitant jet width to the left ventricular outflow tract diameter on the long axis, or jet area to the aortic root area in the short-axis views (Figs. 5-15 and 5-16). A regurgitant ratio of ≤25 percent is considered mild, 25 to 50 percent moderate, and >50

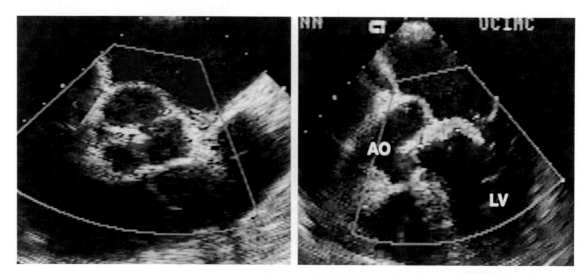

Figure 5-15
Basal short-axis transverse view (left panel) and midesophagus transverse five-chamber view (right panel) of a patient with mild aortic regurgitation. Doppler color flow velocity mapping in the two views allows semiquantitation of the severity based on the ratio of the jet area or height to the left ventricular outflow tract width.

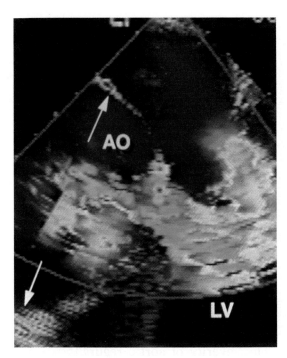

Figure 5-16
Color Doppler flow velocity mapping performed in the midesophagus five-chamber view. In this diastolic frame, flow jet fills the left ventricular outflow tract consistent with severe aortic regurgitation. The aortic regurgitation was due to a dilated aorta (AO, arrows) in a patient with Marfan's syndrome. LV = left ventricle.

percent severe aortic regurgitation.[67] Transthoracic studies have shown an excellent correlation between the color Doppler ratio and the angiographic grade of severity. In a study by Castello et al. the value of transesophageal echocardiography in the assessment of aortic regurgitation was compared to transthoracic echocardiography.[68] There was agreement between the two techniques in the assessment of the presence or absence of aortic regurgitation in 79 percent of 93 patients. In 18 percent of patients, transesophageal echocardiography alone detected the presence of aortic regurgitation. In 3 percent of patients, transthoracic echocardiography alone detected the presence of aortic regurgitation. In all patients in whom there was discordance between the transthoracic and transesophageal echocardiographic techniques, the severity was mild (1 +). In the patients with aortic regurgitation, the severity graded by the two techniques differed in only 16 percent, and in only 3 percent of patients

was the difference as great as two grades. In patients in whom there was an underestimation of aortic regurgitation by transesophageal echocardiography, there was associated aortic root pathology or stenosis that resulted in acoustic shadowing of the left ventricular outflow tract. Thus the advantage of transesophageal echocardiography in the assessment of the presence and severity of aortic regurgitation over transthoracic echocardiography is less clearly defined than is the advantage for mitral regurgitation. Whether biplane transesophageal echocardiography will prove to be of additional value with the added longitudinal imaging planes is not defined.

Right-Sided Valvular Lesions

Imaging Views
Right heart structures can be visualized with the transesophageal probe in the midesophagus and basal positions. The tricuspid valve can be evaluated from the transverse four-chamber midesophagus view and from the basal longitudinal view at the level of the aortic valve. Color flow and continuous-wave Doppler interrogation can be performed to detect the presence and severity of tricuspid regurgitation. The superior and inferior vena caval connections to the right atrium can be recorded in a basal longitudinal view at the level of the superior vena cava.

The pulmonary valve, pulmonary arteries, and right ventricular outflow tract are best examined in the transverse and longitudinal basal views. The longitudinal view is particularly useful in the evaluation of the right ventricular outflow tract, pulmonary valve, and main pulmonary artery (Fig. 5–17).

Tricuspid Valve
The tricuspid valve, since it is an anterior structure, is usually well visualized by a transthoracic echocardiographic study. Transesophageal echocardiography is less useful, therefore, for the assessment of tricuspid valve, as compared with abnormality of the mitral valve. How-

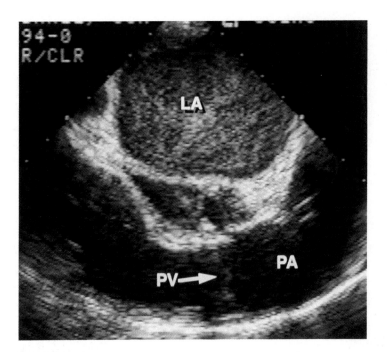

Figure 5-17
Transesophageal longitudinal basal view of the pulmonary outflow tract. In this biplane view, the pulmonary valve (PV) and main pulmonary artery (PA) can be visualized. There are spontaneous contrast echoes in the left atrium (LA).

ever, in patients with technically inadequate studies due to chest deformities, pulmonary disease, or mechanical ventilation, transesophageal echocardiography provides high-resolution images of the tricuspid valve and its chordal attachments. In patients with severe tricuspid regurgitation, the anatomic etiology—including flail leaflets, vegetations, and annular dilatation—can be assessed.[69,70] The severity of the tricuspid regurgitation can be assessed by the area of the regurgitant jet similar to the method used for mitral regurgitation (Fig. 5-18).

Pulmonary Valve

Transthoracic echocardiography is usually reliable in diagnosing pulmonary stenosis. The severity of the stenosis can be evaluated by continuous-wave Doppler flow velocities and the presence and severity of pulmonic regurgitation by color Doppler flow mapping. Nonetheless, transesophageal echocardiography, especially biplane, may be superior in the assessment of the right ventricular outflow tract and the main pulmonary artery with its bifurcation

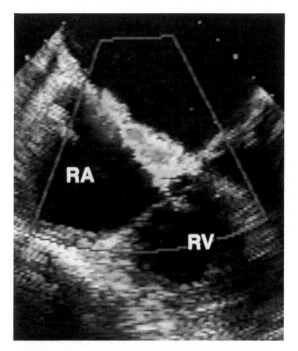

Figure 5-18
Transesophageal imaging in the midesophagus transverse four-chamber view with slight rotation of the probe to visualize the right atrium (RA) and right ventricle (RV). A tricuspid regurgitant jet is directed along the interatrial septum.

(Fig. 5-17). Infundibular stenosis and stenosis of the pulmonary arteries may be more easily visualized in the longitudinal transesophageal echocardiographic basal views.

Summary

Transesophageal echocardiography has greatly increased our ability to evaluate patients with known or suspected native valve disease. Rapid advances in technology, with miniaturization of the probes, improved resolution, and additional planes that may permit three-dimensional reconstruction, will further increase the application of this technique. Proper application of transesophageal echocardiography, however, must be based upon an understanding of its unique contribution and the complementary roles of transesophageal and transthoracic echocardiography.

References

1. Bansal RC, Shah PM: Usefulness of echo-Doppler in management of patients with valvular heart disease. *Curr Probl Cardiol* 14:283, 1989.
2. Stamm RB, Martin RP: Quantification of pressure gradients across stenotic valves by Doppler ultrasound. *J Am Coll Cardiol* 2:707, 1983.
3. Hatle L, Angelson B, Tromsdal A: Noninvasive assessment of atrioventricular pressure half-time by Doppler ultrasound. *Circulation* 60:1096, 1979.
4. Skjaerpe T, Hegrenaes L, Hatle L: Noninvasive estimation of valve area in patients with aortic stenosis by Doppler ultrasound and two-dimensional echocardiography. *Circulation* 72:810, 1985.
5. Otto CM, Pearlman AS, Comess KA, et al: Determination of stenotic aortic valve area in adults using Doppler echocardiography. *J Am Coll Cardiol* 7:509, 1986.
6. Helmcke F, Nanda NC, Hsiung MC, et al: Color Doppler assessment of mitral regurgitation with orthogonal planes. *Circulation* 75:175, 1987.
7. Perry GJ, Helmcke F, Byard C, et al: Evaluation of aortic insufficiency by color Doppler flow mapping. *J Am Coll Cardiol* 9:952, 1987.
8. Seward JB, Khandheria BK, Oh JK, et al: Transesophageal echocardiography: Technique, anatomic correlations, implementation, and clinical applications. *Mayo Clin Proc* 63:649, 1988.
9. Bansal RC, Shah PM: Transesophageal echocardiography. *Curr Probl Cardiol* 15:647, 1990.
10. Seward JB, Khandheria BK, Edwards WD, et al: Biplane transesophageal echocardiography: Anatomic correlations, image orientation, and clinical applications. *Mayo Clin Proc* 65:193, 1990.
11. Fisher EA, Stahl JA, Budd JH, et al: Transesophageal echocardiography: Procedures and clinical application. *J Am Coll Cardiol* 18:1333, 1991.
12. Rusted IE, Schiefley CH, Edwards JE: Studies of the mitral valve: II. Certain anatomic features of the mitral valve and associated structures in mitral stenosis. *Circulation* 14:398, 1956.
13. Reid CL, McKay CR, Chandraratna PAN, et al: Mechanisms of increase in mitral valve area and influence of anatomic features in double-balloon, catheter balloon valvuloplasty in adults with rheumatic mitral stenosis: A Doppler and two-dimensional echocardiographic study. *Circulation* 76:628, 1987.
14. Reid CL. Chandraratna PAN, Kawanishi DT, et al: Influence of mitral valve morphology on double-balloon catheter balloon valvuloplasty in patients with mitral stenosis: Analysis of factors predicting immediate and 3-month results. *Circulation* 80:515, 1989.
15. Herrmann HC, Wilkins GT, Abascal VM, et al: Percutaneous balloon mitral valvotomy for patients with mitral stenosis: Analysis of factors influencing early results. *J Thorac Cardiovasc Surg* 96:33, 1988.
16. Abascal VM, Wilkins GT, Choong CY, et al: Mitral regurgitation after percutaneous balloon mitral valvuloplasty in adults: Evaluation of pulsed Doppler echocardiography. *J Am Coll Cardiol* 1:257, 1988.
17. Marwick TH, Torelli J, Obarski T, et al: Assessment of the mitral valve splitability score by transthoracic and transesophageal echocardiography. *Am J Cardiol* 68:1106, 1991.
18. Reid CL, Otto CM, Davis KB, et al: Influence of mitral valve morphology on mitral balloon

commissurotomy: Immediate and six-month results from the NHLBI balloon valvuloplasty registry. *Am Heart J* 124:657, 1992.

19. Aschenberg W, Schlüter M, Kremer P, et al: Transesophageal two-dimensional echocardiography for the detection of left atrial appendage thrombus. *J Am Coll Cardiol* 7:163, 1986.

20. Bansal RC, Heywood JT, Applegate PM, et al: Detection of left atrial thrombi by two-dimensional echocardiography and surgical correlation in 148 patients with mitral valve disease. *Am J Cardiol* 64:243, 1989.

21. Reid CL, Rahimtoola SH: The role of echocardiography/Doppler in catheter balloon treatment of adults with aortic and mitral stenosis. *Circulation* 84:I240, 1991.

22. Gorcsan J, Kenny WM, Diana P, et al: Transesophageal continuous-wave Doppler to evaluate mitral prosthetic stenosis. *Am Heart J* 121:911, 1991.

23. Keren G, Pardes A, Miller HI, et al: Pulmonary venous flow determined by Doppler echocardiography in mitral stenosis. *Am J Cardiol* 65:246, 1990.

24. Hofmann T, Kasper W, Meinertz T, et al: Determination of aortic valve orifice area in aortic valve stenosis by two-dimensionsl transesophageal echocardiography. *Am J Cardiol* 59:330, 1987.

25. Schlüter M, Kremer P, Hanrath P: Transesophageal 2-D echocardiographic feature of flail mitral leaflet due to ruptured chordae tendineae. *Am Heart J* 108:609, 1984.

26. Hozumi T, Yoshikawa J, Yoshida K, et al: Direct visualization of ruptured chordae tendineae by transesophageal echocardiography. *J Am Coll Cardiol* 16:1315, 1990.

27. Himelman RB, Kusumoto F, Oken K, et al: The flail mitral valve: Echocardiographic findings by precordial and transesophageal imaging and Doppler color flow mapping. *J Am Coll Cardiol* 17:272, 1991.

28. Sochowski RA, Chan K-L, Aschah KJ, et al: Comparison of accuracy of transesophageal versus transthoracic echocardiography for the detection of mitral valve prolapse with ruptured chordae tendineae (flail mitral leaflet). *Am J Cardiol* 67:1251, 1991.

29. Alam M, Sun I: Superiority of transesophageal echocardiography in detecting ruptured mitral chordae tendineae. *Am Heart J* 6:1819, 1991.

30. Yoshida K, Yoshikawa J, Yamawra Y, et al: Valve of acceleration flows and regurgitant jet direction by color Doppler flow mapping in the evaluation of mitral valve prolapse. *Circulation* 81:879, 1990.

31. Patel AM, Miller FA, Khandheria BK, et al: Role of transesophageal echocardiography in the diagnosis of papillary muscle rupture secondary to myocardial infarction. *Am Heart J* 118:1330, 1989.

32. Stoddard MF, Keedy DL, Kupersmith J: Transesophageal echocardiographic diagnosis of papillary muscle rupture complicating acute myocardial infarction. *Am Heart J* 120:690, 1990.

33. Sakai K, Nakamura K, Hosoda S: Transesophageal echocardiographic findings of papillary muscle rupture. *Am J Cardiol* 68:561, 1991.

34. Sprecher DC, Adamick R, Adams D, et al: In vitro color flow, pulsed, and continuous wave Doppler ultrasound masking of flow by prosthetic valves. *J Am Coll Cardiol* 9:1306, 1987.

35. Yoshida K, Yoshikawa J, Yamaura Y, et al: Assessment of mitral regurgitation by biplane transesophageal color Doppler flow mapping. *Circulation* 82:1121, 1990.

36. Kamp O, Dykstra J-W, Huitcnk H, et al: Transesophageal color flow Doppler mapping in the assessment of native mitral valvular regurgitation: Comparison with left ventricular angiography. *J Am Soc Echo* 4:598, 1991.

37. Castello R, Lenzen P, Aguirre F, et al: Quantification of mitral regurgitation by transesophageal echocardiography with Doppler color flow mapping: Correlation with cardiac catheterization. *J Am Coll Cardiol* 19:1516, 1992.

38. Miyatake K, Izumi S, Okamoto M, et al: Semiquantitative grading of severity of mitral regurgitation by real-time two-dimensional Doppler flow imaging techniques. *J Am Coll Cardiol* 7:82, 1986.

39. Helmcke F, Nanda NC, Hsuing MC, et al: Color Doppler assessment of mitral regurgitation with orthogonal planes. *Circulation* 75:175, 1987.

40. Hoit BD, Jones M, Eidbo EE, et al: Sources of variability for Doppler color flow mapping of regurgitant jets in an animal model of mitral regurgitation. *J Am Coll Cardiol* 13:1631, 1989.

41. Utsunomiya T, Ogawa T, King SW, et al: Effect of machine parameters on variance display in Doppler color flow mapping. *Am Heart J* 120:1395, 1990.

42. Utsunomiya T, Ogawa T, King SW, et al: Pitfalls in the display of color Doppler jet areas: Combined variability due to Doppler

angle, frame rate, and scanning direction. *Echocardiography* 7(6):739, 1990.

43. Simpson IA, Sahn DJ: Quantification of valvular regurgitation by Doppler echocardiography. *Circulation* 84:I-188, 1991.

44. Chen C, Thomas JD, Anconina J, et al: Impact of impinging wall jet on color Doppler quantification of mitral regurgitation. *Circulation* 84:712, 1991.

45. Maciel BC, Moises VA, Shandas R, et al: Effects of pressure and volume of the receiving chamber on the spatial distribution of regurgitant jets as imaged by color Doppler flow mapping. *Circulation* 83:605, 1991.

46. Smith MD, Harrison MR, Pinton R, et al: Regurgitant jet size by transesophageal compared with transthoracic Doppler color flow imaging. *Circulation* 83:79, 1991.

47. Yoshida K, Yoshikawa J, Yamaura Y, et al: Assessment of mitral regurgitation by biplane transesophageal color Doppler flow mapping. *Circulation* 82:1121, 1990.

48. Castello R, Lenzen P, Aguirre F, et al: Variability in the quantitation of mitral regurgitation by Doppler color flow mapping: Comparison of transthoracic and transesophageal studies. *J Am Coll Cardiol* 20:433, 1992.

49. Kuecherer HF, Muhuideen IA, Kusumoto FM, et al: Estimation of mean left atrial pressure from transesophageal pulsed Doppler echocardiography of pulmonary venous flow. *Circulation* 82:1127, 1990.

50. Castello R, Pearson AC, Lenzen P, et al: Evaluation of pulmonary venous flow by transesophageal echocardiography in subjects with a normal heart: Comparison with transthoracic echocardiography. *J Am Coll Cardiol* 18:65, 1991.

51. Nishimura RA, Abel MD, Hatle LK, et al: Relation of pulmonary vein to mitral flow velocities by transesophageal Doppler echocardiography: Effect of different loading conditions. *Circulation* 81:1488, 1990.

52. Basnight MA, Gonzalez MS, Kershenoviech SC, et al: Pulmonary venous flow velocity: Relation to hemodynamics, mitral flow velocity and left atrial volume, and ejection fraction. *J Am Soc Echocardiogr* 4:547, 1991.

53. Kuecherer HF, Kusumoto F, Muhiudeen IA, et al: Pulmonary venous flow patterns by transesophageal pulsed Doppler echocardiography: Relation to parameters of left ventricular systolic and diastolic function. *Am Heart J* 122:1683, 1991.

54. Klein AL, Obarski TP, Stewart WJ, et al: Transesophageal Doppler echocardiography of pulmonary venous flow: A new marker of mitral regurgitation severity. *J Am Coll Cardiol* 18:518, 1991.

55. Castello R, Pearson AC, Lenzen P, et al: Effect of mitral regurgitation on pulmonary venous velocities derived from transesophageal echocardiography color-guided pulsed Doppler imaging. *J Am Coll Cardiol* 17:1499, 1991.

56. Masuyama T, Lee J-M, Tamai M, et al: Pulmonary venous flow velocity pattern as assessed with transthoracic pulsed Doppler echocardiography in subjects without cardiac disease. *Am J Cardiol* 67:1396, 1991.

57. Klein AL, Tajik AJ: Doppler assessment of pulmonary venous flow in healthy subjects and in patients with heart disease. *J Am Soc Echocardiogr* 4:379, 1991.

58. Simpson IA, Sahn DJ: Quantification of valvular regurgitation by Doppler echocardiography. *Circulation* 84(suppl I):I-188, 1991.

59. Recusani F, Bargiggia GS, Yoganathan AP, et al: A new method for quantification of regurgitant flow rate using color Doppler flow imaging of the flow convergence region proximal to a discrete orifice (an in vitro study). *Circulation* 83:594, 1991.

60. Gardin JM: Doppler color flow "Proximal isovelocity surface area (PISA)": An alternative method for estimating volume flow across narrowed orifices, regurgitant valves, and intracardiac shunt lesions. *Echocardiography* 9(1):39, 1992.

61. Utsunomiya T, Ogawa T, Tang HA, et al: Doppler color flow mapping of the proximal isovelocity surface area: A new method for measuring volume flow rate across a narrowed orifice. *J Am Soc Echocardiogr* 4:338, 1991.

62. Utsunomiya T, Doshi R, Patel D, et al: Accuracy of regurgitant volume calculation using color Doppler "zero-baseline shift" proximal isovelocity surface area method. *Circulation* 82:III-553, 1990.

63. Utsunomiya T, Ogawa T, Doshi R, et al: Doppler color flow "proximal isovelocity surface area"; method for estimating volume flow rate: Effects of orifice shape and machine factors. *J Am Coll Cardiol* 17:1103, 1991.

64. Utsunomiya T, Doshi R, Patel D, et al: Regurgitant volume estimation in patients with mitral regurgitation: Initial studies using the color Doppler "proximal isovelocity surface area" method. *Echocardiography* 9(1):63, 1992.

65. Mügge A, Daniel WG, Frank G, et al: Echocardiography in infective endocarditis: Reassessment of prognostic implications of vegetation size determined by the transthoracic and transesophageal approach. *J Am Coll Cardiol* 14:631, 1989.

66. Shively BK, Gurule FT, Roldan CA, et al: Diagnostic value of transesophageal compared with transthoracic echocardiography in infective endocarditis. *J Am Coll Cardiol* 18:391, 1991.

67. Perry GJ, Helmcke F, Nanda NC, et al: Evaluation of aortic insufficiency by Doppler color flow mapping. *J Am Coll Cardiol* 9:952, 1987.

68. Castello R, Fagan L Jr, Lenzen P, et al: Comparison of transthoracic and transesophageal echocardiography for assessment of left-sided valvular regurgitation. *Am J Cardiol* 68:1677, 1991.

69. Winslow T, Redberg R, Schiller NB: Transesophageal echocardiography in the diagnosis of flail tricuspid valve. *Am Heart J* 123:1682, 1992.

70. Herrera CJ, Mehlman DJ, Hartz RS, et al: Comparison of transesophageal and transthoracic echocardiography for diagnosis of right-sided cardiac lesions. *Am J Cardiol* 70:964, 1992.

6

Evaluation of Heart Valve Prostheses by Transesophageal Echocardiography

Helmut Baumgartner
Steven Khan
Gerald Maurer

Introduction

Transesophageal echocardiography has dramatically improved the diagnostic abilities of ultrasound techniques in the assessment of heart valve prostheses. Although transthoracic two-dimensional and Doppler echocardiography have been shown to be of potential value in the evaluation of prosthetic valves,[1–14] their use is often limited by poor imaging quality in the far field and by ultrasound attenuation due to shadowing from the synthetic material of the valve.[15] Therefore, the accurate assessment of mitral prostheses has been particularly difficult with transthoracic echocardiography. Transesophageal echocardiography has overcome these limitations. Owing to the proximity of the esophageal probe to the heart without interposition of lung tissue or thoracic wall and to the ability to use higher ultrasound frequencies, imaging resolution has dramatically improved.[16–18] Furthermore, interrogation of the left atrium from its posterior surface avoids "masking" of mitral regurgitant flow by

the prosthetic valve.[15] Therefore, the accurate assessment of mitral prosthetic regurgitation is the most frequently reported major advantage of transesophageal echocardiography.[19–23] In addition, the underlying pathology can be revealed in many instances.[19,21–23] High imaging resolution also allows improved detection of vegetations,[22–24] thrombi,[22,23] abscesses,[22,25,26] and spontaneous echo contrast within the left atrium.[27] Thus transesophageal technique has recently been reported to demonstrate an abnormality in 48 percent who had normal results on transthoracic echo examination and to have an overall sensitivity of 96 percent when compared to catheterization and surgery in patients with mitral prosthetic valves.[23]

Although some authors have reported a similar improvement in the assessment of aortic valve prostheses,[28] others found that the transesophageal approach was not superior to the transthoracic ultrasound examination, particularly in the assessment of prosthetic aortic regurgitation.[19,21,22,29,30] However, single-plane transesophageal echocardiography may still be superior in diagnosing perivalvular abscess, subaortic perforation, valvular dehiscence, and torn or thickened bioprosthetic aortic valve cusps,[22,26,28-30] and in distinguishing perivalvular from valvular aortic regurgitation.[21,29] Nevertheless, the single-plane technique is limited because it allows only cross-sectional or oblique views of the aortic valve. Biplane[31] and the recently developed multiplane technique[32-34] may overcome this drawback and may improve the ability of transesophageal echocardiography to evaluate both aortic and mitral valve prostheses.[35]

Prosthetic Valve Regurgitation

Normal Regurgitation

While transvalvular regurgitation is uncommon in normal bioprosthetic valves, a certain amount of backflow occurs in every mechanical valve.[36] Backflow during valve closure occurs only over a very short time period, does not form a well-defined jet, and is usually not confused with abnormal regurgitation. However, in modern tilting disk and bileaflet valves, some leakage backflow persists throughout systole and diastole for mitral and aortic valves, respectively. With conventional transthoracic Doppler, this normal regurgitation was detected in only 0 to 38 percent of patients.[6-21] Transthoracic color flow imaging has shown an even lower incidence of 0 to 6 percent.[11,13,14] However, because of the higher sensitivity of transesophageal echocardiography and the elimination of flow masking, the normal leakage regurgitation has been observed in 100 percent of patients with tilting disk and bileaflet mitral valve prostheses.[37-42] The frequency of observation of leakage backflow in aortic valve prostheses is considerably lower (0 to 44 percent).[30,41,43] This may be due to acoustic shadowing of the left ventricular outflow tract from a prosthetic mitral valve,[29] to ultrasound attenuation by a thickened native mitral valve, or simply to the greater distance of the ultrasound

probe from the left ventricular outflow tract and the near 90° direction of the jet of aortic regurgitation away from the probe.

Although the actual leakage volumes across normal valves are small,[36,44] typically on the order of 3 to 5 ml per beat, complex regurgitant jets can be imaged by transesophageal echocardiography (Figs. 6-1 to 6-5). Color Doppler patterns of normal regurgitation are characteristic for each valve type and have previously been described for the most commonly implanted bileaflet and tilting disk valves.[37-42,44,45] These patterns should be known to avoid a mistaken diagnosis of valve malfunction:

In St. Jude valves, two to four jets can be imaged simultaneously, depending on the imaging plane (Figs. 6-1 and 6-4). Two converging jets originate from the pivot points; a central jet originates from the gap between the two leaflets; and a variable number of peripheral jets originate from the circumferential gap between the leaflets and the valve housing. The best-defined patterns can be seen in two imaging planes: (1) parallel to the coaptation line of the two disks where two converging jets originate from the pivot points and rarely a third jet is seen from a common origin with one of the converging jets but directed perpendicularly into the chamber; and (2) the plane perpendicular to the coaptation line where one central jet originates from the central coaptation line of the two leaflets and two diverging peripheral jets originate in the circumferential gap between leaflets and the valve housing. A maximal number of four simultaneous jets can be found.

Medtronic-Hall tilting disk valves typically show a large central jet originating from the central hole in the disk (Figs. 6-2 and 6-5). Depending on the transducer orientation, none, one, or two small peripheral jets can be seen. Although the color images show a large central jet with only small peripheral jets, in vitro studies demonstrated that the majority of regurgitation (approximately 70 percent) originates from the circumference of the disk.[44] The central jet in Medtronic-Hall valves may

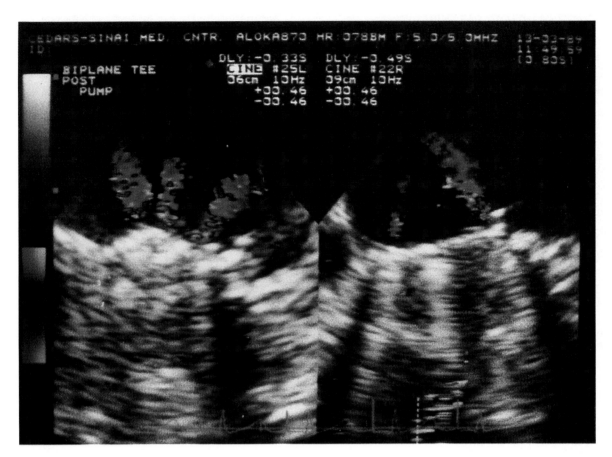

Figure 6-1
Color Doppler image from a biplane transesophageal study in a patient with a normal St. Jude valve in mitral position.

reach the posterior wall of the left atrium and is easily misinterpreted as a pathologic finding. Normal valves have reportedly been explanted by mistake on the basis of this Doppler finding (personal communication, Medtronic, Inc. Minneapolis, MN).

Björk-Shiley tilting disk valves typically show two small jets originating from the small gap between disk and valve housing (Fig. 6-3).

Distinction between Normal and Pathologic Prosthetic Regurgitation

Shape of the Regurgitant Jet
Normal and pathologic regurgitation may frequently be distinguished by the shape of the regurgitant jet. Pathologic regurgitation in me-

chanical valves is most frequently due to paravalvular leakage. These jets usually differ in shape from the normal jets described above. Frequently, they are eccentric and have a crescent-like shape[42] (Fig. 6-6).

Velocity Distribution of the Jet
The velocity distribution has also been found to be an important characteristic of normal prosthetic valve regurgitation.[38,44] St. Jude and Björk-Shiley valves typically show low-velocity jets with aliasing only close to the valve (Figs. 6-1 and 6-3). This is also true for peripheral jets in Medtronic-Hall valves (Fig. 6-5). However, it has to be emphasized that the large central jet in Medtronic-Hall valves may demonstrate aliasing extending far into the atrium (Figs. 6-2 and 6-5).

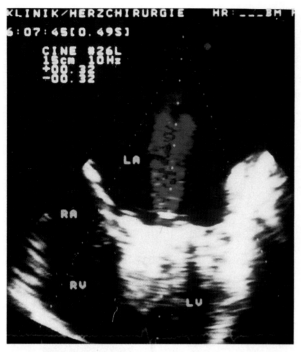

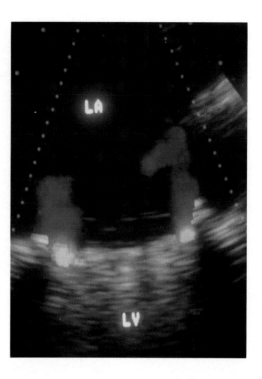

Figure 6-2
Color Doppler image from a transesophageal study in a patient with a normal Medtronic-Hall valve in mitral position. LA = left atrium; LV = left ventricle; RA = right atrium; RV = right ventricle. (Courtesy of Dr. R. De Simone, Department of Surgery, University of Heidelberg, FRG.)

Figure 6-3
Color Doppler image from a transesophageal study in a patient with a normal Bjørk-Shiley valve in mitral position. LA = left atrium; LV = left ventricle.

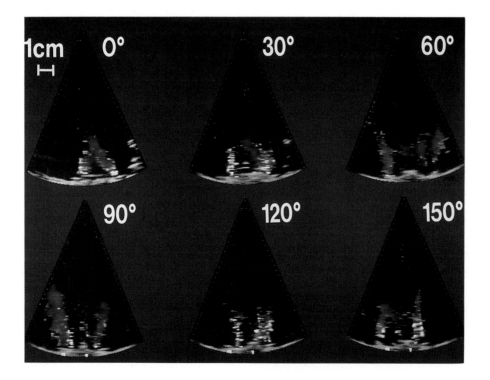

Figure 6-4
In vitro color Doppler images of regurgitation across a closed St. Jude valve (29 mm) at a left ventricular pressure of 130 mmHg. The six panels show the regurgitation in six rotational image planes (0° = image plane parallel to the coaptation line). [Reprinted from Baumgartner et al: Color Doppler regurgitant characteristics of normal mechanical mitral valve prostheses in vitro. *Circulation* 85:323, 1992 (by permission of the American Heart Association, Inc.).]

Figure 6-5
In vitro color Doppler images of regurgitation across a closed Medtronic-Hall valve (29 mm) at a left ventricular pressure of 130 mmHg. The six panels show the regurgitation in six rotational image planes. (0° = image plane parallel to the strut of the valve.) [Reprinted from Baumgartner et al: Color Doppler regurgitant characteristics of normal mechanical mitral valve prostheses in vitro. *Circulation* 85:323, 1992 (by permission of the American Heart Association, Inc.).]

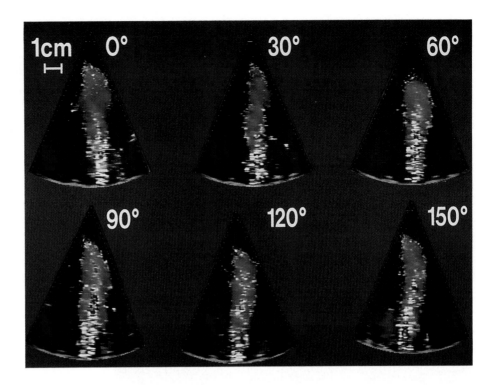

Location of the Jet

These normal central jets can, however, be identified by their central location. The origin of the jet can also be helpful for the distinction between normal and abnormal regurgitation. This is particularly the case when the regurgitant jets can be identified to originate outside the valve ring indicating paravalvular leakage.

Color M-Mode

Color M-mode studies have been reported to be also useful in this scenario.[39] In pathologic paravalvular regurgitation, color M-mode interrogation fails to reveal the two components characteristic of normal transvalvular regurgitation (early systolic closure backflow followed by holosystolic leakage backflow).

Finally, the severity of regurgitation may distinguish normal from pathologic regurgitation (see below).

Underlying Pathomorphology

Transesophageal echocardiography has been found to be of particular value in assessing the underlying mechanism of prosthetic regurgitant lesions.[19,21–23,29]

Paravalvular Regurgitation

Valve dehiscence can be directly visualized by two-dimensional echocardiography in some patients, particularly when lesions are severe (Fig. 6-7). Smaller leakages may not be detected by two-dimensional ultrasound but can still correctly be diagnosed by color Doppler when jets clearly originate outside the valve ring (Fig. 6-8). Transesophageal echocardiography has been shown to be accurate in distinguishing valvular from paravalvular regurgitation for both mitral and aortic prostheses.[21,23,29,46,47] For mitral periprosthetic leaks, good agreement between the site of regurgitation indicated by transesophageal echo and that found by the surgeon has been reported.[48] To define the origin and spatial extent of periprosthetic regurgitation, the mitral annulus should be divided into four quadrants similar to those used in surgery (Fig. 6-9). The location of the leak can be considered medial when the jet is imaged along the interatrial septum and anterior when the jet is imaged along the aortic root. Jets along the free left atrial wall can be considered lateral when imaged in a five-chamber view and posterior when imaged in a

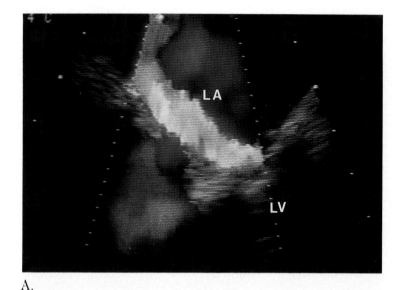

A.

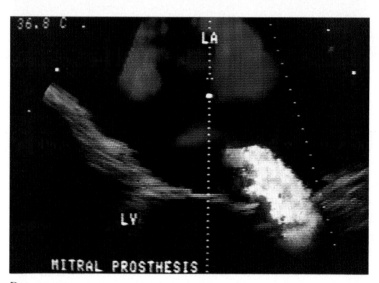

B.

Figure 6-6
Color Doppler images
from a transesophageal
study in a patient with a
Björk-Shiley mitral
valve. *A.* Medial periprosthetic leak; the jet has
the typical crescent-like
shape. *B.* Posterior periprosthetic leak; owing to
eccentricity the jet size
is small and would un-
derestimate the regurgi-
tation as it can be appreciated from the width of
the jet and the flow con-
vergence in the left ven-
tricle. LA = left atrium;
LV = left ventricle.

four-chamber view.[48] Using the single-plane
technique, the probe has to be manipulated up
and down behind the left atrium in order to
carefully scan the entire valve ring. The new
multiplane probes allow rotation of the imaging
plane and may improve the diagnostic accuracy.[35]

Transvalvular Regurgitation

Pathologic transvalvular regurgitation is a
much more common complication in bioprosthetic valves and aortic homografts than in
mechanical valves.[21] The underlying cause is
frequently torn and flail leaflets (Fig. 6-10) or
thickened and shrunken leaflets (Fig. 6-11). A
dramatic improvement in diagnosing torn or
flail leaflets has been shown in studies comparing transthoracic and transesophageal echocardiography.[19,21,23,47] However, it has to be kept
in mind that small tears or unfavorably located
lesions (Fig. 6-12) may still be missed with the
use of single-plane technique as shown by
studies that examined pathologic correlations.[19,21,23,49,50] The sensitivity and accuracy of
transesophageal echocardiography may further

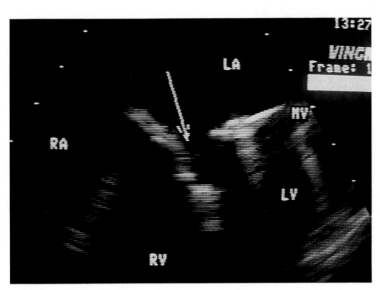

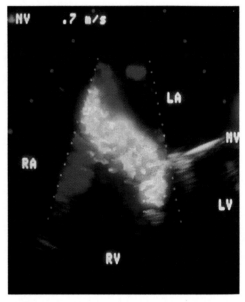

left   right

Figure 6-7
Images from a transesophageal study in a patient with a Björk-Shiley mitral valve. Left panel, 2D image clearly demonstrating medial dehiscence that resulted in severe mitral regurgitation. Right panel, color Doppler image of the periprosthetic regurgitant jet. LA = left atrium; LV = left ventricle; MV = mitral valve; RA = right atrium; RV = right ventricle.

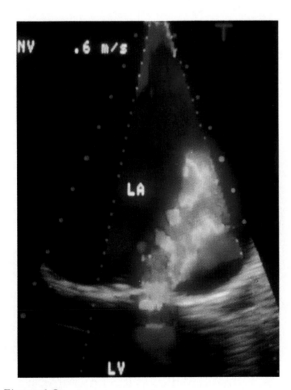

Figure 6-8
Color Doppler image from a transesophageal study in a patient with a Björk-Shiley valve and moderate periprosthetic regurgitation. LA = left atrium; LV = left ventricle.

improve in this respect with the use of multiplane probes.[35]

Quantification of Regurgitation

Transesophageal echocardiography may not offer any advantage over the transthoracic approach in the quantification of prosthetic aortic regurgitation unless the transthoracic image quality is poor.[19,21,22,29,30,47] There may even be disadvantages of the transesophageal approach when the left ventricular outflow tract is shadowed by a mitral prosthetic valve or a thickened and calcified anterior mitral leaflet.[29] Mild regurgitation that is found on transthoracic views may even be missed from a transesophageal approach.[29] Detection and quantification of prosthetic mitral regurgitation, however, is very limited from a transthoracic approach because of flow masking by the synthetic material of the valve.[15] Since transesophageal echocardiography interrogates the left atrium from its posterior surface without shadowing of the jet by the prosthesis, it is not surprising that the transesophageal approach has been reported to be superior to the transthoracic approach in accurate

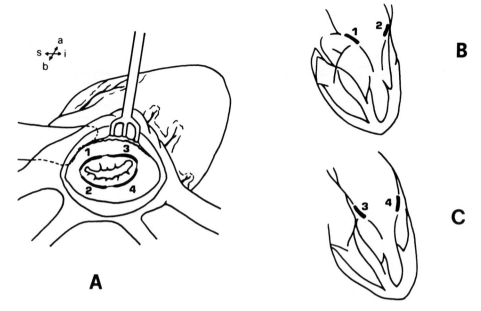

A

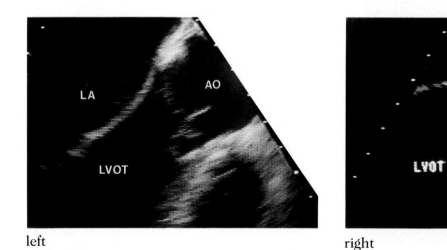

Figure 6-9
Panel A, schematic drawing showing the surgical view of the mitral annulus. a = anterior; b = basal; i = inferior; s = superior; 1 = anterior quadrant; 2 = lateral quadrant; 3 = medial quadrant; 4 = posterior quadrant. Panel B, schematic drawing of transesophageal five-chamber view. Panel C, schematic drawing of transesophageal four-chamber view. [From Meloni et al: Localization of mitral periprosthetic leaks by transesophageal echocardiography. *Am J Cardiol* 69:276, 1992 (by permission of the author and the American Journal of Cardiology).]

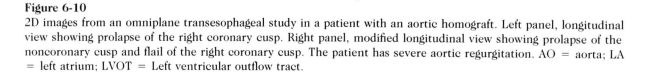

left   right

Figure 6-10
2D images from an omniplane transesophageal study in a patient with an aortic homograft. Left panel, longitudinal view showing prolapse of the right coronary cusp. Right panel, modified longitudinal view showing prolapse of the noncoronary cusp and flail of the right coronary cusp. The patient has severe aortic regurgitation. AO = aorta; LA = left atrium; LVOT = Left ventricular outflow tract.

Figure 6-11
Color Doppler image from a single-plane transesophageal study in a patient with an aortic bioprosthetic valve. Oblique view of the thickened bioprosthesis. The aortic regurgitant jet fills the left ventricular outflow tract. The patient had severe valvular regurgitation and moderate prosthetic stenosis. AVP = aortic valve prosthesis; LA = left atrium; LV = left ventricle; RV = right ventricle.

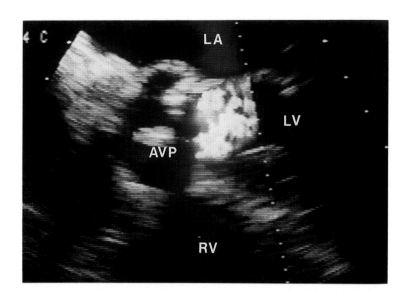

quantification of prosthetic mitral regurgitation.[19–23,47]

Jet Size

Transesophageal grading of the severity of prosthetic regurgitation has been done using criteria similar to the ones used in transthoracic imaging.[19,23,29,30,42] However, both regurgitant jet size and the overall estimate of regurgitant lesion severity have been shown to be greater on transesophageal color Doppler imaging compared with transthoracic imaging.[51] Furthermore, jet area to left atrial area ratios are difficult to calculate in transesophageal imaging owing to foreshortening of the left atrium.[52] The relationship between regurgitant jet size and flow volume is very complex. It is affected not only by multiple physiologic variables in-

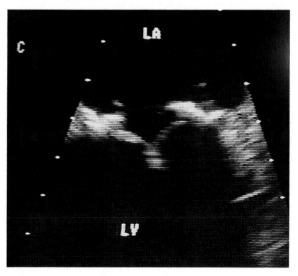

left

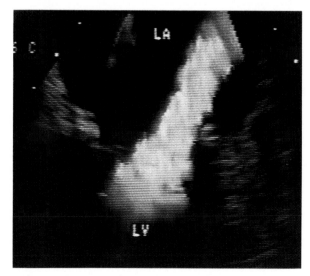

right

Figure 6-12
Images from a single-plane transesophageal study in a patient with a mitral bioprostheses. Although the 2D image (left panel) showed normal cusps, the color Doppler study (right panel) revealed severe valvular regurgitation. The third cusp was torn but could not be adequately visualized with single-plane technique. LA = left atrium; LV = left ventricle.

cluding the driving pressure, regurgitant orifice size, and the size and compliance of the receiving chamber[53,54] but also by the Doppler gain and other instrument settings.[55] Nevertheless, jet size as obtained from transesophageal imaging has been shown to correlate with angiographic grading[56] and may be one helpful parameter for semiquantitative assessment of prosthetic regurgitation.[19,23]

Jet Momentum

Fluid dynamic principles suggest that the single most important physical parameter for determining a free jet's size is the transfer of momentum by the jet into the receiving chamber which is given by the product of the jet flow rate at the orifice multiplied by orifice velocity. Although the Doppler echocardiographic quantification of jet momentum has been validated in vitro,[57,58] its use in clinical studies is not realistic yet.[59] However, it points out the critical importance of measuring blood pressure in patients to establish the driving pressure and permit more consistent serial follow-up. The sensitivity of atrioventricular valve regurgitation to the afterload state has also been shown intraoperatively.[60] Since the increase in color Doppler regurgitant area is highly variable in individual patients when blood pressure is increased, the relationship between jet area and blood pressure is probably a manifestation not only of increasing momentum transfer by the jet but of more complex pathophysiologic changes.

Jet Eccentricity

It should also be considered that prosthetic regurgitant jets are frequently eccentric and impinge on the left atrial wall (Fig. 6-6). These impinging wall jets have been shown to be less predictable and to have smaller color Doppler areas than free jets of comparable regurgitant severity.[46,61,62] In a recent study, eccentric wall jets were only approximately 40 percent of the size of corresponding free jets with the same regurgitant fraction and same flow rates.[61] The reduction in jet size is caused by transfer of jet momentum to the chamber wall and by distortion of the jet caused by its spreading laterally across the adjacent wall. As the jet spreads out over the adjacent wall, it thins out, resulting in a sheet of flow along the wall. Since color Doppler images a two-dimensional slice through this jet, all that is detected is a thin cross section of this sheet of flow resulting in underestimation of the magnitude of regurgitation. Therefore, jet morphology should be considered to avoid underestimation of regurgitant lesions.

Jet Width at the Origin

The width of the jet at its origin has been found to be a valuable indicator of aortic regurgitant severity in transthoracic imaging[63–65] and has been validated in vitro.[66] It has also been used for grading prosthetic aortic regurgitation in transesophageal imaging[26,30] (Fig. 6-11). Measuring regurgitant jet width at its origin has recently been reported to be also helpful for assessing the severity of mitral regurgitation with transesophageal color flow imaging.[67] Although there are few data on the value of this grading criterion for prosthetic regurgitation, this may be an additional parameter to consider (Fig. 6-6).

Proximal Flow Acceleration

Another approach to quantification of valvular regurgitation is analysis of the acceleration of flow proximal to the regurgitant orifice.[68] When flow accelerates toward the regurgitant orifice, it forms a series of concentric, roughly hemispheric, isovelocity surfaces centered at the orifice. According to the continuity principle, the product of the velocity at a certain distance from the orifice and the surface area over which this velocity occurs equals the regurgitant flow and should provide a quantitative estimate of mitral regurgitation.[68] The value of acceleration flow signals proximal to the leaking orifice in assessing the severity of prosthetic mitral regurgitation using transthoracic imaging has recently been reported.[69] Although this approach may have limited applicability in transesophageal imaging owing to shadowing of the left ventricle by the material of the mitral prosthetic valve, it may turn out to be helpful by providing additional information on the regurgitant severity in selected cases (Figs. 6-6 and 6-8).

Pulmonary Venous Flow

Some authors have proposed to combine the appearance of the regurgitant jet and pulmonary venous flow patterns to grade the severity of prosthetic mitral regurgitation.[21-23] Regurgitation may be considered mild if the regurgitant jet reaches up to the midleft atrium, moderate if the regurgitation passes beyond the midleft atrium but does not affect pulmonary venous flow, and severe if the regurgitation produces reversal of systolic pulmonary venous flow or fills the atrial appendage. Normal pulmonary venous flow demonstrates a biphasic forward flow pattern with systolic flow greater than diastolic flow. Mild mitral regurgitation does not significantly alter this flow pattern. As the degree of mitral regurgitation increases, the peak diastolic velocity and proportion of diastolic flow have been shown to increase, whereas the peak systolic velocity and proportion of systolic flow decrease.[70,71] In patients with severe mitral regurgitation, the systolic flow becomes reversed (Fig. 6-13). In two recent studies, the sensitivity of reversed systolic flow for severe regurgitation was 90 and 93 percent, respectively, and the specificity was 100 percent in both studies.[70,71] However, decreased systolic flow is much less specific

for determining the grade of mitral regurgitation.[71] It has also been shown that jet eccentricity and direction do not affect pulmonary venous flow reversal in left and right pulmonary veins in severe mitral regurgitation.[72] However, it should be remembered that pulmonary venous flow patterns may be affected by multiple other factors than the severity of mitral regurgitation including left ventricular performance, afterload, cardiac rhythm, and the type of prosthetic valve.[73-75] For example, systolic flow reversal may be absent in patients with severe mitral regurgitation but with a markedly reduced left ventricular ejection fraction.[73] Systolic forward flow may be reduced by an increase in afterload[74] and may be reduced or even disappear in patients in atrial fibrillation without significant mitral regurgitation. Furthermore, it has to be considered that the presence of a mitral prosthesis itself affects the pulmonary venous flow pattern. Systolic forward flow has been seen to be significantly lower in patients with prosthetic mitral valves.[75] Since the reversal of systolic flow correlates with the v wave,[76] the relationship between flow pattern and regurgitant severity is probably also affected by the size and compliance of the left atrium.

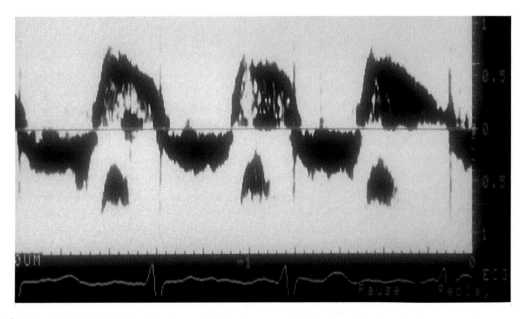

Figure 6-13
Pulsed-wave Doppler recording of pulmonary venous flow showing holosystolic flow reversal (from a transesophageal study in a patient with a St. Jude mitral valve and severe paravalvular regurgitation).

Antegrade Flow Velocity

Finally, a significant increase of the antegrade flow velocity across prosthetic valves due to the regurgitant volume may indicate hemodynamically important regurgitation. In contrast to an increase of forward velocity due to prosthetic stenosis, this velocity increase will occur in combination with a normal pressure half-time.[23] The availability of baseline data for comparison is very helpful in assessing increases in forward flow. For further methods for assessing the severity of regurgitation see the chapter on Valvular Regurgitation.

It has to be emphasized that all these grading criteria are only semiquantitative and do not provide accurate estimates of regurgitant volume or regurgitant fraction. However, the same is true for angiography and all other methods currently used to assess valvular regurgitation. Although each of the above-described criteria has its limitations and pitfalls, their combined use may allow accurate evaluation of prosthetic regurgitation in the majority of patients. Preoperative cardiac catheterization is frequently not necessary unless coronary anatomy has to be assessed.[21,23,77]

Prosthetic Valve Stenosis

Morphology

Mechanical Valves

In the mitral position, leaflet or disk motion can usually be adequately assessed in tilting disk and bileaflet valves (Figs. 6-14 and 6-15). It may often be possible even to measure opening and closing angles, although a multiplane probe may sometimes be necessary to obtain an adequate imaging plane for this measurement. Reduced disk or leaflet excursion indicates prosthetic stenosis (Fig. 6-15) and tissue overgrowth or thrombosis may be visualized.[78] Although some authors have reported adequate evaluation of disk or leaflet motion in the aortic position,[28] this may only be possible with biplane or multiplane probes. With single-plane probes that provide only cross-sectional and oblique views of aortic valve prostheses, opening angles cannot be adequately assessed.[29] It is still not clear whether echocardiography can provide accurate quantitative measurements of disk opening angles. However, transesophageal echocardiography may be very helpful in providing a rapid qualitative assessment of disk motion.

Bioprostheses

Because of ultrasound attenuation by the valve ring and stents, it is often difficult to visualize the valve cusps in transthoracic imaging.[22,23,28,29,79] However, transesophageal two-dimensional echocardiography allows accurate evaluation of mitral bioprosthetic anatomy in the majority of patients (Fig. 6-16).[22,23,79] Although some authors have described similar success rates for the aortic position,[28,29] others have reported difficulties in visualizing the cusps of aortic bioprosthetic valves.[19,21,22,26] The single-plane technique does not always provide precise cross-sectional views of the valve since the ultrasound beam often encounters the valve in an oblique position (Fig. 6-17). This relation may preclude a proper evaluation of bioprosthetic cusp thickness and opening.[22] Biplane and multiplane techniques provide additional longitudinal views of the valve and may overcome these limitations and improve the evaluation of both aortic and mitral prosthetic valves.

Thickened bioprosthetic cusps can also be encountered in patients with subclinical valve degeneration. A cusp thickness of greater than 3 mm and cusp opening of less than 7 mm has been reported to distinguish patients with significant prosthetic stenosis from patients with subclinical degeneration.[79] However, the degree of flow obstruction may often be difficult to assess solely from the two-dimensional image (Fig. 6-17).

Gradient Estimation

Hemodynamic evaluation is indispensable for the quantification of prosthetic stenosis (Fig. 6-18). Transthoracic continuous-wave Doppler ultrasound has clearly demonstrated its usefulness for calculating prosthetic valve gradients.[1-5] With the introduction of new transesophageal probes, it has become possible to

Figure 6-14
2D images from a biplane transesophageal study in a patient with a normal St. Jude mitral valve. Left panel, open position; right panel, closed position.

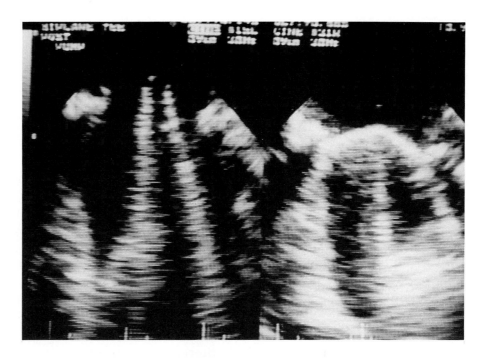

make continuous-wave Doppler measurements applicable from this approach, too. However, owing to the limited variability of the transducer position and orientation within the esophagus, transthoracic Doppler echocardiography may remain superior to the transesophageal examination for estimation of prosthetic valve gradients.[21] Proper alignment of the ultrasound beam and flow direction may often not be possible, particularly in aortic valve

prostheses. For mitral stenoses and mitral prostheses, transesophageal continuous-wave Doppler has recently been shown to provide adequate velocity measurements in the majority of patients[80] (Fig. 6-18). However, some patients in this study had extremely eccentric mitral inflow that precluded acceptable alignment of the ultrasound beam. Thus transthoracic echocardiography may be the procedure of choice for gradient estimation in most cases.

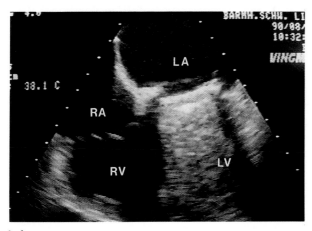

left

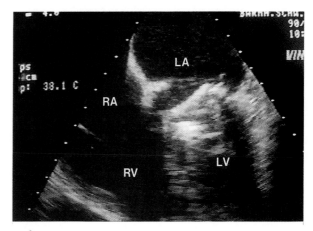

right

Figure 6-15
2D images from a single-plane study in a patient with a tilting disk mitral valve (Bjørk-Shiley). Left panel, closed position; right panel, maximal open position showing that the opening angle is reduced to 38°. LA = left atrium; LV = left ventricle; RA = right atrium; RV = right ventricle.

Figure 6-16
2D image from an omniplane transesophageal study (modified transverse view) in a patient with a normal mitral bioprosthetic valve. LA = left atrium; LV = left ventricle; MVP = mitral valve prosthesis.

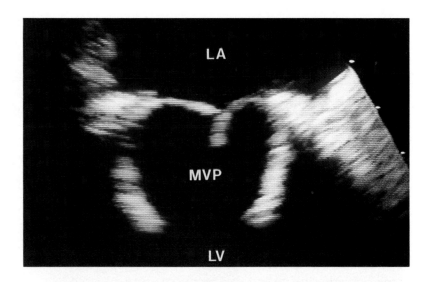

Figure 6-17
2D image from a single-plane study in a patient with a degenerated bioprosthesis in aortic position. With single-plane technique it was only possible to obtain oblique views that show thickening of the valve. Gradient estimation that was only possible with transthoracic echocardiography revealed severe prosthetic valve stenosis. AVP = aortic valve prosthesis; LA = left atrium; LV = left ventricle.

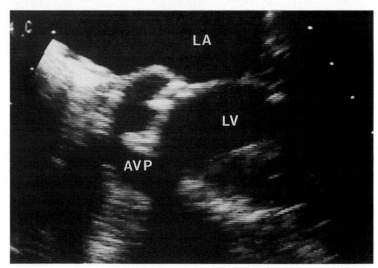

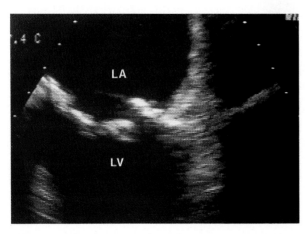

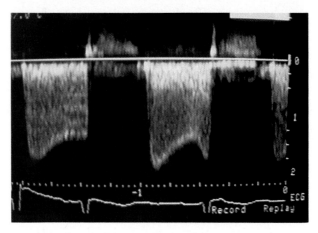

left   right

Figure 6-18
2D image (left panel) and continuous-wave Doppler recording from a single-plane study in a patient with a stenotic bioprosthesis in mitral position. Prosthetic valve orifice area as calculated with the pressure half-time method was 1.0 cm^2 (right panel, CW Doppler recording). LA = left atrium; LV = left ventricle.

The interpretation of Doppler prosthetic valve gradients is complicated by the fact that most normal heart valve prostheses cause some degree of flow obstruction and can demonstrate significant pressure gradients at higher flow rates.[4,5] Doppler gradients vary with valve type and valve size owing to the variation of effective orifice areas. Therefore, valve type and size have to be considered when interpreting Doppler data. Although "normal" values of Doppler gradients have been reported for most of the commonly used valve types and sizes, the normal ranges vary widely, particularly for small sizes.[4] This is due to the marked flow dependence of Doppler velocities and gradients across prosthetic valves.[81] At high flow rates, gradients may reach values that are ordinarily considered to reflect prosthetic valve stenosis. Therefore, accurate evaluation of prosthetic valve function from Doppler velocities requires information on the flow rate at which gradients were measured. Furthermore, there are some specific limitations of Doppler gradient estimation across certain heart valve prostheses. For some valve types, such as bileaflet and caged-ball valves, substantial discrepancy between Doppler and catheter gradients has been reported.[82–86] These discrepancies are due to the occurrence of localized high velocities and pressure recovery distal to the valve.[85] Continuous-wave Doppler measures the highest velocity and therefore the highest gradient along the Doppler beam. In contrast, clinical catheterization studies measure the recovered distal pressure that results in a lower catheter gradient compared with the Doppler gradient.

Some of these limitations may be overcome when baseline Doppler examinations are available for comparison,[17,87] although possible changes of other variables including heart rate and flow rate have to be considered.

Prosthetic Valve Orifice Area

Since gradients are highly flow-dependent, calculation of the effective prosthetic orifice area should be the best method for diagnosis of prosthetic valve stenosis. The continuity equation has been used to calculate prosthetic valve areas with transthoracic Doppler echocardiography in both mitral and aortic valves.[5,17,88,89]

Because of the difficulties with beam alignment mentioned earlier, the continuity area may be difficult to measure accurately in aortic valves when transesophageal echocardiography is used. Although there are no reports yet, this measurement could be done in mitral valves since beam alignment is frequently possible for this valve.[80] However, it should be remembered that the continuity equation is not accurate in bileaflet valves where the occurrence of localized high velocities leads to underestimation of the effective orifice area.[5,90] For prosthetic mitral valves, effective orifice area can also be calculated using the pressure half-time method,[2] and normal values have been reported for the most commonly implanted valves.[4] This method has also been used with transesophageal Doppler echocardiography, and good agreement has recently been found compared with transthoracic measurements.[80] Although the pressure half-time method is an easy and convenient way to obtain effective orifice area, it has its limitations including the dependence on left atrial and left ventricular compliance and the initial gradient across the valve.[91,92]

Vegetation, Abscess, Thrombus

Infective Disease

Since echocardiography provides direct visualization of vegetations and myocardial abscesses, it has generally been accepted as the diagnostic method of choice in infective endocarditis. The diagnosis of endocarditis has been dramatically improved by transesophageal echocardiography.[22–24,26,46,93–95] An increase of the detection rate of vegetations from 58 to 90 percent has been reported for transesophageal imaging when compared with transthoracic imaging in a group of patients with native and prosthetic valves.[24] Although the detection rate was smaller for prosthetic valves, the improvement in diagnosis with transesophageal echocardiography was even more significant, with only 27 percent of lesions detected by transthoracic echo versus 77 percent by transesophageal echo. It has to be emphasized, however, that accurate echocardiographic differentiation between true vegetations and other valve lesions such as ruptured leaflets or chordae is sometimes impossible.[24] False-positive results have also been reported in bioprosthetic valves with degenerated cusps.[96]

The diagnosis of abscesses associated with endocarditis has been difficult with transthoracic imaging and has been substantially improved by transesophageal echocardiography.[22,25,26,28,96,97] In one series, transesophageal echocardiography had a sensitivity of 87 percent for the detection of abscesses while the sensitivity for transthoracic imaging was only 28 percent.[25] Many of these patients had heart valve prostheses. Transesophageal echocardiography has also been shown to be of value in the detection of other endocarditis-associated abnormalities including fistulas[28,26,98] and involvement of the anterior mitral leaflet in association with aortic endocarditis.[99,100]

Despite the significant impact of transesophageal echocardiography on the diagnosis and overall management of patients with suspected infective endocarditis, it should be remembered that the detection of vegetations and other endocarditis-associated lesions is still more difficult in patients with prosthetic valves than it is in patients with native valves. While a negative transesophageal echocardiogram has been reported to virtually exclude infective endocarditis in native valves, this has not been the case in prosthetic valves.[101]

Echocardiographic differentiation between vegetation and sterile thrombus is not possible. Although the clinical presentation of the patient and blood cultures are of major importance, repeated transesophageal studies may sometimes help to make correct diagnosis.

For further detail and examples see also the chapter on Endocarditis.

Thrombi and Other Indicators of Embolic Risk

Prosthetic valve thrombosis is a serious complication primarily encountered in mechanical valve prostheses. Although the potential value of transesophageal echocardiography in detecting thrombi in patients with prosthetic valves has been demonstrated[22,23,28,78,96,102]

(Fig. 6-19), there are no reported studies showing the sensitivity and specificity of the method. Thrombi may cause either obstruction of prosthetic valves with hemodynamic compromise or embolic events.[102] In obstructed prosthetic valves, disk or leaflet opening may be restricted and can also be detected by transesophageal echocardiography.[78]

Pathologic correlations of transesophageal echocardiography have shown that small thrombi can be missed, particularly when located on the ventricular side of mitral prosthetic valves.[23,96] However, the transesophageal echocardiography is highly sensitive for abnormalities on the atrial side of mitral valves. Very small, fibrinous-like attachments (strands) have been detected and appear more common on mechanical than on bioprosthetic valves. These strands may represent a potential source of emboli that has previously not been recognized.[103] Two forms of spontaneous echo con-

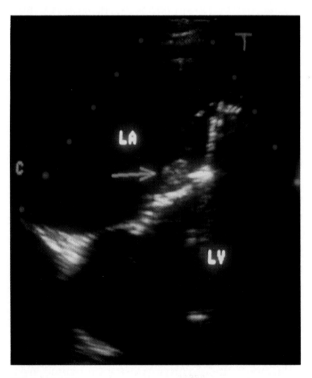

Figure 6-19
2D image from a transesophageal study in a patient with a St. Jude mitral valve. The thrombus on the left atrial surface of the valve disappeared after one week of improved anticoagulation without any signs of embolism. LA = left atrium; LV = left ventricle.

trast are also associated with prosthetic valves. The first type, left atrial spontaneous echo contrast, is best visualized by transesophageal echocardiography and has been found in 37 percent of patients after mitral valve replacement.[27] Left atrial spontaneous echo contrast is seen as swirling smokelike structures in the left atrium. This finding has been shown to be associated with an increased incidence of left atrial thrombi and a history of arterial embolic episodes. This smokelike echo contrast has to be differentiated from a second type of spontaneous left atrial contrast that may be encountered in patients with mechanical valves.[104] These are bright reflective bubblelike echos emanating from the valve during closure of the disk or leaflet and closely resemble microbubbles produced by agitated saline. The cause of these bubbles is not clear; however, they may be caused by the phenomenon of cavitation on prosthetic valves.[105]

References

1. Wilkins GT, Gillam LD, Kritzer GL, et al: Validation of continuous-wave Doppler echocardiographic measurements of mitral and tricuspid prosthetic valve gradients: A simultaneous Dopper-catheter study. *Circulation* 74:786, 1986.

2. Sagar KB, Wann S, Paulsen WHJ, et al: Doppler echocardiographic evaluation of Hancock and Bjørk-Shiley prosthetic valves. *J Am Coll Cardiol* 7:681, 1986.

3. Burstow DJ, Nishimura RA, Bailey KR, et al: Continuous-wave Doppler echocardiographic measurements of prosthetic valve gradients—A simultaneous Doppler-catheter correlative study. *Circulation* 80:504, 1989.

4. Reisner SA, Meltzer RS: Normal values of prosthetic valve Doppler echocardiographic parameters: A review. *J Am Soc Echocardiogr* 1:201, 1988.

5. Chafizadeh ER, Zoghbi WA: Doppler echocardiographic assessment of the St. Jude medical prosthetic valve in the aortic position using the continuity equation. *Circulation* 83:213, 1991.

6. Weinstein IR, Marberger JP, Perez JE: Ultrasonic of the St. Jude prosthetic valve: M mode, two-dimensional, and Doppler echocardiography. *Circulation* 68:897, 1983.

7. Williams GA, Labovitz AJ: Doppler hemodynamic evaluation of prosthetic (Starr-Edwards and Bjørk-Shiley) and bioprosthetic (Hancock and Carpentier-Edwards) cardiac valves. *Am J Cardiol* 56:325, 1985.

8. Sagar KB, Wann LS, Paulsen WHJ, et al: Doppler echocardiographic evaluation of Hancock and Bjørk-Shiley prosthetic valves. *J Am Coll Cardiol* 7:681, 1986.

9. Panidis IP, Ross J, Mintz GS: Normal and abnormal prosthetic valve function as assessed by Doppler echocardiography. *J Am Coll Cardiol* 8:317, 1986.

10. Cooper DM, Stewart WJ, Schiavone WA, et al: Evaluation of normal prosthetic valve function by Doppler echocardiography. *Am Heart J* 114:576, 1987.

11. Dittrich H, Nicod P, Hoit B, et al: Evaluation of Bjørk-Shiley prosthetic valves by real-time two-dimensional Doppler echocardiographic flow mapping. *Am Heart J* 115:133, 1988.

12. Pye M, Weerasana N, Bain WH, et al: Doppler echocardiographic characteristics of normal and dysfunctioning prosthetic valves in the tricuspid and mitral position. *Br Heart J* 63:41, 1990.

13. Kapur KK, Fan P, Nanda NC, et al: Doppler color flow mapping in the evaluation of prosthetic mitral and aortic valve function. *J Am Coll Cardiol* 13:1561, 1989.

14. Alam M, Rosman HS, McBroom D, et al: Color flow Doppler evaluation of St. Jude Medical prosthetic valves. *Am J Cardiol* 64:1387, 1989.

15. Sprecher DL, Adamick R, Adams D, et al: In vitro color flow, pulsed and continuous wave Doppler ultrasound masking of flow by prosthetic valves. *J Am Coll Cardiol* 9:1306, 1987.

16. Matsuzaki M, Toma Y, Kusukawa R: Clinical applications of transesophageal echocardiography. *Circulation* 82:709, 1990.

17. Nanda NC, Cooper JW, Mahan III EF, et al: Echocardiographic assessment of prosthetic valves. *Circulation* 84(suppl I):I-228, 1991.

18. Fisher EA, Stahl JA, Budd JH, et al: Transesophageal echocardiography: Procedures and clinical application. *J Am Coll Cardiol* 18:1333, 1991.

19. Nelessen U, Schnittger I, Appleton CP, et al: Transesophageal two-dimensional echocardiography and color Doppler flow velocity

mapping in the evaluation of cardiac valve prostheses. *Circulation* 78:848, 1988.

20. Labovitz AJ: Assessment of prosthetic heart valve function by Doppler echocardiography. *Circulation* 80:707, 1989.

21. Chaudhry FA, Herrera C, DeFrino PF, et al: Pathologic and angiographic correlations of transesophageal echocardiography in prosthetic heart valve dysfunction. *Am Heart J* 122:1057, 1991.

22. Herrera CJ, Chaudhry FA, DeFrino PF, et al: Value of limitations of transesophageal echocardiography in evaluating prosthetic or bioprosthetic valve dysfunction. *Am J Cardiol* 69:697, 1991.

23. Khandheria BK, Seward JB, Oh JK, et al: Value and limitations of transesophageal echocardiography in assessment of mitral valve prostheses. *Circulation* 83:1956, 1991.

24. Mügge A, Daniel WG, Frank G, et al: Echocardiography in infective endocarditis: Reassessment of prognostic implications of vegetation size determined by the transthoracic and the transesophageal approach. *J Am Coll Cardiol* 14:631, 1989.

25. Daniel WG, Mügge A, Martin RP, et al: Improvement in the diagnosis of abscesses associated with endocarditis by transesophageal echocardiography. *N Engl J Med* 321:795, 1991.

26. Pinto FJ, Wranne B, Schnittger I: Transesophageal echocardiography for study of bioprostheses in the aortic valve position. *Am J Cardiol* 69:274, 1992.

27. Daniel WG, Nellessen U, Schröder E, et al: Left atrial spontaneous echo contrast in mitral valve disease: An indicator for an increased thromboembolic risk. *J Am Coll Cardiol* 11:1204, 1988.

28. Dittrich HC, McCann HA, Walsh TP, et al: Transesophageal echocardiography in the evaluation of prosthetic and native aortic valves. *Am J Cardiol* 66:758, 1990.

29. Karalis DG, Chandrasekaran K, Ross JJ, et al: Single-plane transesophageal echocardiography for assessing function of mechanical or bioprosthetic valves in the aortic valve position. *Am J Cardiol* 69:1310, 1992.

30. Alam M, Serwin JB, Rosman HS, et al: Transesophageal color flow Doppler and echocardiographic features of normal and regurgitant St. Jude medical prostheses in the aortic valve position. *Am J Cardiol* 66:873, 1990.

31. Omoto R, Kyo S, Matsumura M, et al: Evaluation of biplane color Doppler transesophageal echocardiography in 200 consecutive patients. *Circulation* 85:1237, 1992.

32. Pandian N, Hsu TL, Weintraub A, et al: Realtime multiplane transesophageal echocardiography using a prototype phased array TEE probe with 180 degree scan plane steering capability: Method, echo-anatomic correlations and early clinical experience. *J Am Coll Cardiol* 19(suppl A):235A, 1992.

33. Daniel WG, Pearlman AS, Hausman D, et al: Multiplane transesophageal echocardiography: Initial experience and potential applications. *J Am Coll Cardiol* 19(suppl A):235A, 1992.

34. Flachskampf FA, Hoffmann R, Hanrath P: Experience with a transesophageal echotransducer allowing full rotation of the viewing plane: The omniplane probe. *J Am Cardiol Coll* 17(suppl A):34A, 1991.

35. Flachskampf FA, Hoffmann R, Hanrath P: Improved evaluation of prosthetic valve regurgitation with a new multiplanar transesophageal echo-transducer. *Circulation* 84(suppl II):II-706, 1991.

36. Rashtian MY, Stevenson DM, Allen DT, et al: Flow characteristics of four commonly used mechanical heart valves. *Am J Cardiol* 58:743, 1986.

37. Van den Brink RBA, Visser CE, Basart DCG, et al: Comparison of transthoracic and transesophageal color Doppler flow imaging in the patients with mechanical prostheses in the mitral valve position. *Am J Cardiol* 63:1471, 1989.

38. Taams MA, Gussenhoven EJ, Cahalan MK, et al: Transesophageal Doppler color flow imaging in the detection of native and Bjørk-Shiley mitral valve regurgitation. *J Am Coll Cardiol* 13:95, 1989.

39. Lange HW, Olson JD, Pedersen WR, et al: Transesophageal color Doppler echocardiography of the normal St. Jude medical mitral valve prosthesis. *Am Heart J* 122:489, 1991.

40. Flachskampf FA, O'Shea JP, Griffin BP, et al: Patterns of normal transvalvular regurgitation in mechanical valve prostheses. *J Am Coll Cardiol* 18:1493, 1991.

41. Mohr-Kahaly S, Kupferwasser I, Erbel R, et al: Regurgitant flow in apparently normal valve prostheses: Improved detection and semiquantitative analysis by transesophageal

two-dimensional color-coded Doppler echocardiography. *J Am Soc Echocardiogr* 3:187, 1990.

42. Alam M, Serwin JB, Rosman HS, et al: Transesophageal color flow Doppler and echocardiographic features of normal and regurgitant St. Jude medical prostheses in the mitral valve position. *Am J Cardiol* 66:871, 1990.

43. Kyo S, Takamoto S, Matsumura M, et al: Immediate and early postoperative evaluation of results of cardiac surgery by transesophageal two-dimensional Doppler echocardiography. *Circulation* 76(suppl V): V-113, 1987.

44. Baumgartner H, Khan S, DeRobertis M, et al: Color Doppler regurgitant characteristics of normal mechanical mitral valve prostheses in vitro. *Circulation* 85:323, 1992.

45. Hixson CS, Smith MD, Mattson MD, et al: Comparison of transesophageal color flow Doppler imaging of normal mitral regurgitant jets in St. Jude medical and Medtronic Hall cardiac prostheses. *J Am Soc Echocardiogr* 5:57, 1992.

46. Vandenberg BF, Dellsperger KC, Chandran KB, et al: Detection, localization, and quantitation of bioprosthetic mitral valve regurgitation. An in vitro two dimensional color-Doppler flow-mapping study. *Circulation* 78:539, 1988.

47. Mulhern K, Mehlman D, O'Rourke RA, Zabalgoitia M: Value and limitations of transesophageal echocardiography for evaluation of prosthetic valve dysfunction. *J Am Coll Cardiol* 19(suppl A):182A, 1992.

48. Meloni L, Aru GM, Abbruzzese PA, et al: Localization of mitral periprosthetic leaks by transesophageal echocardiography. *Am J Cardiol* 69:276, 1992.

49. Chan KL, Walley VM: Pathologic correlations of transesophageal echocardiographic findings in degenerated bioprosthetic valves. *Circulation* 82(suppl III):III-44, 1990.

50. Chan KL, Walley VM: Accuracy of transesophageal echocardiographic detection of cusp tears in degenerated bioprosthetic valves. *J Am Cardiol Coll* 17(suppl A):371A, 1991.

51. Smith MD, Harrison MR, Pinton R, et al: Regurgitant jet size by transesophageal compared with transthoracic Doppler color flow imaging. *Circulation* 83:79, 1991.

52. Kleinman JP, Czer LSC, DeRobertis M, et al: A quantitative comparison of transesophageal and epicardial color Doppler echocardiography in the intraoperative assessment of mitral regurgitation. *Am J Cardiol* 64:1168, 1989.

53. Bolger AF, Eigler NL, Pfaff JM, et al: Computer analysis of Doppler color flow mapping images for quantitative assessment of in vitro fluid jets. *J Am Coll Cardiol* 12:450, 1988.

54. Simpson IA, Valdez-Cruz LM, Sahn DJ, et al: Doppler color flow mapping of simulated in vitro regurgitant jets: Evaluation of the effects of orifice size and hemodynamic variables. *J Am Coll Cardiol* 13:1195, 1989.

55. Baumgartner H, Schima H, Kühn P: Importance of technical variables for quantitative measurements by color Doppler imaging. *Am J Cardiol* 67:314, 1991.

56. Yoshida K, Yoshikawa J, Yamaura Y, et al: Assessment of mitral regurgitation by biplane transesophageal color Doppler flow mapping. *Circulation* 82:1121, 1990.

57. Cape EG, Skoufis EG, Weyman AE, et al: A new method for noninvasive quantitation of valvular regurgitation based on conservation of momentum—In vitro validation. *Circulation* 79:1343, 1989.

58. Thomas JD, Liu CM, Flachskampf FA, et al: Quantification of jet flow by momentum analysis—An in vitro color Doppler flow study. *Circulation* 81:247, 1990.

59. Thomas JD: Theory of regurgitant jets and their imaging by color flow Doppler: Is there hope for quantification? *ACC Learning Center Highlights* 7:15, 1992.

60. Maurer G, Siegel RJ, Czer LSC: The use of color flow mapping for intraoperative assessment of valve repair. *Circulation* 84(suppl I):I-250, 1991.

61. Chen C, Thomas JD, Anconina J, et al: Impact of impinging wall jet on color Doppler quantification of mitral regurgitation. *Circulation* 84:712, 1991.

62. Chao K, Moises VA, Shandas R, et al: Influence of the coanda effect on color Doppler jet area and color encoding. In vitro studies using color Doppler flow mapping. *Circulation* 85:333, 1992.

63. Perry GJ, Helmcke F, Nanda NC, et al: Evaluation of aortic insufficiency by Doppler color flow mapping. *J Am Coll Cardiol* 9:952, 1987.

64. Baumgartner H, Kratzer H, Helmreich G, et

al: Quantitation of aortic regurgitation by colour coded cross-sectional Doppler echocardiography. *Eur Heart J* 9:380, 1988.

65. Baumgartner H, Kratzer H, Helmreich G, et al: Evaluation of aortic regurgitation by color-coded two dimensional Doppler echocardiography—Usefulness of different jet parameters for quantification. *Am J Noninvas Cardiol* 3:185, 1989.

66. Baumgartner H, Schima H, Kühn P: Value and limitations of proximal jet dimensions for the quantitation of valvular regurgitation: An in vitro study using Doppler flow imaging. *J Am Soc Echocardiogr* 4:57, 1991.

67. Tribouilloy C, Shen WF, Quéré JP, et al: Assessment of severity of mitral regurgitation by measuring regurgitant jet width at its origin with transesophageal Doppler color flow imaging. *Circulation* 85:1248, 1992.

68. Bargiggia GS, Tronconi J, Sahn DJ, et al: A new method for quantitation of mitral regurgitation based on color flow Doppler imaging of flow convergence proximal to regurgitant orifice. *Circulation* 84:1481, 1991.

69. Yoshida K, Yoshikawa J, Akasaka T, et al: Value of acceleration flow signals proximal to the leaking orifice in assessing the severity of prosthetic mitral valve regurgitation. *J Am Coll Cardiol* 19:333, 1992.

70. Castello R, Pearson AC, Lenzen P, et al: Effect of mitral regurgitation on pulmonary venous velocities derived from transesophageal echocardiography color-guided pulsed Doppler imaging. *J Am Coll Cardiol* 17:1499, 1991.

71. Klein AL, Obarski TP, Stewart WJ, et al: Transesophageal Doppler echocardiography of pulmonary venous flow: A new marker of mitral regurgitation severity. *J Am Coll Cardiol* 18:518, 1991.

72. Pearson AC, Alton ME, Whyles RJ, et al: Jet direction does not affect pulmonary venous flow reversal in left and right pulmonary veins in severe mitral regurgitation. *Circulation* 84(suppl II):II-105, 1991.

73. Jain S, Helmcke F, Fan PH, et al: Limitations of pulmonary venous flow criteria in the assessment of mitral regurgitation severity by transesophageal echocardiography. *Circulation* 82(suppl III):III-551, 1990.

74. Konstadt SN, Loule EK, Black S, et al: Pulmonary venous flow dynamics before and after acute increases in afterload in patients with mitral regurgitation. *J Am Coll Cardiol* 19(suppl A):200A, 1992.

75. Kreis A, Lambertz H, Hanrath P: Variation of pulmonary venous flow pattern in patients with different types of normal mitral valve prostheses. *Circulation* 82(suppl III):III-18, 1990.

76. Klein AL, Stewart WJ, Litowitz H, et al: Pulmonary venous flow assessment of mitral regurgitation: A simultaneous left atrial pressure and transesophageal echo Doppler study. *Circulation* 82(suppl III):III-552, 1990.

77. Diebold B, Laperche T, Raffoul H, et al: Efficacy of TEE for making surgical decisions in valvular prosthesis dysfunction. *Circulation* 82(suppl III):III-43, 1990.

78. Dzvik V, Cohen G, Chan KL: Role of transesophageal echocardiography in the diagnosis and management of prosthetic valve thrombosis. *J Am Coll Cardiol* 18:1829, 1991.

79. Alam M, Rosman HS, Polanco GA, et al: Transesophageal echocardiographic features of stenotic bioprosthetic valves in the mitral and tricuspid valve positions. *Am J Cardiol* 68:689, 1991.

80. Mügge A, Hausmann D, Bargheer K, et al: Continuous-wave Doppler measurement of mitral valve area and gradient from the esophagus: Are monoplane probes sufficient? *J Am Coll Cardiol* 19(suppl A):200A, 1992.

81. Baumgartner H, Khan S, DeRobertis M, et al: Effect of prosthetic aortic valve design on the Doppler-catheter gradient correlation: An in vitro study of normal St. Jude, Medtronic-Hall, Starr-Edwards and Hancock valves. *J Am Coll Cardiol* 19:324, 1992.

82. Yoganathan AP, Jones M, Sahn DJ, et al: Bernoulli gradient calculations for mechanical prosthetic aortic valves: In vitro Doppler study. *Circulation* 74(suppl 2):II-391, 1986.

83. Rothbart RM, Smucker ML, Gibson RS: Over-estimation by Doppler echocardiography of pressure gradients across Starr-Edwards prosthetic valves in the aortic position. *Am J Cardiol* 61:475, 1988.

84. Arabia FA, Talbot TL, Stewart SF, et al: A computerized physiologic pulse duplicator for in-vitro hydrodynamic and ultrasonic studies of prosthetic heart valves. *Biomed Instrum Technol* 23:205, 1989.

85. Baumgartner H, Khan S, DeRobertis M, et al: Discrepancies between Doppler and catheter gradients in aortic prosthetic valves in vitro: A manifestation of localized gradients and pressure recovery. *Circulation* 82:1467, 1990.

86. Geibel A, Kasper W, Konstantinides S, et al: Limitation of Doppler-echocardiography in the judgement of prosthetic valves. *J Am Coll Cardiol* 19(suppl A):39A, 1992.

87. Wiseth R, Hegrenaes L, Rossvoll O, et al: Validity of an early postoperative baseline Doppler recording after aortic valve replacement. *Am J Cardiol* 67:869, 1991.

88. Dumesnil JG, Honos GN, Lemieux M, et al: Validation and applications of mitral prosthetic valvular areas calculated by Doppler echocardiography. *Am J Cardiol* 65:1443, 1990.

89. Miller FA, Khanderia BK, Freeman WK, et al: Mitral prosthesis effective orifice area by a new method using continuity of flow between left atrium and prosthesis. *J Am Coll Cardiol* 19(suppl A):214A, 1992.

90. Baumgartner H, Khan S, DeRobertis M, et al: Doppler assessment of prosthetic valve orifice area: An in vitro study. *Circulation* 85:2275, 1992.

91. Thomas JD, Weyman AE: Doppler mitral pressure half-time: A clinical tool in search of theoretical justification. *J Am Coll Cardiol* 10:923, 1987.

92. Thomas JD, Wilkins GT, Choong CYP, et al: Inaccuracy of mitral pressure half-time immediately after percutaneous mitral valvulotomy. *Circulation* 78:980, 1988.

93. Sanfilippo AJ, Picard MH, Newell JB, et al: Echocardiographic assessment of patients with infectious endocarditis: Prediction of risk for complications. *J Am Coll Cardiol* 18:1191, 1991.

94. Taams MA, Gussenhoven EJ, Bos E, et al: Enhanced morphological diagnosis in infective endocarditis by transesophageal echocardiography. *Br Heart J* 63:109, 1990.

95. Culver DL, Cacchione J, Stern D, et al: Diagnosis of infective endocarditis on a Starr-Edwards prosthesis by transesophageal echocardiography. *Am Heart J* 119:972, 1990.

96. Diebold B, Cormier B, Roudaut R, et al: Value and limitations of transesophageal echocardiography for assessing prosthesis dysfunctions: Surgical correlates in a series of 184 operated prosthetic valves. *J Am Coll Cardiol* 19(suppl A):201A, 1992.

97. Cormier B, Bertrand S, Roger V, et al: Transesophageal echocardiography for the detection of prosthetic complications. *Circulation* 82(suppl III):III-17, 1990.

98. Dick CD, Skopal J, Ulstad V, et al: Aortic perivalvular defects: Characterization by transesophageal echocardiography. *Circulation* 84(suppl II):II-128, 1991.

99. Karalis DG, Chandrasekaran K, Wahl JM, et al: Transesophageal echocardiographic recognition of mitral valve abnormalities associated with aortic valve endocarditis. *Am Heart J* 119:1209, 1990.

100. Trakhtenbroit AD, Desir R, Smith M, et al: Detection of unusual complications of prosthetic valves by transesophageal echocardiography. *Circulation* 82(suppl III):III-17, 1990.

101. Lowry RW, Zoghbi WA, Baker WB, et al: Clinical impact of transesophageal echocardiography in the diagnosis and management of infective endocarditis: Significance of a negative finding. *J Am Coll Cardiol* 19(suppl A):237A, 1992.

102. Chan K, Sochowski R: Management and outcome of patients with prosthetic valvular thrombosis diagnosed by transesophageal echocardiography. *J Am Coll Cardiol* 19(suppl A):39A, 1992.

103. Isada L, Klein AL, Torelli J, et al: "Strands" on mitral valve prostheses by transesophageal echocardiography—Another potential embolic source. *J Am Coll Cardiol* 19(suppl A):32A, 1992.

104. Taylor D, Chan KL: Transesophageal echocardiographic identification of two types of left atrial spontaneous contrast in patients with mitral mechanical prosthetic valves. *Circulation* 84(suppl II):II-161, 1991.

105. Graf T, Fischer H, Reul H, et al: Cavitation potential of mechanical heart valve prostheses. *Int J Arif Organs* 14:169, 1991.

7

Arterial Emboli and Cardiac Masses: Role of Transesophageal Echocardiography

Frederick A. Dressler
Arthur J. Labovitz

Introduction

Stroke leads to nearly 700,000 hospitalizations and 125,000 fatalities in the United States per year.[1] Its direct health care costs are over $3 billion annually and are growing steadily as the population ages. Although the burden of stroke on already limited resources is great, it is a far greater tragedy for the patient, often signaling an abrupt end to productivity, vitality, and autonomy.

Despite the gravity of this disease, the etiology of cerebral ischemia often remains unknown after thorough medical evaluation. Before computed tomography (CT), cerebral angiography, and carotid ultrasound the classification of strokes was apparently simple: bloody spinal fluid indicated hemorrhage; the presence of atrial fibrillation or rheumatic heart disease, embolism; and in the absence of either, cerebral artery thrombosis was assumed. Although the introduction of CT and angiography might have been expected to decrease uncertainty in these patients, quite the opposite has occurred. These diagnostic tests have revealed a wide variety of findings in the stroke population. In some patients, such as those with hemorrhagic stroke, the etiology is frequently identified by CT scan and angiogram. However, in patients with ischemic stroke the cause often remains unknown.

Although carotid artery atherothrombotic narrowing or occlusion is the most often identified abnormality, its frequency varies according to the definitions used. It is generally found in only up to one-half of patients presenting with cerebral ischemia.[2-7] Presumably a significant portion of those patients without carotid stenosis have emboli of cardiac or aortic origin as the etiology of cerebral ischemia.

Transthoracic Echocardiography

The heart has long been recognized as a source and conduit for emboli destined for the cerebral vasculature. While most cardiac sources can be suspected by history and/or exam, the echocardiogram is useful in the diagnosis of many. Early studies of cardiac sources of emboli often employed *transthoracic echocardiography* (TTE) because it was the best widely available diagnostic method to evaluate structural cardiac abnormalities. The usefulness of TTE in patients with systemic emboli, however, has varied widely. Although the yield for cardiac abnormalities is reported to be between 10 and 60 percent,[4,8–17] those studies with stricter criteria found TTE to be of little help in finding cardiac sources of emboli.[14–17] If only cardiac findings *well recognized* to cause systemic emboli are included, the frequency is generally low. For example, of patients with cerebral ischemia (n = 97) reported by Fogelholm and coworkers,[13] echocardiographic abnormalities were seen in 60 percent. Included among these, however, were left ventricular hypertrophy, left atrial and ventricular enlargement, and aortic valve cusp thickening without stenosis. None of these by itself has been clearly associated with systemic emboli. If only definite embolic sources are considered, the frequency falls to 11 percent in this study. The yield of TTE is somewhat higher when patients with cerebral ischemia and normal cerebral angiograms are considered. Of 138 patients presenting in this fashion, Lovett and colleagues[14] reported a potential cardiac source of emboli in 30 percent. However, if patients with no history of cardiac illness were considered, a source was identified in only 4 percent. Similarly, Come et al.[9] reported that of patients "referred for possible cardiac source of embolism" (n = 280), TTE found a possible etiology in 35 percent. However, a far lower frequency (14 percent) was identified in those without a history of cardiac disease. Other authors have reported similar findings.[8,15,18] Thus, in suspected embolic, noncerebrovascular ischemia, TTE identifies potential cardiac sources in approximately one-third. However, most of these findings are suspected by history. In patients without a cardiac history, the yield is low. Overall, the etiology remains unknown after TTE in approximately two-thirds of patients. With the introduction of transesophageal echocardiography (TEE), this group of patients is being reexamined.

Transesophageal Echocardiography

Hisanoga and coworkers first entered the esophagus with an ultrasonic probe in 1977.[19] Since then our ability to view the heart has changed. The retrocardiac position of the probe, its juxtaposition to the heart, and the use of a higher-frequency probe (5 vs. 3.5 MHz) allows TEE greater near-field resolution compared with TTE. Thus exquisite anatomic and functional detail are commonly obtained. This has had a great impact in the evaluation of cerebral ischemia. TEE's ability to view the known sources of systemic emboli, such as left atrial thrombi, is unsurpassed (Table 7-1), and several structures epidemiologically tied to systemic emboli are virtually invisible to other imaging techniques.

Encouraged by its high yield in this setting,[17,20,22] cardiac source of embolus is presently the most common indication for TEE in most laboratories (Fig. 7-1). This is mainly attributable to its greater sensitivity (compared with TTE) for atrial abnormalities. Several studies verify the superior sensitivity of TEE in detecting left atrial (LA) thrombus,[17,22–29] atrial septal aneurysm (ASA),[17,22,24,25,27,29,30,31,34–36] patent foramen ovale (PFO),[32,33] and LA spontaneous contrast (LASC).[20,23,31] In addition, atheroma in the thoracic aorta, a finding well recognized as an embolic source and virtually hidden from TTE (and most other imaging methods), is often easily seen by TEE.[37–39] Each of these atrial and aortic findings is thought to predispose to systemic emboli. This is suggested by the high prevalence of each in patients with systemic (especially cerebral) emboli compared with those receiving TEE for other indications. For example, of 270 patients with unexplained cerebral ischemia studied in this laboratory (Fig. 7-2), a potential source was found in 51 percent compared with only 8 percent in patients studied for other reasons (n = 772). Of the potential sources or findings associated with systemic emboli, LA thrombus was most commonly found (17 percent), followed by ASA (15 percent), LASC (14 percent), PFO (14 percent), aortic atheroma (4 percent), and aortic or mitral

TABLE 7-1   Unexplained Systemic Arterial Emboli; Yield of TTE and TEE for Cardiac Sources of Emboli (CSE)

Author	Ref	Year	No. Pts.	Embolic Site		Potential CSE	
				Cerebral (%)	Peripheral (%)	TTE (%)	TEE (%)
Pop	21	1990	72	100	0	8	61
Hoffmann	20	1990	153	55	45	36	58
Pearson	17	1991	79	100	0	15	57
Lee	22	1991	50	100	0	*	52

TEE = transesophageal echocardiography; TTE = transthoracic echocardiography.

* Patients with CSE on TTE excluded.

Figure 7-1
Indications for transesophageal echocardiography; Saint Louis University Hospital (n = 1402). *Native = 15 percent; prosthetic = 10 percent.

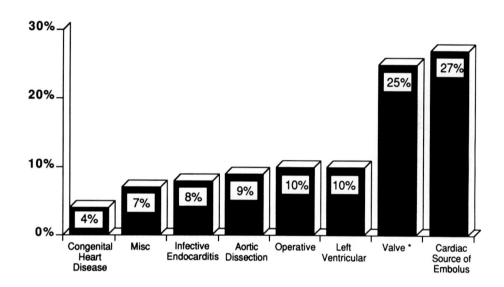

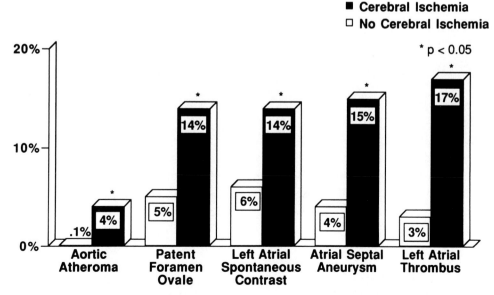

Figure 7-2
Potential embolic sources in patients with (n = 270) and without (n = 700) cerebral ischemia.

valve vegetation (2 percent). The previously cited authors have described similar findings. Some suggest that the greatest improvement in TEE's sensitivity for these cardiac abnormalities is in patients without suspected cardiac illness. Of patients with systemic emboli unassociated with significant cerebral artery narrowing that were reported by Hofmann et al.[20] 36 percent had a source identified by TTE compared with 58 percent by TEE. However, if only patients without clinical heart disease were considered, an embolic source was seen by TTE in only 19 percent compared with 46 percent by TEE. Likewise, Lee and colleagues,[22] reporting a similar cohort ($n = 50$), found no cardiac sources by TTE while in 52 percent one or more were discovered by TEE. Furthermore, a potential source was found in 33 percent of patients without a history of cardiac illness. Thus the value of TEE in patients with unexplained systemic emboli and especially in those without clinical cardiac disease is well described.

Sources of Systemic Arterial Emboli

Although TEE has proved to be of great utility for the evaluation of most potential sources of emboli, there are some for which an advantage has not been proved. For example, no study thus far has described increased sensitivity of TEE in viewing left ventricular thrombus or mitral valve prolapse. Of course in patients with technically difficult surface echocardiography, TEE might be the best remaining method to evaluate these entities. As mentioned above, however, TEE's superior abilities have been well established for several findings. In the following sections, each of the known and suspected sources of systemic arterial emboli best seen by TEE will be reviewed.

Left Atrial Thrombus

Although thrombus in the left atrium (LA) is a well-recognized source of systemic emboli, it is rarely seen by surface echocardiography. Even in patients at high risk for LA thrombi, such as those with chronic atrial fibrillation (AFib) in the presence of mitral stenosis, LA thrombus can rarely be identified with confidence by surface echocardiography. It may be expected that the difficulties in visualizing LA thrombus by TTE are due to the distance between the probe and the atria and the decreased ability to define the LA endocardium. Both of these limitations are somewhat overcome by TEE. The recognition of thrombus

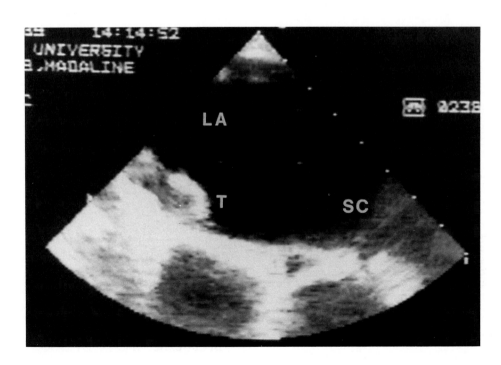

Figure 7-3
Left atrial (LA) thrombus (TEE No. 16-5). This 66-year-old woman with repaired atrial septal defect and chronic atrial fibrillation had several transient ischemic neurologic events. A horizontal-axis TEE view showed spontaneous contrast (SC) and a large sessile thrombus (T) in the left atrium (LA).

during TEE depends on close scrutiny of the interface between endocardium and blood. One should recall that the endocardial lining of the LA chamber (unlike the right atrium) is entirely smooth while ridges of pectinate muscles cross the appendage along its short axis. Thrombus attached to the endocardium appears as an echogenic mass clearly protruding into the main chamber (Fig. 7-3) and/or appendage cavity. While it is most often widest at the base, pedunculated thrombi are not uncommon (Fig. 7-4). Although generally not mobile, hy-

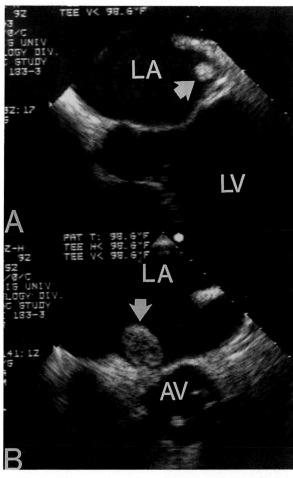

Figure 7-4
Left atrial (LA) thrombus (TEE No. 183-3). This 52-year-old man with mitral stenosis and new-onset atrial fibrillation received TEE prior to planned electrical cardioversion. Horizontal-axis views show two mobile protruding thrombi (arrows), one (1.0 × 1.0 cm) just above the lateral portion of the mitral annulus (A) and another (1.9 × 2.7 cm) adjacent to the aortic valve (AV) (B). LV = left ventricle.

permobility does occur on occasion and suggests but does not confirm the diagnosis of thrombus. While the diagnosis is often simple, subtle abnormalities are difficult to assess. This is especially true in the atrial appendage, where great care must be taken in distinguishing pectinate muscle ridges from thrombi. Confirmation and further anatomic description should be obtained in both longitudinal- and transverse-axis planes if possible. The distinction between LA thrombus and neoplastic tumor is at times difficult and is somewhat influenced by the setting in which a mass is identified. In the presence of the appropriate risk factors for stasis (e.g., mitral stenosis, AFib), a left atrial mass is more likely to represent thrombus. Likewise, the location of the mass within the left atrium may suggest an etiology. For example, while the appendage is the most frequent site for thrombus, neoplasms rarely occur there. Conversely, when present in the left atrium, thrombi most often involve the appendage. Thus a mass in the left atrial appendage associated with the appropriate risk factors suggests thrombus while a mass in the main left atrial chamber that is unassociated with risk factors is more likely to be neoplastic. Using the anatomic findings and clinical setting, the likely etiology of LA mass may be determined.

Prevalence in Subgroups at Risk
Mitral stenosis (MS) and concomitant atrial fibrillation (AFib) have long been known to be risk factors for systemic emboli and are presently the major indication for long-term anticoagulation. These recommendations are based on the high incidence of systemic emboli in this setting. Although several surgical and autopsy reports have appeared, LA thrombus has been difficult to study clinically. The strength of TEE for atrial abnormalities has been used to better understand the clinical settings that predispose to this condition. For example, the incidence of LA thrombus in patients with unexplained systemic emboli is high. Several studies examining patients with cerebral ischemia have reported the prevalence of LA thrombus to be between 4 and 19 percent.[17,20–22] In our experience, LA thrombus

is the most common cardiac source of systemic emboli, accounting for 17 percent. Thus LA thrombus is a relatively common finding in patients presenting with unexplained cerebral ischemia.

Mitral valve function and cardiac rhythm have a strong influence on the formation of LA thrombi. Mitral stenosis (MS) and AFib appear to provide the appropriate environment to produce atrial thrombus. The low-flow state that accompanies this combination of abnormalities is especially thrombogenic. Thus the frequency of MS and AFib are strong determinants of the prevalence of LA thrombi. For example, in patients studied prior to balloon mitral valvuloplasty in whom AFib was present in the majority of patients,[23,25] LA thrombus is described in approximately one-quarter to one-third of patients. In contrast, the incidence of LA thrombus is only between 5 and 10 percent in studies where MS or AFib were present in the minority of those studied.[17,22,24,26,29,34,35]

Patients with LA Thrombus

If only patients with LA thrombus are considered, the strong influence of mitral valve function and atrial rhythm is underscored. Of the patients with TEE-confirmed LA thrombus, reported by several authors (141 patients),[17,22–29,32,34,35] nearly 75 percent are in AFib, while MS is seen in approximately 50 percent. Both of these conditions, individually and especially together, predispose to stasis in the atria. Accordingly, LA spontaneous contrast (LASC), which is strongly associated with low blood flow, also is seen in the vast majority of patients with LA thrombi. It is important to consider, however, that although most patients with LA thrombi have a mitral valve or rhythm abnormality, 5 to 10 percent of LA thrombi occur in patients with sinus rhythm and no mitral valve dysfunction. Thus, in the appropriate clinical setting, a search for LA thrombus should not be abandoned because MS and/or AFib are absent. It should also be noted that LA thrombus is rarely associated with significant mitral regurgitation. None of the patients with LA thrombus in the aforementioned studies had significant mitral regurgitation. It has been suggested that the presence of a regurgitant jet into the atrium greatly diminished stasis and hence thrombus.

Thrombus Location

As stated above, the LA is divided into the main smooth-walled chamber and the small anteriorly located appendage. Although blood drains into the main chamber from the four

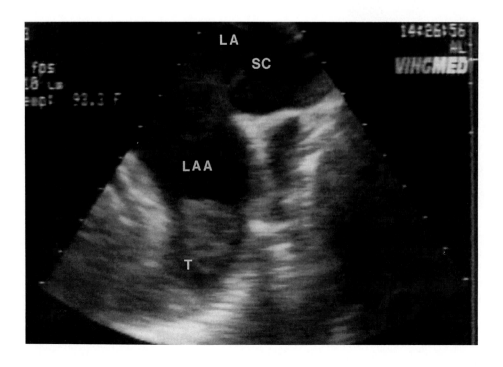

Figure 7-5
Left atrial appendage thrombus (TEE). This was a 60-year-old man with lone atrial fibrillation who presented with stroke. Close-up horizontal-axis TEE views showed a large (2.5 cm × 1.8 cm) thrombus (T) in left atrial appendage (LAA) and spontaneous contrast (SC) in the main left atrial (LA) chamber.

pulmonary veins, no such drainage is present for the appendage. The circulation of blood in the appendage largely depends on its own contraction and relaxation during normal atrial systole. Thus it has been suggested that when AFib occurs, the stagnation of blood in the atrial appendage is greater than in the main chamber. This has been supported by TEE studies, where the LA appendage is the only site of thrombus in nearly 75 percent of patients (Figs. 7-5 and 7-6). Further, when LA thrombi are found in the main chamber, they are often associated with thrombi in the appendage. Once again, it is suggested that the thrombotic threshold is first reached in the appendage and only at times is severe enough in the main chamber to also promote thrombosis there. It is likely that thrombus once formed in the appendage may remain limited or extend into the LA chamber, depending on the intensity of the predisposing factors.

Thus TEE is one of the only widely available and sensitive methods to evaluate LA thrombus. This is due to its unique ability to view the LA and especially the appendage. In patients with unexplained cerebral ischemia, LA thrombus is one of the most common sources of embolus found in approximately 4 to 19 percent of patients and up to one-third of patients with concomitant MS and AFib. The location of thrombus is most often limited to the appendage; however, if the predisposing factors are severe enough, the LA chamber may also be involved.

Left Atrial Spontaneous Contrast

Spontaneous contrast was first described by two-dimensional surface echocardiography, where it was reminiscent of the agitated saline contrast often used in the detection of shunts. Although the clinical settings in which it may be found have been well described, our understanding of the basic mechanism of this phenomenon is lacking. TEE has revealed the "contrast" to be composed of much finer constituents than the microbubbles seen with agitated saline (Fig. 7-6). The spontaneous contrast is more aptly described as "smokelike." Until the underlying pathophysiology is better delineated, we will continue to use these descriptive terms. What is known is that stasis is common to nearly all situations in which spontaneous contrast is seen. A variety of settings, all with slow, nearly stagnant blood flow in common, have been associated with spontaneous contrast. These include left ventricular aneurysm, the false lumen of a dissecting aorta, and the inferior cava in constric-

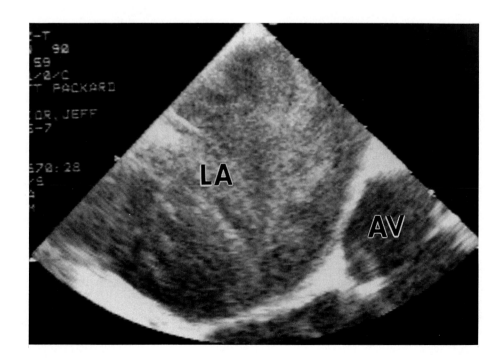

Figure 7-6
Left atrial (LA) spontaneous contrast (TEE No. 65-7). This 27-year-old man with congenital heart disease had TEE to evaluate a prosthetic atrioventricular valve implanted 18 months previously. A horizontal-axis TEE view shows a massively enlarged LA with extensive spontaneous contrast. AV = aortic valve.

tive pericarditis. It should be noted, however, that spontaneous contrast has also been described in the normal descending aorta.[39] In the heart, spontaneous contrast is most often seen in the left atrium in patients with AFib and/or MS.

The diagnosis of LASC is entirely limited to echocardiographic techniques. Although surface echocardiography was the first to diagnose LASC, its yield is exceedingly low compared with TEE. Several studies have reported the yield of both TEE and TTE for LASC.[17,22,24,25,27,29,34] Of all the patients with TEE-confirmed LASC in these studies ($n =$ 210) in only 2 percent was it seen by TTE. It would appear that TTE is quite insensitive for this finding. Although the specific therapeutic implications of LASC have not as yet been determined, this finding suggests a strongly thrombogenic environment and should be sought by TEE in the appropriate clinical setting.

Risk Factors for LASC

The prevalence of LASC depends on the population studied. In this way, it is somewhat similar to LA thrombus where mitral valve function and cardiac rhythm have a strong influence. For example, in studies where MS and/or AFib was present in a majority of patients,[25,34,35] LASC was detected in 35 to 74 percent of patients. In contrast, studies where MS and/or AFib occurred in the minority of patients,[24,27,29] LASC occurred in only 16 to 19 percent of patients. Likewise, in patients presenting with unexplained cerebral ischemia[17,22] the incidence of LASC has been reported to be between 15 and 20 percent.

Systemic Emboli

Both thrombogenesis and spontaneous contrast share slowed blood flow as a precursor. Thus thrombi and spontaneous contrast might be expected to commonly be seen together. Since nearly all emboli originate from thrombi, it also might be expected that spontaneous contrast and embolism often occur concomitantly. This is supported by the previously cited studies where prevalence of LASC in patients presenting with systemic emboli was increased (15 and 20 percent in studies of unexplained cerebral ischemia). Furthermore, the finding of LA thrombus does not increase the risk of systemic emboli in patients with LASC. It appears that LASC, even when unassociated with clearly visible thrombi, identifies a highly thrombogenic milieu. The therapeutic implications of LASC are yet to be defined.

Atrial Fibrillation and Left Atrial Spontaneous Contrast

It has long been recognized that AFib leads to blood stasis in the atria. Accordingly, up to 80 percent of patients in the cited studies with LASC have chronic AFib. It also appears that the influence of this rhythm on the presence of LASC is stronger than that of mitral valve function. This is suggested by the 30 to 50 percent prevalence of MS in patients with LASC. Moreover, since MS predisposes to AFib, its independent role in causing LASC is likely to be less than observed. Furthermore, LASC appears to identify a subgroup of patients with AFib that are at increased embolic risk. Of patients with AFib unassociated with mitral valve dysfunction ($n = 60$) reported by Black and colleagues,[27] systemic emboli and/or LA thrombus was present in the majority (75 percent) with LASC compared with only 38 percent of those without this finding. These findings suggest that thromboembolic risk is not uniform throughout the AFib population, and those patients most requiring anticoagulation may be identified with TEE.

Atrial Septal Aneurysm

Atrial septal aneurysm (ASA) is defined as a redundant, hypermobile atrial septum, usually located in the region of the fossa ovalis (Fig. 7-7), although at times involving the entire atrial septum. Diagnostic criteria include a base width of ≥ 1.5 cm and cyclic or continuous displacement into LA or right atrium of ≥ 1.1 to 1.5 cm (Fig. 7-8).

The role of ASA in systemic embolic events remains controversial. Earlier reports described pathologic and/or surface echocardiographic findings only. ASA has at once been described as an incidental finding and, alternatively, implicated as a source of stroke. The

Figure 7-7
Atrial septal aneurysm (ASA) (TEE No. 13-2). This was a 62-year-old man with transient ischemic neurologic events and normal cerebrovascular Doppler. A horizontal-axis, four-chamber TEE view shows an ASA protruding into the right atrium (RA). LA = left atrium.

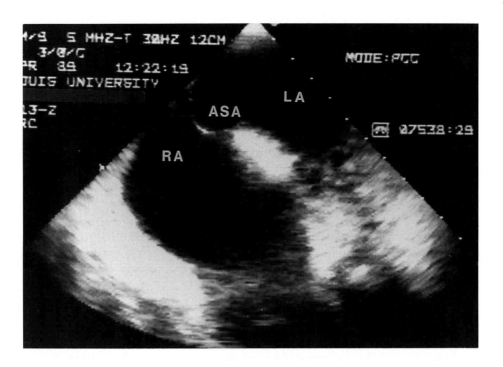

prevalence of this entity, however, is difficult to describe with TTE owing to its low sensitivity for this finding. Whereas it is seen by TTE in less than 1 percent,[40] ASA is present in 3 to 16 percent of TEEs,[17,30,31] depending on the population studied. The preliminary TEE studies identifying ASAs have described an epidemiologic link with cerebral emboli. Although thrombi have been identified in the aneurysm,[31] this is a rare event and one that has not been sufficiently documented. Notwithstanding, the prevalence of ASA in patients with cerebral ischemia is significantly greater than that found in normal controls. Conversely, patients with ASA have an increased frequency of cerebral ischemic events. It has been suggested that this association may be attributable to the large number of TEEs that are done for a cardiac source of embolus. However, when TEEs performed for reasons other than systemic emboli are examined, the incidence of ASA is much lower. Although these data suggest that the relationship between ASA and systemic emboli is real, several cardiac abnormalities frequently seen with ASA confound the issue. Nearly 80 percent of patients reported to have ASA also have one or more other cardiac findings that possibly account for systemic emboli including PFO (>50 percent) and mitral valve prolapse (20 percent). Pure ASA (unassociated with other possible sources) has been described in approximately 20 percent of patients. A relationship between ASA and cerebral vascular events is suggested in these patients, but further studies are needed to describe the clinical implications and the relative risk of this finding.

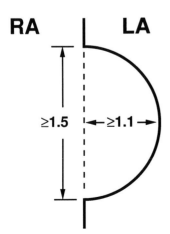

Figure 7-8
Diagnostic criteria for atrial septal aneurysm: (1) Base width (longitudinal distance between hinge points of aneurysm) ≥1.5 cm; and (2) continuous or cyclic excursion into either atria ≥1.1 cm. LA = left atrium; RA = right atrium.

Patent Foramen Ovale

In most individuals the foramen ovale fuses shortly after birth; however, it remains patent in 25 to 30 percent of normal adults.[41,42] Although it will remain asymptomatic in the majority of these, hypoxia and cerebral and peripheral ischemia have been associated with PFO. It has been suggested that these events are due to the right-to-left shunting of venous blood and emboli, respectively. Although these associations have been long debated, the introduction of TEE has allowed further study of PFO in patients with otherwise unexplained embolic events presumably secondary to "paradoxical" emboli.

Diagnosis

Whether by transesophageal or surface echocardiography, the technique of contrast echocardiography for the diagnosis of PFO is similar. Typically, saline (10 ml) and air (1 ml) are vigorously agitated between two syringes via a three-way stopcock. This process creates microbubbles which are then injected intravenously. Oftentimes maneuvers to temporarily increase right atrial pressure (cough, Valsalva) are performed. A complete examination requires full opacification of the right atrium with a dense cloud of contrast while provocative maneuvers are performed. The appearance of contrast in the left atrium within three cycles of complete opacification is a generally accepted criterion for patency (Fig. 7-9). The rapidity and degree of shunting have been reported to correlate with adverse events. Additional color flow evidence of left-to-right shunting and visible septal discontinuity suggest atrial septal defects rather than PFO.

Surface vs. Transesophageal Echocardiography

The diagnosis of PFO has long depended on TTE. It was once thought that surface echocardiography was quite sensitive for PFO; however, several studies comparing TTE and TEE have shown the latter to be superior for PFO.[32,33,43–45] These studies suggest that TTE is falsely negative for PFO in as many as two-thirds of patients. It is not clear whether this is due to better imaging of the atria or whether the procedures followed during TEE are more stringent. In clinical practice, however, it is suggested that PFO cannot be completely excluded until TEE is performed.

Systemic Emboli

Several studies using TTE and/or TEE have found the prevalence of PFO greater in patients

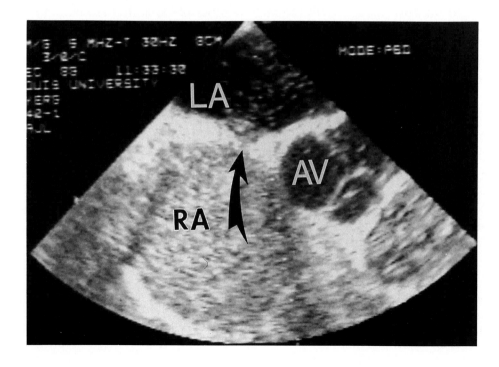

Figure 7-9
Patent foramen ovale (TEE No. 40-2). This 45-year-old woman had an acute inferior myocardial infarction complicated by hypoxia. A close-up, horizontal-axis TEE view shows extensive shunting of venous contrast across the atrial septum via a patent foramen ovale (arrow) and into the left atrium (LA). AV = aortic valve; RA = right atrium.

with systemic emboli compared with controls[43–45] (Fig. 7-10). While the prevalence of PFO in the general population is approximately between 3 and 15 percent, in young patients with risk factors for stroke who present with unexplained cerebral ischemia, PFO has been found in approximately 25 to 50 percent. In older patients with systemic emboli, association of PFO is less clear. DeBelder and colleagues[32] described a 26 percent prevalence of PFO in older patients (mean age = 57) without other risk for stroke, compared with only 3 percent in controls. Conversely, Hausmann et al.[33] reported a similar prevalence in a cohort of older patients with unexplained stroke (22 percent), compared with controls (21 percent). When patients less than 40 years old were examined, however, the frequency of PFO was significantly increased (31 vs. 11 percent). To summarize, although the prevalence of PFO is affected by the population studied, most echocardiographic studies have shown significantly higher rates in those presenting with systemic emboli of unexplained etiology. This appears especially true in younger patients.

Furthermore, owing to the high false-negative rate of TTE, it may be prudent to perform TEE even when PFO is suspected but not seen by TTE.

Aortic Atheroma

The aorta has been long recognized as a site where atherosclerosis is common and at times extensive. Complicated atherosclerotic plaques are well described potential sources for systemic emboli.[46,47] Despite this knowledge, most studies of embolic arterial ischemia have focused on the heart and cerebrovasculature as potential sources and ignored the aorta. This is mainly due to the inability to image the endoluminal surface of the aorta. Thus sessile, low-risk aortic plaques that are ubiquitous could not be distinguished from mobile, protruding, high-risk plaques that might be expected to be more likely to embolize. Since the introduction of TEE, however, detailed morphologic aspects of the thoracic and adjacent abdominal aorta are obtainable. Accordingly, our understanding of aortic atheroma and systemic emboli has increased. Several

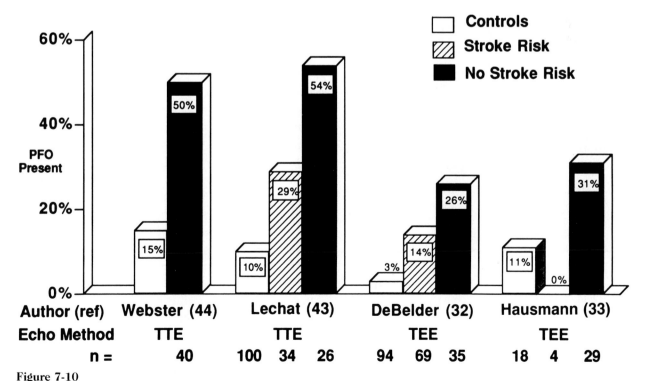

Figure 7-10
Prevalence of patent foramen ovale in young* patients with embolic stroke.
*Mean age of study patients and controls less than 40 years except DeBelder (mean age = 57).

features and associations have been found. First, the finding of aortic atheroma by TEE has been strongly associated with systemic emboli (Fig. 7-11).[37–39,48–52] Of those with aortic atheroma (n = 36) studied by Karalis and coauthors,[50] 31 percent had systemic emboli. Furthermore, of these plaques, those that were mobile were associated with emboli in 73 percent of patients whereas this occurred in 12 percent of those with immobile, layered plaques. Katz and coworkers[51] in a study of patients undergoing cardiopulmonary bypass

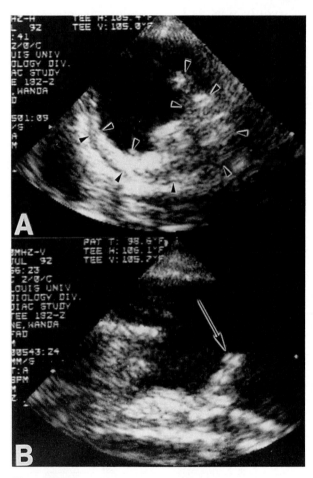

Figure 7-11
Aortic atheroma (TEE No. 182-2). This 59-year-old woman had cerebral emboli after emergent coronary artery bypass grafting. *A*. Close-up, horizontal-axis TEE views of the descending thoracic aorta shows a large (1.5 × 1.8 cm) atheroma (arrowheads) protruding into the lumen. *B*. Longitudinal-axis views of the atheroma reveal a mobile, pedunculated portion (arrow) attached to a sessile base.

found embolic stroke in 25 percent of those with mobile aortic atheroma compared with only 2 percent of those without this finding. Likewise, of patients with unexplained embolic stroke (n = 62) reported by Toyoda and colleagues,[52] 33 percent of those without other identified sources had complicated aortic atheroma. Last, it has been suggested that aortic atheroma may be the single most common potential source of systemic emboli that is identified by TEE alone. Of patients with unexplained stroke or transient ischemia attack (n = 63) described by Tunick and Kronzon,[49] 23 patients had a potential source of systemic emboli identified by TEE that was not seen by TTE. Aortic atheroma represented nearly half of these findings. Thus it appears that aortic atheroma are a significant source of emboli in those patients without other identified sources. Furthermore, although aortic atherosclerosis is ubiquitous in the elderly, certain morphologic features only identified by TEE suggest a high risk for systemic emboli.

Infective Endocarditis and Prosthetic Thrombosis

Infective endocarditis, whether on native or prosthetic heart valves, is a well-recognized source of systemic emboli (Fig. 7-12). Although an in-depth review of TEE's role in these infections appears elsewhere, a few concepts will be reviewed. Several studies of valvular endocarditis suggest that TTE has relatively poor sensitivity for vegetations. It is estimated that approximately 25 to 50 percent of vegetations are missed by TTE. With the introduction of TEE, however, with its superior near-field resolution, a much higher yield has been identified.[53,54] Of patients with infective endocarditis (n = 105) studied by Mügge and coworkers[54] a vegetation was identified in 90 percent by TEE compared with 58 percent by TTE. If only prosthetic valves are considered, the yield for vegetation was 77 percent by TEE compared with only 27 percent by TTE alone. Furthermore, these authors identified the size and mobility of the vegetation as significant determinants of embolic risk. Of patients with vegetations larger than 1 cm, 47 percent had sys-

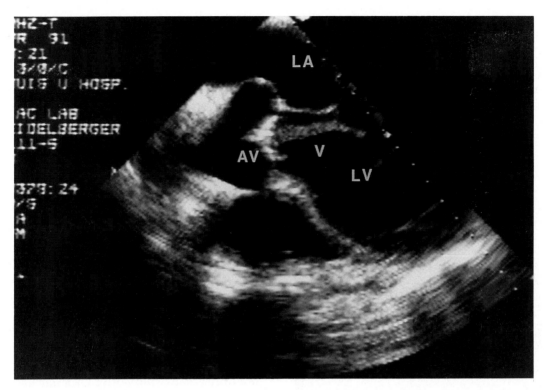

Figure 7-12
Aortic valve (AV) infective endocarditis (TEE No. 111-5). This 76-year-old man with multiple strokes had *Staphylococcus aureus* cultured from blood samples. Horizontal-axis TEE views showed a highly mobile, 4-cm-long vegetation (V) attached to the ventricular aspect of the AV. LA = left atrium; LV = left ventricle.

temic emboli compared with only 19 percent in those with smaller vegetations. Likewise, these authors reported embolic events to be twice as common (38 percent) in those with mobile vegetations compared with those with immobile vegetations (19 percent). Preliminary studies from other authors have suggested similar findings. Thus it appears that infective endocarditis, whether involving a native or prosthetic valve, requires examination with transesophageal echocardiography in order first to make diagnosis of infective endocarditis and second to define the morphologic aspects that are associated with embolic risks and other complications such as ring abscess.

As with prosthetic valve endocarditis, thrombosis of cardiac prostheses is better defined by TEE than with TTE. In patients with left-sided prostheses, who present with systemic emboli, thrombosis is often suspected. The increased sensitivity of TEE over TTE has been described,

as has the association of left atrial spontaneous contrast and prosthetic valve thrombosis by several authors. Of the patients with mitral valve prostheses ($n = 70$) studied by Scott et al.,[55] 15 had had a stroke. A prosthetic thrombus was identified by TEE in 8 (53 percent) of these patients whereas TTE found thrombus in only 1 (7 percent). These and other preliminary studies suggest that TEE is one of the best available methods for direct visualization of thrombus on prostheses and should be performed in nearly all patients suspected of having this diagnosis.

Cardiac Tumors
Of patients with malignancy, approximately 2 to 22 percent have cardiac involvement. Much less frequently (<0.1 percent) tumors are primary to the heart (Fig. 7-13). The most common involvement of the heart is direct pericardial tumor invasion and subsequent pericardial

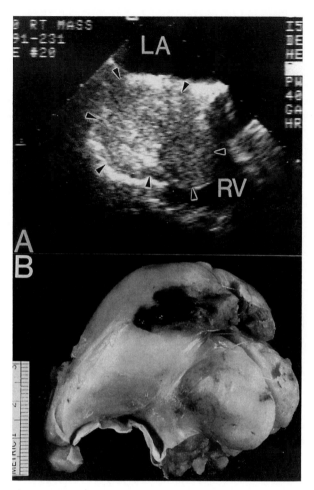

Figure 7-13
Cardiac mass (TEE No. Deac-20). This asymptomatic 71-year-old woman had a right atrial mass found incidentally on surface echocardiography. Although the mass, as seen by TEE (*A*) occupied nearly all of the right atrium, it caused no valvular dysfunction. At surgery (S91-5142) (*B*), the 80-g tumor mass and most of the atrial septum were excised. Histologic exam revealed lipomatous hypertrophy. LA = left atrium; RA = right atrium.

and colleagues,[28] in a study of 32 patients with cardiac masses, found the sensitivity of TTE equal to TEE except for tumors of the right pericardial region, where 36 percent were missed by TTE alone. These authors also found that several relevant morphologic features such as the attachment point and presence of cysts were better evaluated by TEE. They suggest that these morphologic details may distinguish tumor from thrombus. Likewise, of the TEE-identified cardiac tumors (*n* = 25) reported by Reeder and coworkers,[56] 32 percent were not seen by TTE. In this study, it appeared that extracardiac masses were missed by TEE in half of the patients examined. Further, it was determined that TEE led to a change in management in 64 percent of patients. The authors also suggest that tumor site did not determine whether TEE would provide clinically useful information in addition to TTE. Thus these preliminary studies suggest that not only is sensitivity of TEE for cardiac tumors better than TTE but clinically useful morphologic information is also available. It appears that even good-quality TTE identification of a cardiac mass should not deter further evaluation with TEE.

Summary

Transesophageal echocardiography provides high-resolution images of the heart and great vessels. This ability is particularly useful in identifying cardiac masses and other abnormalities associated with emboli of cardiac origin. Transesophageal echocardiography is unique in its ability to identify abnormalities such as left atrial thrombus and spontaneous left atrial contrast, as well as a variety of other abnormalities that have been associated with systemic embolic events. This sensitivity may alter the therapeutic clinical approach to a small but significant number of patients with unexplained cerebral or systemic ischemic events. Accordingly, transesophageal echocardiographic examination should be strongly considered in the evaluation of such patients.

effusion. The evaluation of these metastatic complications by M-mode and two-dimensional TTE has been well described. Although it may be expected that TEE (with its improved resolution) may provide clinically useful information beyond that available by TTE, its effect on management of pericardial tumor is not known. In the setting of endocardial tumors, however, a few preliminary studies suggest increased yield and an influence on management. Mügge

References

1. Wolf PA: An overview of the epidemiology of stroke. *Stroke* 21 (suppl II) II/4-Centers for Disease Control: Progress in chronic disease prevention: Chronic disease reports: Mortality trends—United States, 1979–1986. *MMWR* 38:189, 1989.

2. Sorensen PS, Pedersen H, Marquardsen J, et al: Acetylsalicylic acid in the prevention of stroke in patients with reversible ischemic attacks. A Danish operative study. *Stroke* 4:15, 1983.

3. Caplan LR, Hier DB, D'Cruz I: Cerebral embolism in the Michael Reese stroke registry. *Stroke* 14:530, 1983.

4. Gagliardi R, Benventi L, Froisini F, et al: Frequency of echocardiographic abnormalities in patients with ischemia of the carotid territory—A preliminary report. *Stroke* 16: 118, 1985.

5. Olsen TS, Skriver EB, Herning M: Cause of cerebral infarct in the carotid territory. Its relation to the size and location of the infarct and to the underlying vascular lesion. *Stroke* 16:459, 1985.

6. Ferro JM, Crespo M: Young adult stroke: Neuropsychological dysfunction and recovery. *Stroke* 19:982, 1988.

7. European Carotid Surgery Trialists' Collaborative Group MRC European Carotid Surgery Trial: Interim results for symptomatic patients with severe (70–99%) or with mild (0–29%) carotid stenosis. *Lancet* 337:1235, 1991.

8. Greenland P, Knopman DS, Mikell FL, et al: Echocardiography in diagnostic assessment of stroke. *Ann Intern Med* 95:51, 1981.

9. Come PC, Riley MF, Bivas NK: Roles of echocardiography and arrhythmia monitoring in the evaluation of patients with suspected systemic embolism. *Ann Neurol* 13:527, 1983.

10. The American-Canadian Co-Operative Study Group: Revasture Aspirine trial in cerebral ischemia, part II: Endpoint results. *Stroke* 16:406, 1985.

11. Rem JA, Hachinski VC, Boughner DR, et al: Value of cardiac monitoring and echocardiography in TIA and stroke patients. *Stroke* 16:950, 1985.

12. Good DC, Frank S, Verhulst S, et al: Cardiac abnormalities in stroke patients with negative arteriograms. *Stroke* 17:6, 1986.

13. Fogelholm R, Melin J: Echocardiography in ischemic cerebrovascular disease. *Br Med J* 295:305, 1987.

14. Lovett JL, Sandok BA, Giuliani ER, et al: Two-dimensional echocardiography inpatients with focal cerebral ischemia. *Ann Intern Med* 95:1, 1981.

15. Robbins JA, Sagar KB, French M, et al: Influence of echocardiography on management of patients with systemic emboli. *Stroke* 14:546, 1983.

16. Shuaib A, Hachinski VC, Oczkowski WJ: Transient ischemic attacks and normal cerebral angiograms: A follow-up study. *Stroke* 19: 1223, 1988.

17. Pearson AC, Labovitz AJ, Tatineni S, et al: Superiority of transesophageal echocardiography in detecting cardiac source of embolism in patients with cerebral ischemia of uncertain etiology. *J Am Coll Cardiol* 17:66, 1991.

18. Bogousslavsky J, Hachinski VC, Boughner DR, et al: Cardiac and arterial lesions in carotid transient ischemic attacks. *Arch Neurol* 43:223, 1986.

19. Hisanoga K, Hisanoga A, Nogata K, et al: A new transesophageal realtime two-dimensional echocardiographic system using a flexible tube and its clinical application. *Proc Jpn Soc Ultrason Med* 32:43, 1977.

20. Hofmann T, Kasper W, Meinerty T, et al: Echocardiographic evaluation of patients with clinically suspected arterial emboli. *Lancet* 336:1421, 1990.

21. Pop G, Sutherland GR, Koudstaal PJ, et al: Transesophageal echocardiography in the detection of intracardiac embolic sources in patients with transient ischemic attacks. *Stroke* 21:560, 1990.

22. Lee RJ, Bartzokis T, Yeoh TK, et al: Enhanced detection of intracardiac sources of cerebral emboli by transesophageal echocardiography. *Stroke* 22:734, 1991.

23. Aschenberg W, Schluter M, Kremer P, et al: Transesophageal two-dimensional echocardiography for the detection of left atrial appendage thrombus. *J Am Coll Cardiol* 7:163, 1986.

24. Castello R, Pearson AC, Labovitz AJ: Prevalence and clinical implications of atrial spontaneous contrast in patients undergoing transesophageal echocardiography. *Am J Cardiol* 65:1149, 1990.

25. Kronzon I, Tunick PA, Colossman E, et al: Transesophageal echocardiography to detect atrial clots in candidates for percutaneous

trans-septal mitral balloon valvuloplasty. *J Am Coll Cardiol* 16:1320, 1990.

26. Mügge A, Daniel WB, Hausmann D, et al: Diagnosis of left atrial appendage thrombi by transesophageal echocardiography: Clinical implications and follow-up. *Am J Cardiac Imag* 4:173, 1990.

27. Black IW, Hopkins AP, Lee LCL, et al: Left atrial spontaneous echo contrast: A clinical and echocardiographic analysis. *J Am Coll Cardiol* 18:398, 1991.

28. Mügge A, Daniel WG, Haverich A, et al: Diagnosis of non-infective cardiac mass lesions by two-dimensional echocardiography. Comparison of the transthoracic and transesophageal approaches. *Circulation* 83:70, 1991.

29. Olson JD, Goldenberg IF, Pedersen W, et al: Exclusion of atrial thrombus by transesophageal echocardiography. *J Am Soc Echocardiogr* 5:52, 1992.

30. Schneider B, Hanrath P, Vogel P, et al: Improved morphologic characterization of atrial septal aneurysm by transesophageal echocardiography: Relation to cerebrovascular events. *J Am Coll Cardiol* 16:1000, 1990.

31. Pearson AC, Nagelhout D, Castello R, et al: Atrial septal aneurysm and stroke: A transesophageal echocardiographic study. *J Am Coll Cardiol* 18:1223, 1991.

32. DeBelder MA, Tourikis, Leech G, et al: Risk of patent foramen ovale for thromboembolic events in all age groups. *Am J Cardiol* 69:1316, 1992.

33. Hausmann D, Mügge A, Becht I, et al: Diagnosis of patent foramen ovale by transesophageal echocardiography and association with cerebral and peripheral embolic events. *Am J Cardiol* 70:668, 1992.

34. Manning WJ, Reis GJ, Douglas PS: Use of transesophageal echocardiography to detect left atrial thrombi before percutaneous balloon dilatation of the mitral valve: A prospective study. *Br Heart J* 67:170, 1992.

35. Daniel WG, Nellessen V, Schröder E, et al: Left atrial spontaneous contrast in mitral valve disease: An indicator for an increased thromboembolic risk. *J Am Coll Cardiol* 11:1204, 1988.

36. Karalis DG, Chandrasekaran K, Victor MF, et al: Recognition and embolic potential of intraaortic atherosclerotic debris. *J Am Coll Cardiol* 17:73, 1991.

37. Simons AJ, Carlson R, Hare CL, et al: The use of transesophageal echocardiography in detecting aortic atherosclerosis in patients with embolic disease. *Am Heart J* 123:224, 1992.

38. Tunick PA, Kronzon I: The improved yield of transesophageal echocardiography over transthoracic echocardiography in patients with neurologic events is largely due to the detection of aorta protruding atheroma echocardiography. *J CV Ultrasound Atrial Technol* 9:491, 1992.

39. Castello R, Pearson AC, Labovitz AJ: Spontaneous echocardiogram contrast in the descending aorta. *Am Heart J* 120:915, 1990.

40. Hanley PC, Tajik AJ, Hynes JK, et al: Diagnosis and classification of atrial septal aneurysm by two-dimensional echocardiography: Report of 80 consecutive cases. *J Am Coll Cardiol* 6:1370, 1985.

41. Schrockenstein RF, Wasenda GJ, Edwards JE: Valvular competent patent foramen ovale in adults. *Minn Med* 55:11, 1972.

42. Hagen PT, Scholz DG, Edwards WD: Incidence and size of patent foramen ovale during the first 10 decades of life: An autopsy study of 965 normal hearts. *Mayo Clin Proc* 59:17, 1984.

43. Lechat PH, Mas JL, Lascault G, et al: Prevalence of patent foramen ovale in patients with stroke. *N Engl J Med* 318:1148, 1988.

44. Webster MVI, Smith HJ, Sharpe DN, et al: Patent foramen ovale in young stroke patients. *Lancet* 2:11, 1988.

45. Decoodt P, Kacenelenbogen R, Heuse D, et al: Detection of patent foramen ovale in stroke by transesophageal contrast echocardiography (abstract). *Circulation* 80:II-339, 1989.

46. Fine MJ, Kapoor W, Falanga V: Cholesterol embolization syndrome: A review of 221 cases in the English literature. *Angiology* 38:769, 1987.

47. Amarenco P, Duyckaorts C, Tzouvio C, et al: The prevalence of ulcerated plaques in the aortic arch in patients with stroke. *N Engl J Med* 326:221, 1992.

48. Taams Ma, Gossenhoven WS, Schippens, et al: The value of transesophageal echocardiography for diagnosis of thoracic aorta pathology. *Eur Heart J* 9:1308, 1988.

49. Tunick PA, Kronzon I: Protruding atherosclerotic plaque in the aortic arch of patients with systemic embolization: A new finding seen by transesophageal echocardiography. *Am Heart J* 120:658, 1990.

50. Karalis DG, Chandrasekaran K, Victor MF,

et al: Recognition and embolic potential of intraaortic atherosclerotic debris. *J Am Coll Cardiol* 17:73, 1991.

51. Katz ES, Tunick PA, Rusinek H, et al: Protruding aortic atheromas predict stroke in elderly patients undergoing cardiopulmonary bypass: Experience with intraoperative transesophageal echocardiography. *J Am Coll Cardiol* 20:70, 1992.

52. Toyoda K, Yasaka M, Nagak S, et al: Aortagenic embolic stroke: A transesophageal approach. *Stroke* 23:1056, 1992.

53. Daniel WG, Schröder E, Mügge A, et al: Transesophageal echocardiography in infective endocarditis. *Am J Cardiac Imag* 2:78, 1988.

54. Mügge A, Daniel WG, Frank G, et al: Echocardiography in infective endocarditis: Reassessment of prognostic implications of vegetation size determined by the transthoracic and the transesophageal approach. *J Am Coll Cardiol* 14:631, 1989.

55. Scott PJ, Essop R, Wharton GA, et al: Left atrial clot in patients with mitral prostheses: Increased rate of detection after recent systemic embolism. *Int J Cardiol* 33:141, 1991.

56. Reeder GS, Khandheria BK, Seward JB, et al: Transesophageal echocardiography and cardiac masses. *Mayo Clin Proc* 66:1101, 1991.

8

Transesophageal Echocardiography in Infective Endocarditis

Helmut Baumgartner
Gerald Maurer

Introduction

Because echocardiography provides direct visualization of vegetations and of the complications of endocarditis, such as valvular regurgitation, abscesses, aneurysm formation, and fistulous communications between cardiac chambers, it has become the diagnostic method of choice to evaluate infective endocarditis. Information provided by echocardiography has been shown to be helpful not only for diagnostic purposes but also for patient management and for the prediction of the risk for complications. Owing to enhanced resolution and image quality, transesophageal echocardiography has significantly increased the detection rate of vegetations when compared with transthoracic imaging. In addition, transesophageal imaging has substantially improved the diagnosis of abscesses, mycotic aneurysms, and fistulas. The accurate detection of these complications has an important impact on deciding between medical and surgical treatment and on planning the surgical repair. This information gained from transesophageal echocardiography may have significant effect on patient management and clinical outcome. Therefore, it has become generally accepted that transesophageal echocardiography should routinely be performed not only when infective endocarditis is suspected but also when the diagnosis has already been established by other means, including transthoracic echocardiography.

Vegetation

Definition
Using two-dimensional echocardiography, vegetation has been defined as a sessile or pedunculated mass that is attached to leaflets (cusps), chordae, or chamber walls and typically presents with soft tissue reflectance (distinct echogenicity from the valve or endocardial surface), irregular geometry, and free mobility (Figs. 8-1 to 8-3).[1–3] These echoes should be seen consistently throughout the cardiac cycle and be apparent in multiple views.[4] M-mode echocardiograms may still be helpful in the diagnosis

127

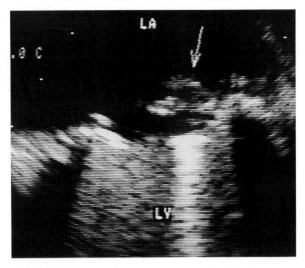

Figure 8-1
Systolic transesophageal transverse view from a patient with prosthetic valve endocarditis showing a vegetation (arrow) attached to the ring of a Björk-Shiley mitral valve prosthesis. LA = left atrium; LV = left venticle.

of vegetations. Shaggy and irregular thickening of valves has been considered as characteristic appearance of vegetations while thickening of other causes usually presents with rather linear echoes.[3]

Detection Rate—Sensitivity

In early echocardiographic studies using M-mode technique, vegetations have been reported in 35 to 75 percent of patients with infective endocarditis.[5–8] Using transthoracic two-dimensional echocardiography, vegetations were detected in 54 to 81 percent of patients with clinical evidence of endocarditis (fever, murmur, and positive blood cultures).[9–14] In one report, compared with findings at surgery or autopsy, a sensitivity of 93 percent has even been reported for transthoracic imaging.[12] However, most of these studies included echo findings that were suggestive for vegetation. In more recent studies that compared transthoracic and transesophageal echocardiography in this setting, "definite" vegetations were detected in only 30 to 58 percent[1,15] and the reported sensitivity ranged from 30 to 63 percent.[2,16–18] Transesophageal echocardiography, however, significantly increased the detection rate of vegetations to 86 to 90 percent[1,15] and

a markedly higher sensitivity of 88 to 100 percent[2,16–18] has been reported. When valves were considered separately,[18] sensitivity was higher for vegetations on the mitral valve (100 percent) than for those on aortic valves (88 percent). Although one explanation for these differences between transthoracic and transesophageal imaging is the poor transthoracic image quality in some patients, the sensitivity improved only slightly from 30 to 36 percent when only echocardiographic studies with good or excellent image quality were analyzed in one study.[18] Differences in image resolution are certainly a major factor. Although vegetations as small as 2 mm have been reported[19] to be detectable by transthoracic echocardiography, the sensitivity of this technique has been shown to be highly size-dependent. Erbel et al.[16] detected only 25 percent of vegetations of less than 5 mm, but 69 and 100 percent of those with 6 to 10 mm and greater than 10 mm when transthoracic echocardiography was used. Most studies primarily refer to left-sided valve endocarditis, whereas few data are available on right-sided valve endocarditis. Nevertheless recent reports suggest that transesophageal echocardiography may be valuable in patients with pulmonic valve endocarditis,[20] particularly when biplane technique[21] is used. Transesophageal echocardiography has particularly improved the diagnostic accuracy in prosthetic valve endocarditis;[1,15,22] an increase of the detection rate from 27 to 77 percent has been reported comparing transthoracic with transesophageal imaging.[1] However, the detection of vegetations and other endocarditis-associated lesions is still more difficult in prosthetic valves and the detection rate is significantly lower than it is in patients with native valves.[1] For this reason, a negative transesophageal echocardiogram has been reported to virtually exclude infective endocarditis in native valves while this may not be the case in prosthetic valves.[23]

Specificity–Potential False-Positive Findings

High specificity has been reported for both transthoracic and transesophageal echocardiography. Specificity ranged from 83 to 100

Figure 8-2
Systolic transesophageal two-dimensional and color Doppler images from a patient with native mitral valve endocarditis. A large vegetation protruding into the left atrium shows an echolucent area (A). Color Doppler imaging demonstrates turbulent flow within this area indicating a communication with the left ventricle (B). AO = aorta; LA = left atrium; LV = left ventricle.

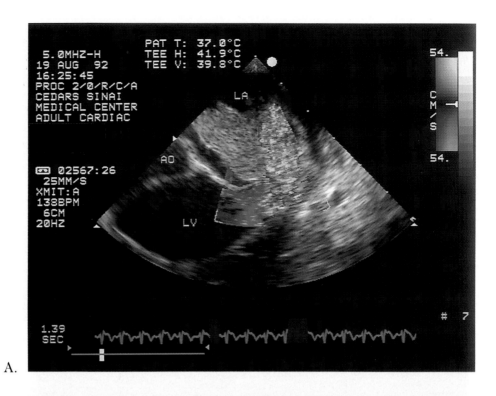

A.

B.

percent using transthoracic imaging[2,9,12,16,17] and was similar for transesophageal imaging (98 to 100 percent).[2,16,17] However, these results may have been significantly affected by patient selection in these studies. Fibrosis and calcification of valvular structures can mimic vegetative endocarditis,[10,11] although their higher echodensity and less mobility and irregularity may usually allow the distinction from vegetations. M-mode echocardiography

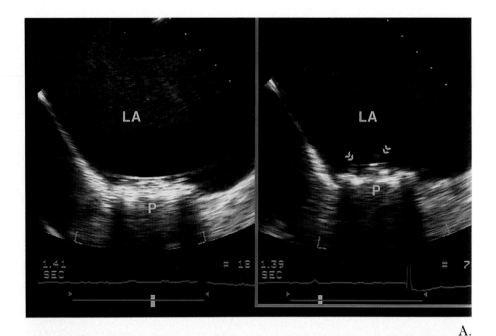

A.

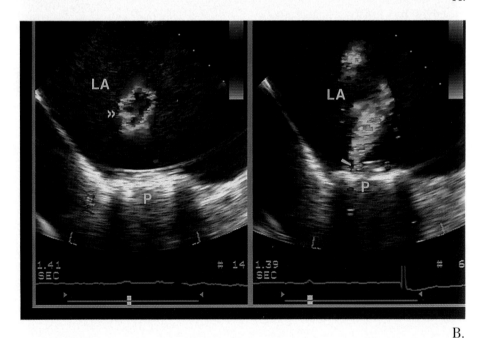

B.

Figure 8-3
Systolic transesophageal two-dimensional (upper panels) and color Doppler images (lower panels) from a patient with a Starr-Edwards mitral valve prosthesis. Left panels were obtained from a first study, right panels were obtained from a follow-up study 8 days later. In the first study, no vegetations were found and color Doppler showed only normal regurgitation due to the closure volume (>>). In the follow-up study, vegetations were detected (>>) and color Doppler imaging revealed pathologic valvular regurgitation (right lower panel). LA = left atrium; P = mitral valve prosthesis.

recorded at high speed is also helpful for evaluation of thickened valve structures. Vegetations typically present with irregular surface and soft echodensity while fibrosis and calcification usually result in smooth parallel lines of echoes with high echogenicity. False-positive examinations may also occur when myxomatous degeneration is present.[10] Tangential views, particularly of the aortic valve, may pretend valve thickening, and this may lead to the mistaken diagnosis of vegetations. Authors comparing anatomic findings as documented at surgery or autopsy and echocardiographic results have also reported that the distinction between vegetations and other endocarditis-induced lesions, such as rupture of leaflets or the valve apparatus, is not always possible.[1] This may also be the case in spontaneous rupture of chordae tendineae. False-positive results have also been reported in bioprosthetic valves with degenerated cusps.[22,24] Hypermobile, redundant chordae tendineae and localized chordal thickening, particularly when accompanied by aortic regurgitation that causes vibration, may easily be misinterpreted as vegetation.[2] Tiny mobile strands below the aortic valve probably representing prominent Lambl's excrescences may also be mistaken for small vegetations.[2] Other potential false-positive findings include strands extending from prosthetic sewing rings and false chordae in the left ventricular outflow tract. Brightly reflectant, transient echoes on the left atrial side of the mitral valve during early systole that have also been observed in healthy volunteers have been reported to be a potential false-positive finding.[2] Furthermore, it has to be emphasized that the appearance of echocardiographically detected vegetations has been reported to remain stable after bacteriologic cure in a high percentage of patients.[7,11] Therefore, it may be impossible to distinguish active from healed vegetations. Serial evaluation of patients with suspected infective endocarditis may be very helpful by detecting changes of preexisting structures or development of new structures (Fig. 8-3). Furthermore, it should be noted that the diagnosis of endocarditis should be based not solely on the echocardiographic visualization of an apparent vegetation but on its demonstration in the appropriate clinical setting, with supportive, although less specific, clinical and laboratory findings.[17]

Prediction of Risk for Complications

Early studies of transthoracic M-mode and two-dimensional echocardiography in infective endocarditis have suggested that the evidence of vegetations by itself indicates an increased risk of congestive heart failure, systemic embolism, death, and more frequent need for surgical intervention.[6,8,11,12,25] Since evidence of vegetations has been reported for the majority of patients with infective endocarditis, these findings may have limited clinical impact. Early attempts to relate vegetation size to complication rate yielded controversial results. Some others found that the risk increased with vegetation size[7,12] while others did not find a significant correlation.[4,11,13] Stafford et al.[12] have

reported that embolism or fatal outcome occurred in their series only in patients with a vegetation of greater than 5 mm in diameter. In more recent studies that used transthoracic and transesophageal echocardiography,[1,26] the prognostic implication of vegetation size has been confirmed. Mügge et al.[1] have reported a significantly higher incidence of embolic events for patients with a vegetation of > 10 mm in diameter than those with a vegetation diameter ≤ 10 mm (47 vs. 19 percent). Although patients with a mobile vegetation had a significantly higher incidence of embolic episodes than did patients with a sessile vegetation, the mobility of vegetations was not a further independent variable to discriminate the risk of patients for embolism because in 85 percent of patients with large vegetations, these were also highly mobile. In this study, vegetation size was not significantly different in patients with or without severe heart failure and in patients surviving or dying during acute endocarditis. In another recent study,[26] vegetation size, extent, mobility, and consistency were all found to be significant univariate predictors of complications (need for surgery, embolism, congestive heart failure, and death). Highly reflective lesions did identify a subgroup in which no complications occurred and may have represented older "healed" lesions or false-positive findings of valve fibrosis or calcification. The other three variables were used to develop a score in order to illustrate the effect of combining variables. A score of 1, 2, 3, or 4 was assigned to a maximal vegetation dimension of ≤6, 7 to 10, 11 to 15, or >15 mm. Extent was graded as follows: grade 1 = single vegetation; grade 2 = multiple vegetations limited to a single valve leaflet; grade 3 = involvement of multiple valve leaflets; grade 4 = extent to extravalvular structure. Vegetation mobility was assessed by grading: grade 1 = fixed lesion; grade 2 = fixed base, free edge; grade 3 = pedunculated; grade 4 = prolapsing vegetation (crossing the coaptation of the leaflets at some point of the cardiac cycle). For mitral valve endocarditis, a score of ≥8 (total possible score 12) predicted the occurrence of complications with a sensitivity of 70 percent and specificity of 92 percent (predictive accuracy of 80 percent). For aortic valve endocarditis, a score of ≥5 provided a predictive accuracy of 71 percent with a sensitivity of 76 percent and specificity of 62 percent. Another important observation of this study was that patients with nonspecific valvular thickening had complication rates roughly equivalent to those with discrete vegetations: 57.1 vs. 52.9 percent and 61.8 percent for mitral vegetation and aortic vegetation, respectively. In patients with nonspecific valve thickening who died, death was clearly attributed to endocarditis, and in some of them autopsy showed small friable vegetations that were, in retrospect, echocardiographically indistinguishable from the irregular, thickened appearance of the aortic cusps that is commonly seen in elderly patients with degenerative changes of valves. Thus, in patients with clinically suspected infective endocarditis, patients with nonspecific thickening of the valves may behave more like those with vegetations than like those with echocardiographically "clean" valves,[26] but these observations may have been biased by the patient selection in this study.

Changes in Vegetation Size and Morphology over Time

There are only few reports in which vegetations were followed by echocardiography during therapy and convalescence. No change, an increase or decrease in size, and complete disappearance of vegetations (with or without embolic event) may be observed. Echodensity may increase over time and M-mode echoes may lose their typical irregularity. In an early M-mode study,[7] little to no change in the echocardiographic size of the vegetations occurred during the first 6 weeks after diagnosis and appropriate antibiotic therapy unless a major systemic embolus occurred and the echocardiogram was of limited value in delineating an active from healed vegetation. Stewart et al.[11] have reported that two-thirds of vegetations detected by transthoracic echocardiography remained stable with respect to size and morphology throughout therapy and for as long as 36 months after bacteriologic cure. Lesion disappearance correlated with embolic events in only two cases of tricuspid valve endocarditis. They also did not find any correlation

between change in lesion size or morphology and the efficacy of medical therapy. In a more recent study using transesophageal echocardiography,[27] patients with increasing or constant size of vegetations (group A) were compared with patients with decreasing vegetation size (group B). Group A patients had a longer duration of fever, need of valve replacement was more frequent (45 vs. 2 percent), embolic events and abscess formation occurred more frequently (45 vs. 17 percent and 13 vs. 2 percent, respectively), and mortality was higher (10 vs. 0 percent). They concluded that an increase in vegetation size during antibiotic treatment predicts a prolonged healing phase of infective endocarditis associated with a significantly increased risk of complications, independent of blood culture results. From the results of this study, complication rate seems to depend not only on vegetation size at first presentation but also on subsequent changes in size. Reduction of vegetation size during antibiotic treatment, however, may indicate a rapid healing phase with an improved prognosis.

Valve Damage and Dysfunction

Valve damage and dysfunction represent major problems in patients with infective endocarditis. Valvular regurgitation is the leading cause of congestive heart failure, and in most patients who need surgical intervention, severe valve dysfunction is present. In a study of 45 necropsy patients with infective endocarditis,[28] 53 percent had no signs of preexisting anatomical abnormalities of their valves. Forty-seven percent of the remaining patients with anatomically abnormal valves had normal valve function before the infection as judged by the absence of signs or symptoms of cardiac dysfunction before the onset of infective endocarditis, and by necropsy evaluation of the involved valve. Thus valve function was normal in 76 percent of patients before the onset of infective endocarditis. After infection, 50 percent had valve dysfunction resulting from infective endocarditis alone, in 9 percent worsening of underlying valve dysfunction had occurred, and 15 percent had dysfunction from underlying disease alone. Doppler echocardiography is more sensitive and has been reported to detect valvular regurgitation in almost every patient with endocarditis. Jaffe et al.[4] in their series found regurgitation ≥2+ in 88 percent. Although rare cases of valvular stenosis due to large vegetations have been reported,[28] most patients with valve dysfunction resulting from infective endocarditis have valvular regurgitation.[28] Cusp perforation, cusp destruction, ruptured chordae tendineae, and ruptured papillary muscles may represent the underlying mechanisms and can accurately be identified by two-dimensional transesophageal echocardiography. Color Doppler flow imaging has improved the detection and localization of valve perforations[29,30] and provides semiquantitative grading of the severity of regurgitant lesions (see Chap. 5). In patients with heart valve prostheses, infective endocarditis frequently results in paravalvular regurgitation, which can also be accurately detected and semiquantified by transesophageal Doppler echocardiography. For further details see Chap. 6.

Cardiac Complications of Infective Endocarditis: Abscess, Aneurysm, Fistula

Definition

Echocardiographically, an abscess has been defined as a definite region of reduced echo density or an echolucent cavity without communication with the circulation (no collapse throughout the cardiac cycle) and located within the valvular annulus or adjacent myocardial structures[15,31] (Figs. 8-4, 8-5). Studies using transthoracic echocardiography have also included abnormal echodense areas in the perivalvular tissue[32] and >10-mm focal aortic root thickening above the annulus.[33] Mycotic aneurysms or pseudoaneurysms present with an abnormal pulsatile echo-free protrusion[15] (Fig. 8-6). Rupture of abscesses and aneurysms may result in leaflet perforation and fistulous communications between cardiac chambers (Figs. 8-7 to 8-9).

Detection Rate, Sensitivity, and Specificity

Presence of abscess formation has been reported in up to 37 percent of patients with

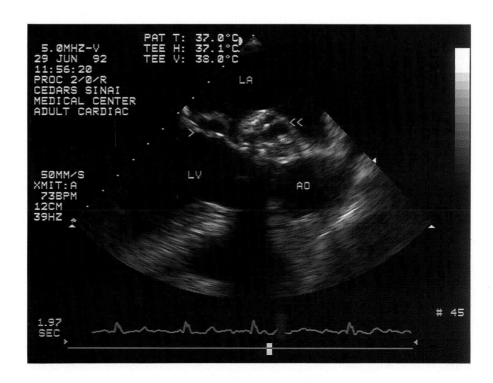

Figure 8-4
Transesophageal longitudinal view from a patient with aortic valve endocarditis with ring abscess (<<) and anterior mitral leaflet abscess (>). AO = aorta; LA = left atrium; LV = left ventricle.

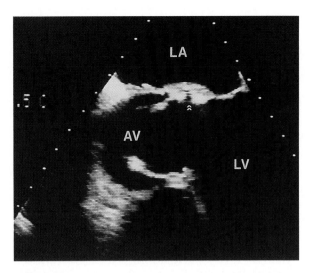

Figure 8-5
Transesophageal transverse view from a patient with aortic valve endocarditis showing a small abscess (>>) of the anterior mitral leaflet. AV = aortic valve; LA = left atrium; LV = left ventricle.

several studies have reported detection of abscesses and mycotic aneurysms with transthoracic echocardiography, most of them are case reports[36-42] or present selected patient groups.[32,33] Thus they do not allow definitive conclusions on detection rates or sensitivity and specificity. Ellis et al.[43] compared transthoracic echocardiographic findings in 22 patients with perivalvular abscess found at surgery or necropsy with those in 24 patients without abscess. A typical echo-free abscess was noted in only one patient in this study. Indirect signs suggestive for abscess were prosthetic valve rocking, sinus of Valsalva aneurysm, anterior aortic root thickening of ≥10 mm, or perivalvular density in a septum of ≥14 mm. Only when combined, these criteria predicted the presence or absence of perivalvular abscess with a sensitivity of 86 percent and specificity of 88 percent in patients with adequate echocardiograms. The diagnosis of abscesses and of aneurysms has been substantially improved by transesophageal imaging.[15,17,18,31,44-46] In 118 prospectively studied patients with infective endocarditis, 37 percent were found to have regions of abscess at surgery or autopsy.[31] Sensitivity and specificity for the detection

native valve infective endocarditis at surgery or at autopsy.[31,34] The incidence of abscess formations in prosthetic valve endocarditis may be substantially higher (100 percent in a necropsy study of 22 patients[35]). Although

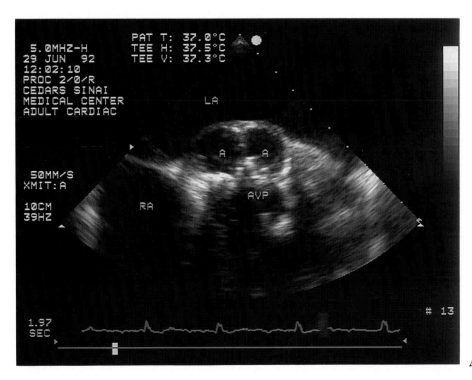

Figure 8-6
Transesophageal cross-sectional views from a patient with aortic prosthetic valve endocarditis. Two mycotic aneurysms (A) can be seen. Systolic expansion (left panel) and diastolic collapse (right panel) indicates communication with the left ventricular outflow tract. AVP = aortic valve prosthesis; LA = left atrium; RA = right atrium.

A.

Figure 8-6
(continued)

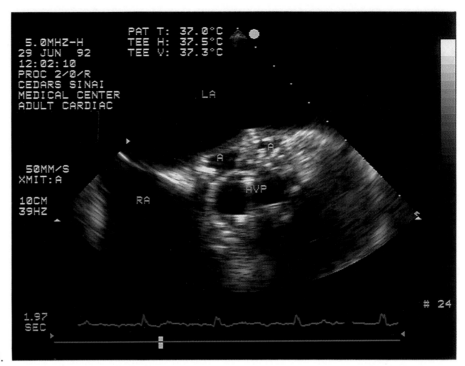

B.

Figure 8-7
Transesophageal longitudinal view from a patient with aortic valve endocarditis complicated by anterior mitral leaflet perforation. A-aortic ring abscess; AML = anterior mitral leaflet; AO = aorta; LA = left atrium; LV = left ventricle.

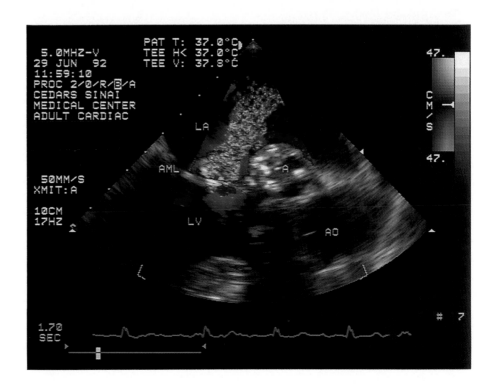

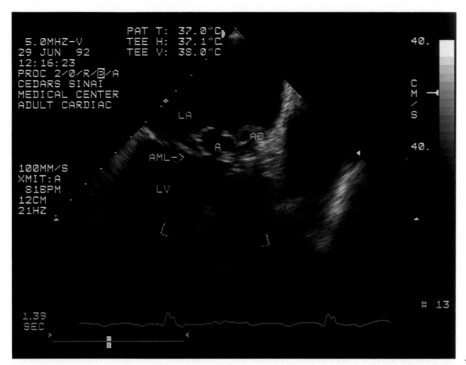

A.

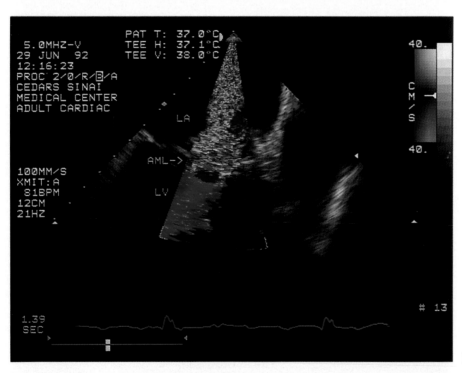

B.

Figure 8-8
Transesophageal oblique view from a patient with aortic valve endocarditis showing an aneurysm (A) of the anterior mitral leaflet that perforated (>) into the left atrium (top panel). Color Doppler imaging demonstrates the flow from the left ventricle through the aneurysm into the left atrium (bottom panel). AO = aortic ring abscess; AML = anterior mitral leaflet; LA = left atrium; LV = left ventricle.

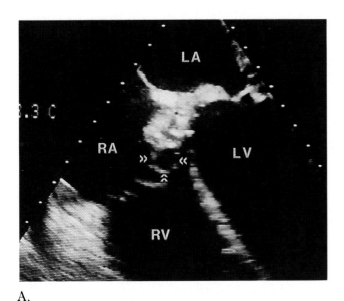

A.

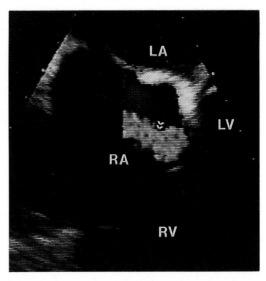

B.

Figure 8-9
Transesophageal four-chamber view from a patient with aortic valve endocarditis. The left panel shows an abscess cavity protruding into the right atrium (>>). Perforation into the left ventricular outflow tract and the right atrium created a fistulous communication between the left ventricle and the right atrium. The right panel shows the jet into the right atrium (>>). LA = left atrium; LV = left ventricle; RA = right atrium; RV = right ventricle.

of abscesses were 28.3 and 98.6 percent for transthoracic imaging but 87.0 and 94.6 percent for transesophageal echocardiography.[31] Positive and negative predictive values were 90.9 and 92.1 percent for the transesophageal approach.

Anatomical Aspects—Extension of the Inflammatory Process

Figure 8-10 schematically demonstrates locations of abscesses, pseudoaneurysms, and possibilities of fistulous communications resulting from rupture of abscesses and aneurysms. The majority of abscess formations and aneurysms have been observed in patients with aortic valve endocarditis.[31,34] In a study of 95 necropsy patients,[34] abscess formation occurred in 28 percent. In 24 of these 27 patients, the aortic valve ring was infected while mitral and tricuspid valve ring abscesses occurred in only 3 patients each. Aortic root abscess and aneurysm formation may lead to aorto–left ventricular discontinuity.[32] From the aortic annulus the infection can extend toward various cardiac structures resulting in several specific complications:

1. From the origin of the left coronary cusp and the adjacent portion of the noncoronary cusp the infection can extend to the mitral-aortic intervalvular fibrosa and to the anterior mitral leaflet[32,44] (Fig. 8-10 A–F). An aneurysm of the mitral-aortic intervalvular fibrosa may rupture into the left atrium, resulting in fistulous communication between left ventricular outflow tract and left atrium.[42,44,49] Even rupture into the pericardial space with consequent pericardial tamponade has been reported.[47] Rupture of the intervalvular fibrosa with consequent fistula between left ventricle and atrium without aneurysm formation has also been echocardiographically documented.[44,48] Extension to the anterior mitral leaflet may result in abscess formation, anterior mitral leaflet aneurysm with or without rupture, and perforation of the anterior leaflet without aneurysm formation. (Figs. 8-4, 8-5, 8-7, 8-8). Detec-

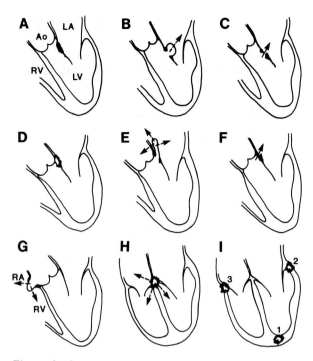

Figure 8-10

Schematic of transesophageal five- and four-chamber views showing various complications of infective endocarditis. Panels a–h: Complications of aortic valve endocarditis (dashed arrows indicate possible fistulous communications due to perforation of aneurysms and abscesses): a, anterior mitral leaflet abscess; b, anterior mitral leaflet aneurysm (→ rupture into the left atrium); c, anterior mitral leaflet perforation without aneurysm formation; d, mitral-aortic intervalvular fibrosa abscess; e, mitral-aortic intervalvular fibrosa aneurysm (→ rupture into the left atrium, the aorta, or the epicardial space); f, rupture of the mitral-aortic intervalvular fibrosa without abscess formation; g, mycotic sinus of Valsalva aneurysm (→ rupture into the right atrium or right ventricle); h, ventricular septum abscess (→ rupture into the left ventricular outflow tract, right ventricle, or right atrium may create an aneurysm and communication between left ventricular outflow tract and the right ventricle or right atrium). Panel i: 1, remote myocardial abscess; 2, mitral ring abscess, and 3, tricuspid ring abscess, rare complications of mitral and tricuspid valve endocarditis.

tion of these complications has been substantially improved by transesophageal echocardiography.[31,44,50–54] The infection may spread from the aortic valve to the mitral valve not only by direct propagation of the infection through the intervalvular fibrosa. It can also be due to secondary infection by regurgitation of blood through an infected aortic valve ("jet lesion"). These secondary mitral valve abnormalities may be overlooked during surgery and cause a complicated postoperative course.[51] This underlines the importance of preoperative evaluation by transesophageal echocardiography that may provide useful information to aid in the decision to repair or replace the mitral valve.[50] The infectious process may also reach the interatrial septum and rupture may create an interatrial fistula.[35,55]

2. From the origin of the right coronary cusp the infection may extend toward the membranous portion of the interventricular septum and farther toward the right atrium [perforation may create a fistulous communication between left ventricular outflow tract and right atrium (Fig. 8-9)], toward the right ventricle or into the muscular ventricular septum and anterobasal left ventricular wall.[3,15,31,35] Rupture of the ventricular septum may create a ventricular septal defect.

3. From the origin of the noncoronary cusp extension into the posterior ventricular septum and propagation to the right ventricular outflow tract or anterior mitral leaflet may occur. A mycotic sinus of Valsalva aneurysm[46] may be complicated by perforation into the right atrium or right ventricular outflow tract.

In prosthetic valve endocarditis, ring abscess formation commonly results in dehiscence and paravalvular regurgitation (Fig. 8-11). Isolated myocardial abscesses (not contiguous to the site of active infection) are rare but have also been documented by echocardiography.[41] They may be due to septic coronary arterial embolism.[28] Acute pericarditis has been reported in 20 percent of patients with infective endocarditis and may present with pericardial effusion. It generally results from extension of the inflammatory process into the pericardium from abscesses[28] but may also be due to a septic embolus to an extramural coronary artery.

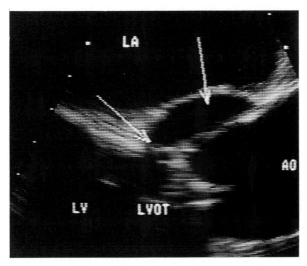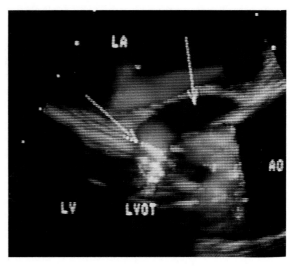

Figure 8-11

Transesophageal longitudinal view from a patient with an aortic homograft. The patient had ring abscesses before surgery. A residual cavity (upper arrow) communicates to aorta and left ventricular outflow tract (lower arrow), resulting in paravalvular aortic regurgitation.

Prognostic Implications—Impact on Surgery and Patient Outcome

Perivalvular infective endocarditis is usually associated with a higher incidence of serious complications, a more complicated surgical procedure, postoperative complications, and death.[3,15,31,56] Appropriately timed surgical treatment can improve patient outcome.[3,56] Therefore, early diagnosis is essential and can be best established by transesophageal echocardiography. The findings may be critical in making surgical decisions, both in deciding on surgery and in defining the type of surgical repair.[57]

Rohmann et al.[3] compared patients with abscess formation documented by transesophageal echocardiography (group A) with patients with proven endocarditis but no evidence of abscess (group B). Group A patients had a higher rate of embolic events (64 vs. 30 percent), need of surgery (64 vs. 19 percent), and death (50 vs. 3.7 percent). Furthermore, 68 percent of group A patients survived when treated surgically, in contrast to only 20 percent who survived undergoing medical therapy. Early abscess diagnosis and early surgery may limit the extent of surgical procedure and lower the risk.

Echocardiographic evaluation may guide the surgical approach for the repair. In case of extensive degrees of aortic–left ventricular discontinuity, for example, primary implantation of an aortic root graft with reimplantation of the coronary arteries may be necessary. In a limited series,[32] presence of an aortic–left ventricular discontinuity of more than 1 cm either anteriorly at the membranous ventricular septum or posteriorly at the intervalvular fibrosa and circumferential involvement of the aortic root by more than 90° necessitated reconstruction of the aortic root using complicated surgical procedures.

Mitral valve aneurysms or perforations associated with aortic valve endocarditis are also frequently overlooked during surgery.[51] Accurate recognition of this complication by transesophageal echocardiography may result in mitral valve repair or replacement and improves the postoperative prognosis.

References

1. Mügge A, Daniel WG, Frank G, et al: Echocardiography in infective endocarditis: Reassessment of prognostic implications of vegetation size determined by the transthoracic and the

transesophageal approach. *J Am Coll Cardiol* 14:631, 1989.

2. Shively BK, Gurule FT, Roldan CA, et al: Diagnostic value of transesophageal compared with transthoracic echocardiography in infective endocarditis. *J Am Coll Cardiol* 18:391, 1991.

3. Rohmann S, Seifert T, Erbel R, et al: Identification of abscess formation in native valve infective endocarditis using transesophageal echocardiography: Implication for surgical treatment. *Thorac Cardiovasc Surg* 39:273, 1991.

4. Jaffe WM, Morgan DE, Pearlman AS, et al: Infective endocarditis 1983–1988: Echocardiographic findings and factors influencing morbidity and mortality. *J Am Coll Cardiol* 15:1227, 1990.

5. Wann LS, Dillon JC, Weyman AE, et al: Echocardiography in bacterial endocarditis. *N Engl J Med* 295:135, 1976.

6. Hickey AJ, Wolfers J, Wilcken DEL: Reliability and clinical relevance of detection of vegetations by echocardiography in bacterial endocarditis. *Br Heart J* 46:624, 1981.

7. Sheikh MU, Covarrubias EA, Ali N, et al: M-Mode echocardiographic observations during and after healing of active bacterial endocarditis limited to the mitral valve. *Am Heart J* 101:37, 1981.

8. Sheikh MU, Covarrubias EA, Ali N, et al: M-Mode echocardiographic observations in active bacterial endocarditis limited to the aortic valve. *Am Heart J* 102:66, 1981.

9. Martin RP, Meltzer RS, Chia BL, et al: Clinical utility of two-dimensional echocardiography in infective endocarditis. *Am J Cardiol* 46:379, 1980.

10. O'Brien JT, Geiser EA: Infective endocarditis and echocardiography. *Am Heart J* 108:386, 1984.

11. Stewart JA, Silimperi D, Harris P, et al: Echocardiographic documentation of vegetative lesions in infective endocarditis: Clinical implications. *Circulation* 61:374, 1980.

12. Stafford WJ, Petch J, Radford DJ: Vegetations in infective endocarditis: Clinical relevance and diagnosis by cross sectional echocardiography. *Br Heart J* 53:310, 1985.

13. Lutas EM, Roberts RB, Devereux RB, et al: Relation between the presence of echocardiographic vegetations and the complication rate in infective endocarditis. *Am Heart J* 112:107, 1986.

14. Rubenson DS, Tucker CR, Stinson EB, et al: The use of echocardiography in diagnosing culture negative endocarditis. *Circulation* 64:641, 1981.

15. Taams MA, Gussenhoven EJ, Bos E, et al: Enhanced morphological diagnosis in infective endocarditis by transesophageal echocardiography. *Br Heart J* 63:109, 1990.

16. Erbel R, Rohmann S, Drexler M, et al: Improved diagnostic value of echocardiography in patients with infective endocarditis by transesophageal approach: A prospective study. *Eur Heart J* 9:43, 1988.

17. Pedersen WR, Walker M, Olson JD, et al: Value of transesophageal echocardiography as an adjunct to transthoracic echocardiography in evaluation of native and prosthetic valve endocarditis. *Chest* 100:351, 1991.

18. Birmingham GD, Rahko PS, Ballantyne F III: Improved detection of infective endocarditis with transesophageal echocardiography. *Am Heart J* 123:774, 1992.

19. Dillon JC, Feigenbaum H, Konecke LL, et al: Echocardiography in bacterial endocarditis. *Am Heart J* 86:698, 1973.

20. Shapiro SM, Young E, Ginzton LE, et al: Pulmonic valve endocarditis as an underdiagnosed disease: Role of transesophageal echocardiography. *J Am Soc Echocardiogr* 5:48, 1992.

21. Winslow T, Foster E, Adams JR, et al: Pulmonary valve endocarditis: Improved diagnosis with biplane transesophageal echocardiography. *J Am Soc Echocardiogr* 5:206, 1992.

22. Alam M, Rosman HS, Sun I: Transesophageal evaluation of St. Jude Medical and bioprosthetic valve endocarditis. *Am Heart J* 123:236, 1992.

23. Lowry RW, Zoghbi WA, Baker WB, et al: Clinical impact of transesophageal echocardiography in the diagnosis and management of infective endocarditis: Significance of a negative finding. *J Am Coll Cardiol* 19(suppl A):237A, 1992.

24. Diebold B, Cormier B, Roudant R, et al: Value and limitations of transesophageal echocardiography for assessing prosthesis dysfunctions: Surgical correlates in a series of 184 operated prosthetic valves. *J Am Coll Cardiol* 19(suppl A):201A, 1992.

25. Buda AJ, Zotz RJ, LeMire MS, et al: Prognostic significance of vegetations detected by two-dimensional echocardiography in infective endocarditis. *Am Heart J* 112:1291, 1986.

26. Sanfilippo AJ, Picard MH, Newell JB, et al:

Echocardiographic assessment of patients with infectious endocarditis: Prediction of risk for complications. *J Am Coll Cardiol* 18:1191, 1991.

27. Rohmann S, Erbel R, Darius H, et al: Prediction of rapid versus prolonged healing of infective endocarditis by monitoring vegetation size. *J Am Soc Echocardiogr* 4:465, 1992.

28. Buchbinder NA, Roberts WC: Left-sided valvular active endocarditis: A study of forty-five necropsy patients. *Am J Med* 53:20, 1972.

29. Miyatake K, Yamamoto K, Park YD, et al: Diagnosis of mitral valve perforation by real-time two-dimensional Doppler flow imaging technique. *J Am Coll Cardiol* 8:1235, 1986.

30. Ballal RS, Mahan EF III, Nanda NC, et al: Aortic and mitral valve perforation: Diagnosis by transesophageal echocardiography and Doppler color flow imaging. *Am Heart J* 121:241, 1991.

31. Daniel WG, Mügge A, Martin RP, et al: Improvement in the diagnosis of abscesses associated with endocarditis by transesophageal echocardiography. *N Engl J Med* 324:795, 1991.

32. Saner HE, Asinger RW, Homans DC, et al: Two-dimensional echocardiographic identification of complicated aortic root endocarditis: Implications for surgery. *J Am Coll Cardiol* 10:859, 1987.

33. Byrd BF III, Shelton ME, Wilson BH III, et al: Infective perivalvular abscess of the aortic ring: Echocardiographic features and clinical course. *Am J Cardiol* 66:102, 1990.

34. Arnett EN, Roberts WC: Valve ring abscess in infective endocarditis: Frequency, location, and clues to clinical diagnosis from the study of 95 necropsy patients. *Circulation* 54:140, 1976.

35. Arnett EN, Roberts WC: Prosthetic valve endocarditis: Clinicopathologic analysis of 22 necropsy patients with comparison of observations in 74 necropsy patients with active endocarditis involving natural left-sided cardiac valves. *Am J Cardiol* 38:281, 1976.

36. Griffiths BE, Petch MC, English TAH: Echocardiographic detection of subvalvular aortic root aneurysm extending to mitral valve annulus as complication of aortic valve endocarditis. *Br Heart J* 47:392, 1982.

37. Nakamura K, Suzuki S, Satomi G, et al: Detection of mitral ring abscess by two-dimensional echocardiography. *Circulation* 65:816, 1982.

38. Scanlan JG, Seward JB, Tajik AJ: Valve ring abscess in infective endocarditis: Visualization with wide angle two dimensional echocardiography. *Am J Cardiol* 49:1794, 1982.

39. Agatston AS, Asnani H, Ozner M, et al: Aortic valve abscess: Two-dimensional echocardiographic features leading to valve replacement. *Am Heart J* 109:171, 1985.

40. Pollak SJ, Felner JM: Echocardiographic identification of an aortic valve ring abscess. *J Am Coll Cardiol* 7:1167, 1986.

41. Zeineddin M, Stewart JA: Echocardiographic detection of non-valve-ring myocardial abscess complicating aortic valve endocarditis. *Am J Med* 85:97, 1988.

42. Fisher EA, Estioko MR, Stern EH, et al: Left ventricular to left atrial communication secondary to a paraaortic abscess: Color flow Doppler documentation. *J Am Coll Cardiol* 10:222, 1987.

43. Ellis SG, Goldstein J, Popp RL: Detection of endocarditis-associated perivalvular abscesses by two-dimensional echocardiography. *J Am Coll Cardiol* 5:647, 1985.

44. Karalis DG, Bansal RC, Hauck AJ, et al: Transesophageal echocardiographic recognition of subaortic complications in aortic valve endocarditis—Clinical and surgical implications. *Circulation* 86:353, 1992.

45. Polak PE, Gussenhoven EJ, Roelandt JRTC: Transesophageal cross-sectional echocardiographic recognition of an aortic valve ring abscess and a subannular mycotic aneurysm. *Eur Heart J* 8:664, 1987.

46. Gussenhoven EJ, van Herwerden LA, Roelandt J, et al: Detailed analysis of aortic valve endocarditis: Comparison of precordial, esophageal and epicardial two-dimensional echocardiography with surgical findings. *J Clin Ultrasound* 14:209, 1986.

47. Pirani CL: Erosive (mycotic) aneurysm of the heart with rupture. *Arch Pathol* 36:579, 1943.

48. Bansal RC, Graham BM, Jutzy KR, et al: Left ventricular outflow tract to left atrial communication secondary to rupture of mitral-aortic intervalvular fibrosa infective endocarditis: Diagnosis by transesophageal echocardiography and color flow imaging. *J Am Coll Cardiol* 15:499, 1990.

49. Giannoccaro P, Ascah JK, Sochowski RA, et al: Spontaneous drainage of paravalvular abscess diagnosed by transesophageal echocardiography. *J Am Soc Echocardiogr* 4:397, 1991.

50. Karalis DG, Chandrasekaran K, Wahl JM, et al: Transesophageal echocardiographic recog-

nition of mitral valve abnormalities associated with aortic valve endocarditis. *Am Heart J* 119:1209, 1990.

51. Reid CL, Chandraratna PAN, Harrison E, et al: Mitral valve aneurysm: Clinical features, echocardiographic-pathologic correlation. *J Am Coll Cardiol* 2:460, 1983.

52. Teskey RJ, Chan KL, Beanlands DS: Diverticulum of the mitral valve complicating bacterial endocarditis: Diagnosis by transesophageal echocardiography. *Am Heart J* 118:1083, 1989.

53. Cziner DG, Rosenzweig BP, Katz ES, et al: Transesophageal versus transthoracic echocardiography for diagnosing mitral valve perforation. *Am J Cardiol* 69:1495, 1992.

54. Nomeir AM, Downes TR, Cordell AR: Perforation of the anterior mitral leaflet caused by aortic valve endocarditis: Diagnosis by two-dimensional, transesophageal echocardiography and color flow Doppler. *J Am Soc Echocardiogr* 5:195, 1992.

55. Sheppard RC, Chandrasekaran K, Ross J, et al: An acquired interatrial fistula secondary to para-aortic abscess documented by transesophageal echocardiography. *J Am Soc Echocardiogr* 4:271, 1992.

56. Croft CH, Woodward W, Elliott A, et al: Analysis of surgical versus medical therapy in active complicated native valve infective endocarditis. *Am J Cardiol* 51:1650, 1983.

57. Shapiro SM, Bayer AS: Transesophageal and Doppler echocardiography in the diagnosis and management of infective endocarditis. *Chest* 100:1125, 1991.

9

Transesophageal Echocardiographic Imaging of Coronary Arteries

Elizabeth O. Ofili
Navin C. Nanda

Introduction

Two-dimensional echocardiography is unique among noninvasive imaging techniques in that it provides detailed endocardial visualization and assessment of the impact of coronary artery disease on segmental and global left ventricular function. However, imaging of the coronary arteries has been fraught with difficulties. In 1976, Weyman et al. described the noninvasive visualization of the left main coronary artery by transthoracic echocardiogram.[1] Despite further technologic improvements with tissue differentiation,[2] Doppler interrogation,[3,4] digital techniques,[5] and use of high-frequency annular array transducers,[6] transthoracic echocardiographic visualization of coronary arteries has met with varying degrees of success. Although visualization rates of 58 to 90 percent have been described for the left main and anterior descending coronary arteries,[2,6–9] the left circumflex and right coronary arteries are visualized in only 30 and 40 percent of cases, respectively.[7] Inconsistent specificity and predictive accuracy of transthoracic echocardiographic imaging of coronary arteries is, in part, due to an inability to detect flow and therefore reliably differentiate obstructive from normal vessels. Furthermore, excessive cardiac motion coupled with poor image resolution results in limited visualization of normal coronary arteries (diameter 2 to 4 mm); diseased coronary arteries (<1 mm diameter) are even more difficult to visualize.

Technical Considerations and Image Acquisition

Transesophageal echocardiography utilizes a high-frequency 5-MHz phased-array transducer in the esophagus; high-resolution images of the proximal coronary arteries, in addition to color flow and pulsed Doppler interrogation, can be readily performed.[10] Most current transesophageal echocardiographic probes have biplane imaging capability with the incorporation

144

of a longitudinal scanning plane in addition to the traditional transverse imaging plane. Color flow and pulsed Doppler technologies available on all transesophageal echocardiographic probes are crucial to the successful and expedient imaging of the coronary arteries.[10] Adequate sedation and additional examination time (at least 3 to 5 min) are necessary for a complete evaluation. Considerable operator experience is a prerequisite for successful and complete visualization of all four coronary arteries. Owing to cardiac motion, the coronary arteries are usually not imaged in the entire cardiac cycle. Digital image acquisition with cineloop and frame-by-frame playback may help to alleviate this problem by selecting a few frames for analysis.[11]

Coronary artery imaging is performed in the basal short-axis view of the transverse imaging plane, just above the aortic valve leaflets. Superior and leftward tilt of the probe tip from the basal short-axis view usually reveals the ostium of the left main coronary artery; minor adjustments (inferior tilt, leftward rotation) permit visualization of the entire length of the left main including its bifurcation. Further inferior tilt of the transducer reveals the left anterior descending artery, which may be followed for up to 10 to 25 mm along its course; the left circumflex is imaged as it runs leftward and posteriorly along the atrioventricular groove by leftward and superior tilt of the probe from the left main imaging plane. The right coronary ostium is located rightward and inferior to the left ostium at the basal short-axis level of the transverse scanning plane. It is usually visualized between 6 and 7 o'clock with the probe tip tilted rightward and inferiorly. The course of the right coronary artery may be immediately rightward or more downward from the ostium.[12] The longitudinal scanning plane provides cross-sectional views, thus potentially allowing a more reliable assessment of luminal narrowing, particularly of the left main coronary artery. Because of the small size of the coronary arteries and the highly reflective surrounding tissues, careful adjustment of the two-dimensional gain settings is necessary; excessive gain will destroy resolution and limit coronary artery visualization. Color flow imaging is performed with color gain optimization, keeping the Nyquist limit in the range of 0.41 to 0.72 m/s.[13] Narrow sector width ensures high frame rates. Color flow imaging frequently helps to identify and follow the course of each coronary artery. Pulsed Doppler interrogation requires careful positioning of the sample volume within the arterial lumen; the audible signals, vessel image, as well as color flow appearance are helpful in sample volume placement. Using a 2- by 2-mm sample volume and a 4- to 16-kHz pulse repetition frequency, satisfactory flow signals are obtained in the proximal left anterior descending artery of most successfully imaged subjects.[14] Pulsed Doppler interrogation of the right coronary and left circumflex artery are less successful owing to the less parallel course of these arteries with respect to the ultrasound beam.

Normal Coronary Findings

Successful coronary artery imaging comprises good visualization of the arterial wall and lumen. Both coronary ostia, the entire length of the left main to its bifurcation; 10 to 20 mm of the left anterior descending and right coronary arteries, and 10 to 34 mm of the left circumflex may be seen.[11–15] Reported visualization rates are highest for the left main (85 to 95 percent) and left circumflex (80 to 90 percent), but more variable for the right coronary (50 to 80 percent) and the left anterior descending arteries (55 to 80 percent).[11–15] Normal arteries appear echolucent without luminal irregularities or ultrasound "shadowing" from calcific plaques (Fig. 9-1). When a vessel is inadequately visualized, it may be due to an obstructive but noncalcific plaque.[12] Transesophageal echocardiographic color flow appearance of normal coronary arteries has been less well described. Normal arteries usually have a laminar flow appearance with maintenance of the width of the color flow channel along the visualized segment (Fig. 9-2A and B). Pulsed Doppler interrogation shows antegrade flow in both systole and diastole with diastolic predominance. Pulsed Doppler mapping is most

Figure 9-1
The left main coronary artery bifurcates into the circumflex and left anterior descending arteries in the short-axis view (left panel); the right panel shows the details of the circumflex artery; the arterial lumen (thin arrow) is free of obstruction, and the arterial walls (thick arrows) are free of atherosclerotic plaques. (Reproduced with permission from Ofili EO, Labovitz AJ, *J Crit Illness* 7:99, 1992.)

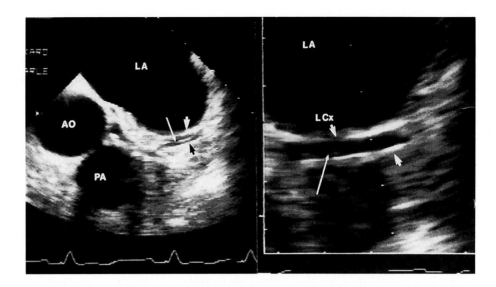

Figure 9-2
Transesophageal echocardiographic identification of proximal left-sided coronary arteries. *A.* The aortic short-axis view demonstrates the left main coronary artery (LMCA) originating from the aorta (AO) at approximately the 1 o'clock position and coursing to the left and somewhat anteriorly before its bifurcation into the left anterior descending (LAD) and left circumflex (LCX) branches. There is no evidence of lumen narrowing. *B.* Transesophageal echocardiographic identification of the proximal right coronary artery. The aortic short-axis view demonstrates the right coronary artery (RCA) originating from the aorta at about the 6 or 7 o'clock position. There is no evidence of lumen narrowing. LA = left atrium. (Reproduced with permission from Samdarshi et al, Usefulness and limitations of transesophageal echocardiography in the assessment of proximal coronary artery stenosis. *J Am Coll Cardiol* 19:572, 1992.)

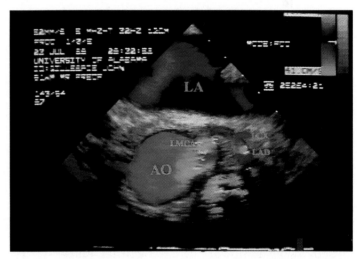

A.

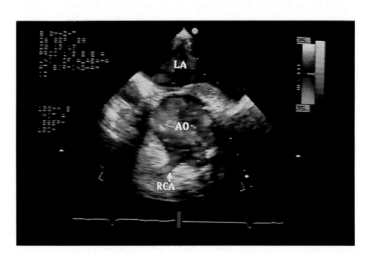

B.

readily accomplished at the distal left main bifurcation, and in the proximal left anterior descending artery.

Despite limited data on transesophageal pulsed Doppler patterns of coronary arteries, measured velocity and Doppler patterns are similar to data obtained using more invasive Doppler techniques. Yamagishi et al.[14] described baseline flow velocity in the normal left anterior descending artery of 39 patients following coronary artery bypass grafting, and found a diastolic predominant pattern with a peak diastolic velocity of 40 ± 20 cm/s. Right coronary artery flow velocity was obtained in only 26 percent of the study group but appeared to have a different pattern with less diastolic predominance. In our experience with the more invasive intracoronary Doppler spectral flow wire, we found baseline peak diastolic velocity of 49 ± 20 cm/s and 37 ± 12 cm/s for the left anterior descending and right coronary arteries, respectively;[16,17] the right coronary artery has less diastolic predominance and a significantly lower peak diastolic to peak systolic velocity ratio compared with the left anterior descending artery.

Diastolic predominance of coronary blood flow is supported by in vitro experiments that show that the higher myocardial wall tension and intramyocardial resistance cause decreased coronary flow in systole; coronary blood flow during diastole is relatively unimpeded owing to lower intramyocardial resistance.[18] Because the right ventricle has a significantly lower compressive force in systole, there is less systolic impedance of the right coronary flow, and thus less diastolic predominance.

Assessment of Coronary Artery Stenosis

Several investigators have reported on the ability of transesophageal echocardiography to correctly identify coronary obstruction, particularly of the proximal left main or ostium[13,15,19–23] (Table 9-1). Although different

criteria were used by these authors, visualization of the arterial lumen was considered adequate if linear images with a relatively echo-free space within them were seen. Stenosis has been defined as an area of apparent luminal narrowing, usually as a result of high-intensity echoes, with visualization of a normal lumen just beyond that area[8] (Figs. 9-3 and 9-4). Color flow imaging typically produces narrowing of the flow channel in addition to a mosaic flow pattern or "aliasing" at the site of stenosis or in the poststenotic segment.[13–21] This flow turbulence results in high baseline velocities by pulsed Doppler interrogation.

Samdarshi et al.[13] performed intraoperative transesophageal echocardiograms on 111 consecutive patients and compared their findings with coronary angiography. Each echocardiographically visualized coronary artery was measured as follows: the length of the left main coronary artery from its origin at the aortic root to the bifurcation; for the left anterior descending and left circumflex arteries, the maximal length was from the bifurcation to the most distal portion of the visualized segment, while the right coronary artery was measured from its origin at the aortic root to the distal portion of the visualized segment. Multiple measurements of the internal diameter of the left main and right coronary arteries were obtained, and the largest diameter of each artery determined the maximal lumen width. The stenosis area was obtained by measuring the smallest diameter and comparing it with the width of the vessel just proximal to the stenosis, expressed as a percentage. Luminal diameter reduction of ≥50 percent was considered significant. The segment of the coronary artery distal to each stenosis was identified, thus excluding the possibility of an artifactual narrowing due to angulation of the artery or cardiac motion away from the scan plane. Angiographic measurements of maximum length and width of each coronary artery were performed by digital calipers, in the projections with minimal or no foreshortening of the segment of interest. Criteria for stenoses were as defined above for echocardiography (≥50 percent reduction in luminal diameter was considered hemodynamically significant).

TABLE 9-1 Reported Studies on the Evaluation of Proximal Coronary Artery Stenosis by Transesophageal Echocardiography

First author (no. of pts.)	Coronary Artery Visualization				Stenosis				
	LM (%)	LAD (%)	LCX (%)	RCA (%)	LM ≥50%	Proximal LAD≥50%	Proximal LCX≥50%	Proximal RCA≥50%	Comments
Zwicky (50 pts.)	100	—	—	—	—	—	—	—	Awake
Yamagishi (39 pts.)	77	77	54	26	—	—	—	—	Postoperative
Pearce (138 pts.)	79	62	57	50	—	—	—	—	Intraoperative
Yoshida (67 pts.)	90	—	—	—	88%(10/12)	—	—	—	Awake
Yamagishi (52 pts.)	90	—	—	—	94%(16/17)	—	—	—	Awake
Schrem (4 pts.)	100	—	—	—	100%(4/4) (al ostial)	—	—	—	Awake
Reichert (25 pts.)	88	52	88	—	100%(4/4)	71%(5/7)	50%(2/4)	—	Postoperative
Taams (83 pts.)	95	14	68	—	65%(15/23)	—	64%(9/14)	—	Awake
Samdarshi (111 pts.)	93	93	93	49	96%(23/24)	82%(11/14)	80%(6/8)	100%(7/7)	Intraoperative

Source Adapted with permission, Samdarshi et al, *J Am Coll Cardiol* 19:572, 1992.

pts. = patients. Abbreviations as in Tables 9-2 and 9-3.

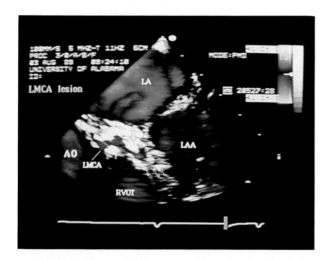

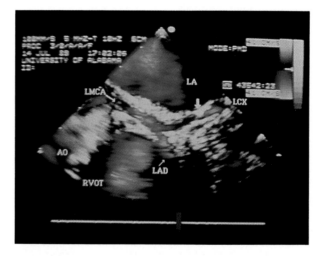

Figure 9-3

Transesophageal echocardiographic identification of left main coronary artery stenosis. The aortic (AO) short-axis view demonstrates an eccentric highly reflectile echo density (arrow), producing marked narrowing of the left main coronary artery (LMCA) lumen. LA = left atrium; LAA = left atrial appendage. (Reproduced with permission from Samdarshi et al, Usefulness and limitations of transesophageal echocardiography in the assessment of proximal coronary artery stenosis. *J Am Coll Cardiol* 19:572, 1992.)

Figure 9-4

Transesophageal echocardiographic identification of proximal left circumflex coronary artery (LCX) stenosis. The aortic (AO) short-axis view demonstrates a prominent eccentric echo density (arrow), producing marked narrowing of the left circumflex coronary artery approximately 1 cm from its origin. The left circumflex artery is identified by its posterior course in contrast to the left main coronary artery (LMCA), which courses somewhat anteriorly. The left main and proximal left anterior descending (LAD) coronary arteries do not show significant narrowing. LA = left atrium; RVOT = right ventricular outflow tract. (Reproduced with permission from Samdarshi et al, Usefulness and limitations of transesophageal echocardiography in the assessment of proximal coronary artery stenosis. *J Am Coll Cardiol* 19:572, 1992.)

TABLE 9-2   Transesophageal Two-Dimensional Echocardiography in the Assessment of Angiographically Defined Proximal Coronary Artery Stenosis, Irrespective of Whether These Coronary Segments Were Visualized by Echocardiography (Total Number of Stenoses = 75)

TEE	ANG	LMC +	LMC −	LAD +	LAD −	LCX +	LCX −	RCA +	RCA −
+		23	1	11	1	6	0	7	0
−		1	78	12	79	3	94	12	36
Sensitivity, %		96		48		67		37	
Specificity, %		99		99		100		100	

Source   Adapted with permission, Samdarshi et al, *J Am Coll Cardiol* 19:572, 1992.

ANG: angiography; LAD: left anterior descending artery; LCX: left circumflex artery; LMC: left main coronary artery; RCA: right coronary artery; TEE: transesophageal two-dimensional echocardiography; +: $\geq$ 50% stenosis; −: < 50% stenosis.

Proximal coronary artery stenosis was defined as an area of narrowing in the left main coronary artery, the proximal one-third of the right coronary artery, the proximal left anterior descending up to the first septal perforator, and the proximal circumflex up to the obtuse marginal.

Because of some variation in the echocardiographically visualized lengths of the proximal coronary arteries among study participants, data were analyzed by comparing the echocardiographically visualized arterial segment with the corresponding angiographic segment; that is, if only 1.5 cm of the left descending coronary artery was visualized by transesophageal echocardiography, the corresponding proximal 1.5 cm obtained on angiography was analyzed. Since this method assumes that the transesophageal echocardiographically visualized segments were identical to angiographic segments, comparison was also made based on the angiographic findings, regardless of whether the segments were visualized by transesophageal echocardiography. There was complete visualization of the left main in 103 of the 111 patients (93 percent); lengths varied from 0.2 to 2.2 cm. Mean lengths of the left anterior descending and left circumflex arteries visualized in these 103 patients were 0.82 ± 0.08 cm and 0.67 ± 0.09 cm, respectively. The right coronary artery was visualized in only 55 patients (49 percent). There was good correlation between transesophageal echocardiography and coronary angiography regarding assessment of the length of the left main ($r = 0.94$), width of the left main ($r = 0.87$), and width of the right coronary artery ($r = 0.77$). When the echocardiographically visualized segments were compared with the corresponding angiographic segments, a correct diagnosis of significant stenosis was made in 88 percent of the 53 lesions: 23 of the 24 (96 percent) with left main stenosis including all 7 ostial lesions (5 left ostial and 2 right ostial stenosis); 11 of the 14 (78 percent) with left anterior descending; 6 of 8 (75 percent) with left circumflex and all the right coronary lesions. There was excellent agreement between 2 independent observers regarding the presence or absence of significant stenosis. There was similar agreement between the same observers 2 months apart. When all angiographically visualized proximal lesions were included (Table 9-2), the respective diagnostic sensitivity and specificity of transesophageal echocardiography for the detection of stenosis were 96 and 99 percent for the left main, 48 and 99 percent for the left anterior descending, 67 and 100 percent for the left circumflex, 37 and 100 percent for the right coronary artery. When the analysis was based only on transesophageal echocardiographically visualized segments, sensitivity for the left anterior descending and right coronary artery were significantly en-

TABLE 9-3 Transesophageal Two-Dimensional Echocardiography in the Assessment of Proximal Coronary Artery Stenosis, Taking into Account Only the Segments Visualized by Echocardiography and Comparing Them with the Corresponding Angiographic Segments (Total Number of Stenoses = 53)

TEE	ANG	LMC +	LMC −	LAD +	LAD −	LCX +	LCX −	RCA +	RCA −
+		23	1	11	1	6	0	7	0
−		1	78	3	88	2	95	0	48
Sensitivity, %		96		79		75		100	
Specificity, %		99		99		100		100	

Source   Adapted with permission, Samdarshi et al, *J Am Coll Cardiol* 19:572, 1992.

ANG: angiography; LAD: left anterior descending artery; LCX: left circumflex artery; LMC: left main coronary artery; RCA: right coronary artery; TEE: transesophageal two-dimensional echocardiography; +: ≧ 50% stenosis; −: < 50% stenosis.

hanced to 78 and 100 percent, respectively (Table 9-3).

Mosaic signals or narrowing of the color flow channel was less useful than two-dimensional echocardiography in detecting stenosis, because flow signals were not observed in 24 percent of the visualized stenoses.[13] When present, however, the mosaic color flow feature or flow channel narrowing served to enhance the confidence with which the diagnosis of stenosis was made, particularly with ostial lesions. Color flow was highly sensitive and specific (92 and 100 percent, respectively) for the detection of left main lesions but was significantly less sensitive in the detection of stenosis in the other coronary arteries, even when only the transesophageal echocardiographically visualized segments were included in the analysis (Table 9-4). Despite the high sensitivity and specificity of transesophageal echocardiography for detection of left main stenosis in other published reports[15,19–23] (see Table 9-1), adequacy of arterial length visualization is not as well described in some of these studies. Of note is that transesophageal echocardiography was able to detect ostial stenosis involving both the left and right ostia in all 7 patients in the study (Fig. 9-5). The accuracy of transesophageal echocardiography to detect ostial lesions has also been reported by other authors[20] and could potentially contribute to the diagnostic evaluation of patients with suspected ostial lesions, in whom catheter positioning precludes accurate diagnosis at cardiac catheterization.

In a study of 55 awake patients, Yamagishi et al[19] reported that mosaic pattern on color flow helped to identify the site of significant left main stenosis. This color flow pattern was seen in 16 of the 20 patients with left main stenosis and in only 3 of 30 patients with normal arteries. Sensitivity and specificity for left main obstruction by transesophageal two-dimensional imaging were 71 and 87 percent, respectively. Adding the Doppler criteria of mosaic color flow pattern significantly enhanced the sensitivity to 94 percent with a specificity of 90 percent. Pulsed Doppler interrogation of the stenosed left main revealed a high velocity of 116 ± 28 cm/s compared with 29 ± 12 cm/s for normal arteries.

Using biplane transesophageal echocardiography, Yoshida et al.[20] described the detection rate of left main stenosis in 67 awake patients. Studies were performed in the cardiac catheterization laboratory with digital image acquisition and cineloop display format. Blood flow in the left main was detected by color Doppler in 85 percent of the study subjects. Transesophageal color Doppler had a sensitivity of 91 percent, specificity of 100 percent, positive predictive accuracy of 100 percent, and negative predictive accuracy of 98 percent for the diagnosis of ≥50 percent left main obstruction.

TABLE 9-4 Transesophageal Color Doppler Echocardiography in the Assessment of Proximal Coronary Artery Stenosis, Taking into Account Only the Segments Visualized by Two-Dimensional Echocardiography and Comparing Them with the Corresponding Angiographic Segments (Total Number of Stenoses = 53)

CD	ANG LMC +	LMC −	LAD +	LAD −	LCX +	LCX −	RCA +	RCA −
Flow channel narrowing	22	0	9	0	6	0	3	0
No flow channel narrowing	0	79	0	76	0	79	0	39
Color signals not seen	2	0	5	12	2	15	4	9
Sensitivity, %	92		64		75		43	
Specificity, %	100		86		84		81	

Source   Adapted with permission, Samdarshi et al, *J Am Coll Cardiol* 19:572, 1992.

ANG: angiography; CD: transesophageal color Doppler echocardiography; LAD: left anterior descending artery; LCX: left circumflex artery; LMC: left main coronary artery; RCA: right coronary artery; + ≧ 50% stenosis: − < 50% stenosis.

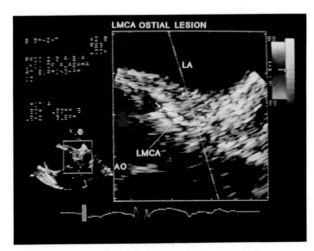

Figure 9-5
Transesophageal echocardiographic identification of left main coronary ostial stenosis. Aortic (AO) short-axis view demonstrates stenosis at the ostium of the left main coronary artery (LMCA) indicated by marked narrowing of the flow channel with widening distally. (Reproduced with permission from Samdarshi et al, Usefulness and limitations of transesophageal echocardiography in the assessment of proximal coronary artery stenosis. *J Am Coll Cardiol* 19:572, 1992.)

Limitations

1. Except for the left main coronary artery, transesophageal echocardiography does not consistently visualize long segments of the coronary arteries. Thus the sensitivity for the detection of angiographically diagnosed coronary stenosis may be quite variable. This is especially problematic in the right coronary artery where visualization rates average 50 percent.

2. Although the sensitivity for diagnosis of stenotic lesions is much higher when adequate lengths of the coronary arteries are visualized, the echocardiographic scan planes may be different from the angiographic views, resulting in discrepancies regarding the severity of stenosis, particularly in eccentric lesions. Furthermore, the small luminal diameter of the coronary arteries makes it difficult to obtain accurate measurements by echocardiography, which has limited resolution in the axial and lateral planes. Some angiographically documented lesions may be missed by transesophageal echocardiography, even when the segments are adequately imaged. This failure to detect a stenotic lesion may be related to the presence of calcific

plaques that could cause acoustic shadowing. Multiplane transesophageal echocardiography may produce a more reliable estimate of luminal narrowing; the additional scan planes may also help to avoid some of the aforementioned problems related to false-negative diagnosis by monoplane and biplane transesophageal echocardiography due to eccentric lesions and calcific plaques.

3. The presence of mosaic flow pattern or narrowed flow channel on color flow adds to the diagnostic sensitivity of transesophageal echocardiography without a significant reduction in specificity; color flow signals may, however, be absent in a significant number of visualized segments. This is, in part, related to the nonparallel orientation of the vessel in relation to the transesophageal ultrasound beam. Preliminary investigation with contrast-enhanced transesophageal color Doppler studies suggests significant improvement in the length and width of color flow channels following contrast injection with resultant improvement in diagnostic sensitivity.[24]

4. The pulsed Doppler sample volume may move in and out of the vessel lumen with cardiac motion; this coupled with respiratory variation makes it difficult to measure flow velocity throughout the cardiac cycle.

Assessment of Coronary Vasodilator Reserve

Normal coronary arteries typically respond to a potent vasodilator infusion by marked increase in flow, up to 3 to 5 times baseline flow[25,26] (Fig. 9-6). This hyperemic response or

Baseline

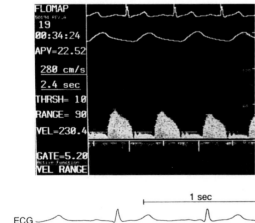

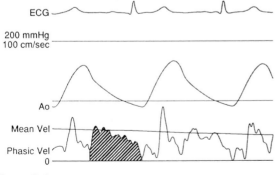

Hyperemia

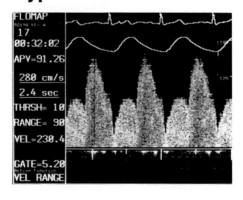

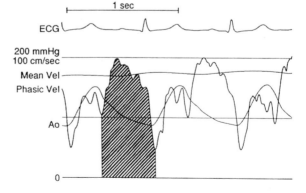

Figure 9-6
Baseline (left) and hyperemia (right) normal left main coronary flow velocity pattern using an intracoronary spectral Doppler wire (top) and zero cross Doppler catheter (bottom). (Reproduced with permission from Ofili et al, *J Am Coll Cardiol* 1993, in press.)

TABLE 9-5   Transesophageal Coronary Doppler Flow Velocity Parameters at
Baseline and During Hyperemia Induced by Dipyridamole (0.56 mg/kg)

Parameter	Group A (Normal) n = 9		Group B (LAD Stenosis ≥ 75%) n = 6	
	Baseline	Hyperemia	Baseline	Hyperemia
PDV, cm/s	35 ± 11	104 ± 21	54 ± 14	76 ± 20
MDV, cm/s	28 ± 9	79 ± 17	41 ± 9	59 ± 18
PSV, cm/s	24 ± 7	48 ± 7	29 ± 10	40 ± 19
MSV, cm/s	20 ± 6	39 ± 5	24 ± 9	33 ± 15

Source   Adapted with permission: Iliceto et al, *Circulation* 83:61, 1991.

PDV = peak diastolic velocity; MDV = mean diastolic velocity; PSV = peak systolic velocity; MSV = mean systolic
velocity; LAD = left anterior descending coronary artery.

vasodilator reserve is impaired in subjects with epicardial coronary artery disease. Furthermore, patients with systemic hypertension, diabetes mellitus, hypertrophic cardiomyopathy, and syndrome X have impaired coronary vasodilator reserve thought secondary to microvascular disease.

Previous studies of coronary vasodilator reserve assessment required cardiac catheterization with measurement of velocity in proximal coronary arteries.[25–27] The ability of transesophageal echocardiography to reliably measure coronary blood flow velocity could potentially provide a much less invasive means to study the coronary microvasculature and assess the effect of pharmacologic interventions. Only a few studies have evaluated this potential role of transesophageal echocardiography.

Iliceto et al. performed pulsed Doppler studies of the left anterior descending artery at baseline, and following coronary vasodilation with intravenous dipyridamole.[28] Twelve out of 39 subjects (31 percent) were excluded owing to technically inadequate studies; 15 patients met the study criteria, that is, technically adequate Doppler studies, angiographically normal arteries, or ≥75 percent proximal left anterior descending coronary artery stenosis without detectable collaterals. There were 9 normal and 6 significantly stenosed arteries. Doppler velocity measurements were performed at baseline and following coronary vasodilation with intravenous dipyridamole (0.56 mg/kg). Abnormal arteries showed no signifi-

cant increase in flow velocity parameters during hyperemia. Velocity parameters in normal arteries, on the other hand, increased significantly during hyperemia (Table 9-5). A problem in this study relates to the high exclusion rate due to technically inadequate echocardiograms and the overall small sample size; use of contrast enhancement may improve Doppler signal quality in future investigations.[29] Despite these limitations the impaired coronary vasodilator reserve in abnormal arteries is similar to previous reports in experimental and human studies of coronary artery disease.[25,26,30] Data from our laboratory using the intracoronary Doppler flow wire showed significant blunting of hyperemic response in abnormal arteries compared with normal arteries[30] (Fig. 9-7A). Abnormal arteries with ≥70 percent reduction in luminal diameter had lower baseline peak diastolic velocities ≥1 cm proximal to the lesion, compared with normal arteries (41 ± 26 vs. 64 ± 26 cm/s, $p < 0.003$). The higher absolute velocities obtained by transesophageal echo Doppler techniques (Fig. 9-7B) may be related to placement of the sample volume within the lesional flow turbulence, since the small segments of the visualized arteries may limit sample volume positioning. Flow reserve determination by transesophageal echocardiography is further limited to the proximal left anterior descending artery owing to the nonparallel orientation of the ultrasound beam to the other coronary arterial segments. Thus the promise of transesophageal echocardiography as a less invasive means to reliably deter-

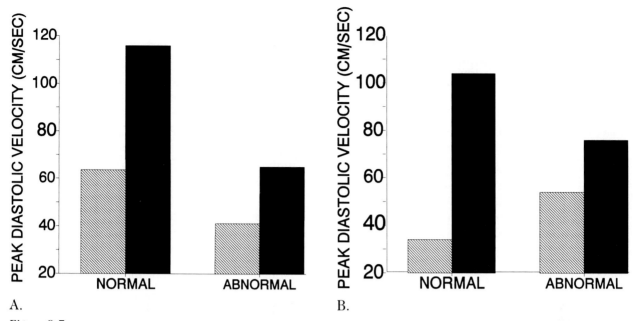

Figure 9-7
A. Peak diastolic velocity at baseline and during hyperemia in normal and abnormal (>70 percent stenosis) proximal coronary arteries using an intracoronary spectral Doppler flow wire. (Adapted with permission from Ofili et al, *J Am Coll Cardiol* 1993, in press.) *B.* Peak diastolic velocity at baseline and during hyperemia in normal and abnormal (≥75 percent stenosis) proximal coronary arteries during transesophageal echocardiographic imaging. (Adapted with permission from Iliceto et al, *Circulation* 83:61, 1991.)

mine coronary flow reserve in coronary arteries other than the proximal left anterior descending artery must await further technologic advances such as rotating or multiplane transducers and pulsed Doppler sample volume tracking devices, in addition to Doppler signal enhancement by contrast injections.

Assessment of Congenital Coronary Artery Anomalies

Anomalous Origin
Anomalous origins of coronary arteries are found in 0.3 to 1 percent of patients undergoing coronary angiography.[31] Clinical recognition is important because of associated risk of myocardial ischemia, infarction, syncope, and sudden cardiac death. In the past, coronary angiography has usually been necessary for diagnostic confirmation in almost all cases. Coronary anomalies presenting the greatest risk to adults

are origin of the left main coronary artery from the right coronary sinus and origin of the right coronary artery from the left coronary sinus when the anomalous vessel passes between the aorta and the pulmonary trunk. Origin of the left main from the right coronary sinus represents the most common anomaly associated with sudden cardiac death in young adults.[32] Acute takeoff of these vessels with a resultant slitlike opening in addition to compression of the coronary artery between the great vessels may result in myocardial ischemia.[33,34] Patients may present with angina (42 percent), atypical chest pain (29 percent), syncope (18 percent), and palpitations (42 percent); there is a high incidence of associated systemic hypertension (40 percent) and valvular heart disease (31 percent) in one of the reported series.[35] Failure to identify an anomalous coronary artery preoperatively in patients undergoing open heart procedures may result in failure to perfuse the aberrant artery during surgery, with subsequent myocardial necrosis.[35] Limited resolution of transthoracic echocardiography significantly hampers its usefulness in the detection of coronary artery anomalies.

Gaither et al.[36] described five patients with anomalous coronary arteries documented by coronary angiography. Anomalous coronary ostia were visualized by transesophageal echocardiography in all five but in none of the four who underwent transthoracic studies. A proximal segment of the anomalous artery was identified in all five patients by transesophageal approach but in only two of the four by transthoracic echocardiography. Transesophageal echocardiographic images were of superior diagnostic quality; however, the acute takeoff of the tortuously coursing arteries meant that only short segments could be visualized at any one time. Included in the series were two anomalous left circumflex arteries originating from the right sinus of Valsalva, one anomalous right coronary artery originating from the left sinus of Valsalva, one anomalous left main from the right sinus of Valsalva, and one anomalous right coronary artery from the pulmonary trunk. Several other case reports in the literature describe transesophageal echocardiographic identification of anomalous origin of the left circumflex artery from the right sinus of Valsalva[37] and directly from the left coronary sinus,[38] and anomalous origin of the right coronary artery from the left sinus of Valsalva[39,40] (Figs. 9-8 and 9-9). Meticulous operator technique, careful identification of the coronary ostia, and color flow tracking of the anomalous artery helped to confirm the diagnosis in these cases.

Fistulous Communications

Coronary fistulas involve the right coronary artery in 50 to 55 percent of patients, the left coronary artery in 35 percent, and both arteries in 5 percent of cases. Communication is usually to the low-pressure right-sided chambers: the right ventricle (40 percent), right atrium (25 percent), pulmonary artery (20 percent), coronary sinus (7 percent), and superior vena cava (1 percent).[41] Most patients are asymptomatic. Angina and myocardial infarction may result from a "steal phenomenon." The extent of coronary artery dilatation depends on the

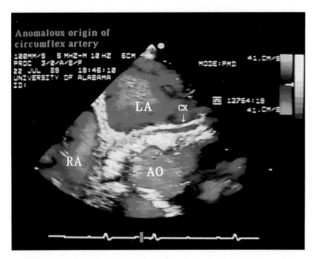

Figure 9-8
Anomalous origin of the left circumflex coronary artery from the right sinus of Valsalva. Transesophageal color Doppler examination. Oblique aortic short-axis view demonstrates the right-sided origin of the anomalous vessel (CX), which then angles sharply posteriorly and subsequently takes on a leftward course between the aorta (AO) and the left atrium (LA). Note the presence of color flow signals within the vessel lumen. RA = right atrium. (Reproduced with permission from Samdarshi et al, *Am Heart J* 122:571, 1991.)

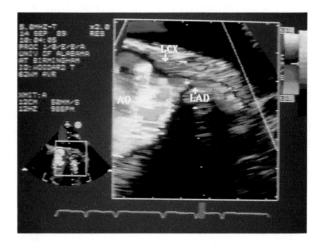

Figure 9-9
Transesophageal color Doppler echocardiogram. Aortic short-axis view. Both the left circumflex (LCX) and left anterior descending (LAD) coronary arteries arise from adjacent but separate orifices. AO = aorta. (Reproduced with permission from Boogaerts et al, Anomalous separate origin of left circumflex coronary artery from a separate ostium in the left coronary sinus: Identification by transesophageal color Doppler echocardiography, *Echocardiography* 7:165, 1990.)

shunt fraction. Congestive heart failure may be present in up to 53 percent of patients with fistulous communication to the coronary sinus or right atrium. Although transthoracic echocardiography has been useful in the detection of coronary fistulas, the distal fistulous communications are usually not identified.[42] Also, the exact site of communication may not be apparent by transthoracic echocardiography and occasionally even by angiography. On the other hand, using transesophageal echocardiography, Samdarshi et al. identified the communication between a coronary artery and the coronary sinus near its entrance into the right atrium in two patients and between the coronary artery and the coronary sinus near the left atrial appendage in one patient[43] (Fig. 9-10). Similar case reports have been presented by other investigators.[44,45]

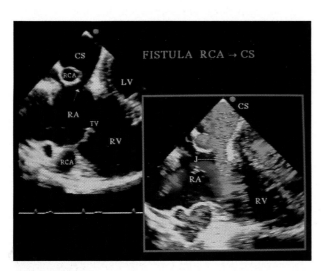

Figure 9-10
Transesophageal color Doppler echocardiogram in right coronary artery to coronary sinus fistula. The right ventricular inflow view demonstrates several large, bounded echo-free spaces containing mosaic-colored signals indicating turbulent blood flow. These structures represent segments of the enlarged and tortuous right coronary artery (RCA). Mosaic flow signals from one of these structures are seen moving through an area of discontinuity into the grossly enlarged adjacent coronary sinus, near its entrance into the right atrium (RA). CS = coronary sinus; LV = left ventricle; RV = right ventricle; TV = tricuspid valve. (Reproduced with permission from Samdarshi et al, Transesophageal echocardiographic assessment of congenital coronary artery to coronary sinus fistulas in adults, *Am J Cardiol* 68:263, 1991.)

Thus transesophageal echocardiography may have a useful role to play in the evaluation of these entities, especially since the surgeon needs delineation of the exact site of communication, which can then be ligated.

Conclusion and Future Directions

Transesophageal echocardiography has provided significant improvement in our ability to visualize the coronary arteries. Variable visualization rates of arterial segments other than the left main and acoustic shadowing from calcific plaques are some factors that limit diagnostic sensitivity in patients with significant stenosis. Future advances in transducer technology including multiplane systems may enhance visualization rates of stenotic lesions. Furthermore, techniques such as contrast echocardiography may improve diagnostic sensitivity by enhancing color flow signals. The addition of flow reserve determination helps to differentiate normal from abnormal vessels. Further investigation is necessary in order to establish the diagnostic role of transesophageal echocardiography relative to more traditional tools for detection of coronary artery disease and the assessment of myocardial ischemia, such as coronary angiography and thallium myocardial perfusion imaging.

References

1. Weyman AE, Feigenbaum H, Dillon JC, et al: Non-invasive visualization of the left main coronary artery by cross-sectional echocardiography. *Circulation* 54:169, 1976.
2. Rogers EW, Feigenbaum H, Weyman AE, et al: Possible detection of atherosclerotic coronary calcification by two-dimensional echocardiography. *Circulation* 62:1046, 1980.
3. Nanda NC, Hodsden J, Santelli S: Pulse Doppler echocardiography of coronary arteries: Methodology and clinical usefulness. *Am J Cardiol* 49:932, 1982.
4. Nanda NC, Saini VD, Maulik D: Characterization of coronary blood flow obtained by pulse

Doppler echocardiography using off-line computer analysis. *Clin Res* 31:208A, 1983.

5. Presti CF, Feigenbaum H, Armstrong WF, et al: Digital two-dimensional echocardiographic imaging of the proximal left anterior descending coronary artery. *Am J Cardiol* 60:1254, 1987.

6. Ross JJ Jr, Mintz GS, Chandrasekaran K: Transthoracic two-dimensional high frequency (7.5 MHz) ultrasonic visualization of the distal left anterior descending coronary artery. *J Am Coll Cardiol* 15:373, 1990.

7. Douglas PS, Fiolkoski J, Berko B, et al: Echocardiographic visualization of coronary artery anatomy in the adult. *J Am Coll Cardiol* 11:565, 1988.

8. Block PJ, Popp RL: Detecting and excluding significant left main coronary artery narrowing by echocardiography. *Am J Cardiol* 55:937, 1985.

9. Ryan T, Armstrong WF, Feigenbaum H: Prospective evaluation of the left main coronary artery using digital two-dimension echocardiography. *J Am Coll Cardiol* 807, 1986.

10. Ofili EO, Labovitz AJ: The technique of transesophageal echocardiography. *J Critical Illness* 7:99, 1992.

11. Iliceto S, Memmola C, De Martico G, et al: in Illiceto S et al (eds): Evaluation of proximal left coronary artery anatomy and blood flow using digital transesophageal echocardiography ultrasound in coronary artery disease. Netherlands, Kluwer Academic Publishers, 1991, p 269.

12. Pearce FB, Sheikh KH, de Bruijn NP, et al: Imaging of the coronary arteries by transesophageal echocardiography. *J Am Soc Echocardiogr* 2:276, 1989.

13. Samdarshi TE, Nanda NC, Gatewood RP, et al: Usefulness and limitations of transesophageal echocardiography in the assessment of proximal coronary artery stenosis. *J Am Coll Cardiol* 19:572, 1992.

14. Yamagishi M, Miyatke K, Beppu S, et al: Assessment of coronary blood flow by transesophageal two-dimensional pulsed Doppler echocardiography. *Am J Cardiol* 15:641, 1988.

15. Reichert SLA, Visser CA, Koolen JJ, et al: Transesophageal examination of the left coronary artery with a 7.5 MHz annular array two-dimensional color flow Doppler transducer. *J Am Soc Echocardiogr* 3:118, 1990.

16. Ofili EO, St Vrain JA, Labovitz AJ, et al: Doppler flow dynamics in angiographically normal proximal and distal coronary arteries. *Eur J Cardiol* 13:272, 1992.

17. Ofili EO, Labovitz AJ: Coronary flow velocity dynamic in normal and diseased arteries. *Am J Cardiol* 71:1D, 1993.

18. Braunwald E, Ross J, Sonnenblick EH: *Regulation of Coronary Blood Flow in Mechanisms of Contraction of Normal and Failing Heart.* 2d ed. Boston, Little, Brown 1976, p 200.

19. Yamagishi M, Yasu T, Ohara K, et al: Detection of coronary blood flow associated with left main coronary artery stenosis by transesophageal Doppler color flow echocardiography. *J Am Coll Cardiol* 17:87, 1991.

20. Yoshida K, Yoshikawa J, Hozvmi T, et al: Detection of left main coronary artery stenosis by transesophageal color Doppler and two-dimensional echocardiography. *Circulation* 81:1271, 1990.

21. Zwicky P, Daniel WG, Mügge A, et al: Imaging of coronary arteries by color coded transesophageal Doppler echocardiography. *Am J Cardiol* 62:639, 1988.

22. Schrem SS, Tunick PA, Slater J, et al: Transesophageal echocardiography in the diagnosis of ostial left coronary artery stenosis. *J Am Soc Echocardiogr* 3:367, 1990.

23. Taams MA, Gussenhoven EJ, Cornel JH, et al: Detection of left coronary artery stenosis by transesophageal echocardiography. *Eur Heart J* 9:1162, 1988.

24. Aggarwal KK, Gatewood R, Nanda NC, et al: Improved transesophageal echocardiographic assessment of proximal coronary artery stenosis using echo contrast enhancement (abstract). *J Am Coll Cardiol* 21:448A, 1993.

25. Wilson RF, White CW: Intracoronary papaverine: An ideal coronary vasodilator for studies of the coronary circulation in conscious humans. *Circulation* 73:444, 1986.

26. Marcus ML, White CW: Coronary flow reserve in patients with normal coronary angiograms. *J Am Coll Cardiol* 6:1254, 1985.

27. Kern MJ: A simplified method to measure coronary blood flow velocity in patients: Validation and application of a Judkins-style Doppler tipped angiographic catheter. *Am Heart J* 120:1202, 1990.

28. Iliceto S, Marangelli V, Memmola C, et al: Transesophageal Doppler echocardiography evaluation of coronary blood flow velocity in

baseline conditions and during dipyridamole induced coronary vasodilation. *Circulation* 83:61, 1991.

29. Iliceto S, Caiatic, Schlief R, et al: Enhanced Doppler signal intensity in coronary artery after intravenous injection of a lung crossing echo contrast agent (SHU 508A). *J Am Coll Cardiol* 19:3, 1992.

30. Ofili EO, Kern MJ, Labovitz AJ: Analysis of coronary blood flow velocity dynamics in angiographically normal and stenosed arteries before and after endoluminal enlargement by angioplasty. *J Am Coll Cardiol* 21:308, 1993.

31. Baltaxe HA, Wixson D: The incidence of congenital anomalies of the coronary arteries in the adult population. *Radiology* 122:47, 1977.

32. Maron BJ, Epstein SE, Roberts WC: Causes of sudden death in competitive athletes. *J Am Coll Cardiol* 7:204, 1986.

33. Cheitlin MD, DeCastro CM, McAllister HA: Sudden death as a complication of anomalous left coronary origin from the anterior sinus of Valsalva: A not-so-minor congenital anomaly. *Circulation* 50:780, 1974.

34. Kimbris D, Iskandrian AS, Segal BL, et al: Anomalous aortic origin of coronary arteries. *Circulation* 58:606, 1978.

35. Click RL, Holmes DR, Vliestra RE, et al: Anomalous coronary arteries: Location, degree of atherosclerosis and effect on survival— A report from the coronary artery surgery study. *J Am Coll Cardiol* 13:531, 1989.

36. Gaither NS, Rogan KM, Stajduhar K, et al: Anomalous origin and course of coronary arteries in adults: Identification and improved imaging utilizing transesophageal echocardiography. *Am Heart J* 122:69, 1991.

37. Samdarshi TE, Hill DL, Nanda NC: Transesophageal color Doppler diagnosis of anomalous origin of left circumflex coronary artery. *Am Heart J* 122:571, 1991.

38. Boogaerts J, Samdarshi TE, Nanda NC, et al: Anomalous separate origin of left circumflex coronary artery from a separate ostium in the left coronary sinus: Identification by transesophageal color Doppler echocardiography. *Echocardiography* 7:165, 1990.

39. Koh KK, Kyonggi-do: Confirmation of anomalous origin of the right coronary artery from the left sinus of Valsalva by means of transesophageal echocardiography. *Am Heart J* 122:851, 1991.

40. Smolin MR, Gorman PD, Gaither NS, et al: Origin of the right coronary artery from the left main coronary artery identified by transesophageal echocardiography. *Am Heart J* 123:1062, 1992.

41. Liberthson RR, Sagar K, Berkoben JP, et al: Congenital coronary arteriovenous fistula. *Circulation* 59:849, 1979.

42. Velvis H, Schmidt KG, Silverman NH, et al: Diagnosis of coronary artery fistula by two-dimensional echocardiogram, pulsed Doppler ultrasound and color flow imaging. *J Am Coll Cardiol* 14:968, 1989.

43. Samdarshi TE, Mahan EF, Nanda NC, et al: Transesophageal echocardiographic assessment of congenital coronary sinus fistulas in adults. *J Cardiol* 68:263, 1991.

44. Sunaga Y, Taniichi Y, Okubo N, et al: Biplane transesophageal echocardiographic study of left coronary artery to right atrium fistula. *Am Heart J* 123:1058, 1992.

45. Kuo CT, Chiang CW, Fang BR, et al: Coronary artery fistula: Diagnosis by transesophageal two-dimensional and Doppler echocardiography. *Am Heart J* 123:218, 1992.

10

The Application of Transesophageal Echocardiography in the Adult with Congenital Heart Disease

John S. Child
Ariane J. Marelli

Introduction

The last three decades have witnessed an exponential growth in the diagnostic, surgical, and medical management of infants and children with congenital heart disease. Congenital heart disease now must be considered not only in terms of the age of onset but also in terms of the age range that survival currently permits. Each year, about 20,000 open operations for congenital heart disease (an approximate minimum) are performed in the United States.[1-3] Of an estimated 25,000 infants currently born with congenital malformations of the heart and circulation, over 85 percent will reach adulthood. In the United States alone, there are presently approximately 600,000 adults with congenital heart disease.[1-3]

The UCLA Adult Congenital Heart Disease program currently has a registry of over 700 patients, of whom two-thirds have had surgical palliation or repair. The underlying congenitally malformed heart together with its pulmo-nary circulation and systemic venous and arterial circulations coexist with postoperative residua and sequelae. It is the nature of this interaction that determines the anatomic and hemodynamic issues anticipated with diagnostic imaging techniques. Advances in refined noninvasive cardiovascular imaging and hemodynamic assessment have revolutionized the management of congenital heart disease.[4] Precise delineation of intracardiac anatomy and hemodynamics has been made possible by the combination of high-quality two-dimensional echocardiography (2DE) and color flow imaging with pulsed and continuous-wave Doppler.[4] Cardiac catheterization has assumed a more focused complementary diagnostic and therapeutic role.

In this chapter, we focus on the application, contributions, and limitations of single-plane and biplane transesophageal echocardiography (TEE) in adults with congenital heart disease. This is considered in three phases: first, in general terms, technical and analytical considerations particular to the congenital patient are highlighted; second, the role of TEE in diagnosis in the in- or outpatient, and in monitoring the patient intraoperatively and during interventional catheterization, is outlined; and, third, segmental anatomic assessment in the context of simple and complex unoperated and operated anatomy is described.

The Esophageal View

The UCLA Adult Echocardiographic Imaging and Hemodynamics Laboratories perform approximately 7000 echocardiograms each year with 3 percent of noncongenital heart disease patients versus 18 percent of adults with congenital heart disease requiring TEE.[6] These proportions are similar to other laboratories who follow adolescents and adults with congenital heart defects and reflects the value of detailed anatomic imaging available by TEE.[5] The indications for transesophageal echocardiographic imaging include diagnosis of anatomy and function in the unoperated patient, intraoperative evaluation and monitoring during surgery for congenital heart disease and in the follow-up of the operated patient, and as an adjunct to therapeutic catheter intervention for congenital lesions (Table 10-1).[5-20]

Preparation of the Adult Congenital Patient

The protocol used for the adult congenital patient undergoing a transesophageal examination is similar to that used for other cardiac patients with some added precautionary measures.[6] We do not recommend antibiotic prophylaxis except for patients with prosthetic valves or a history of infective endocarditis.[3,6,13] Automated blood pressure and pulse oximetry are monitored, particularly in cyanotic patients in whom a decrease in systemic vascular resistance in response to intravenous sedatives can cause an increase in right-to-left shunting and a decrease in systemic oxygen saturation. After local oropharyngeal anesthesia with viscous xylocaine, we administer intravenous midazolam in 0.5- to 1-mg increments. The average

young adult usually requires between 3 and 8 mg to achieve comfortable, moderate sedation. The rate of intravenous delivery of sedatives must be slower in patients with right-to-left shunts because rapid delivery results in prompt appearance of high concentrations in the systemic arterial and therefore cerebral circulation. Respiratory arrest can ensue. In addition, macrobubbles should be eliminated to avoid the risk of paradoxical emboli to the central nervous system in the presence of right-to-left intracardiac shunting. Because anticholinergic agents may cause deleterious effects on heart rate, secretions are managed with mechanical suction.

Data Acquisition and Analysis

The principle of segmental analysis of anatomy underlies the echocardiographic examination of congenital heart disease in patients of all ages, regardless of whether the examination is performed from a transthoracic or a transesophageal window.[4,13] Using the segmental approach, visceral situs, systemic and pulmonary venous return, atrial situs and anatomy, atrioventricular concordance, ventricular morphology and septal anatomy, ventriculoarterial concordance, and aortic and pulmonary anatomy at each level are sought during echocardiographic examination.[6,13] To maximize the gain from the transesophageal study, previous transthoracic studies, as well as other noninvasive and invasive examinations yielding anatomic and hemodynamic information, should be reviewed. At times, limitations, particularly of the transverse plane, may preclude documentation of hemodynamic gradients because of poor alignment. Accordingly, information obtained from the TEE may require completion of spectral Doppler assessment with a transthoracic examination.

What follows is a description of the biplane transesophageal study as we perform it, enabling us to assess most of the segmental information required.[6] Though the examination must, of necessity, be goal-oriented, a complete anatomic and hemodynamic assessment is important provided the patient can tolerate such a complete procedure. To achieve these goals efficiently and accurately, the ex-

TABLE 10-1   Adult Congenital Heart Disease: Indications for TEE

Inpatient or outpatient diagnosis:
  Atrial situs and anatomy
  Anomalies of systemic and pulmonary veins
  ASD size and location, particularly venosus septal defects
  Atrial baffle complications
  Suspected obstruction of Fontan anastomosis
  Assessment of Glenn shunt, pulmonary arteriovenous fistula
  Abnormalities of atrioventricular junction
  Candidacy for surgical atrioventricular valvuloplasty
  Ventricular anatomy (including VSDs) and function
  Anatomy of right and left ventricular outflow tracts
  Assessment of intra- and extra-cardiac conduits
  Suspected prosthetic valvular function
  Coronary artery anomalies
  Aortic pathology (including aortic coarctation)
  Systemic arterial-to-pulmonary shunts
Intraoperative monitoring and assessment:
  Refine anatomic definition of cardiac malformation
  Detect unsuspected details
  Evaluate adequacy of repair
  Establish presence and degree of postoperative residua and sequelae
Facilitate interventional cardiac catheterization:
  Aortic valvuloplasty
  Pulmonary valvuloplasty
  Aortic coarctation balloon dilatation
  Dilatation of atrial baffle obstruction
  Device closure of intracardiac shunts
  Direct catheter puncture of atrial septum
  Guide radiofrequency ablation of arrhythmogenic focus, AV node

Source   Used by permission and modified from Marelli AJ et al, *Cardiol Clin*, in press.[6]

aminer must be thoroughly versed in the spectrum of anatomic variations for each lesion, simple or complex, operated or unoperated.[6] Our on-screen orientation of the image is as described by Nanda and colleagues, although other recommendations for image visualization are equally helpful.[21–25] After intubation of the esophagus, echocardiographic imaging, color flow imaging, and spectral Doppler are usually obtained in sequence. The basal horizontal (transverse) and vertical (longitudinal) views are used to determine atrial situs, systemic and pulmonary venous connections and atrial septal anatomy, ventricular outflow anatomy, the aortic valvular apparatus, and origins of the coronary arteries.[6,13,21–23] The probe is then advanced to the horizontal plane "four-chamber view" (not all patients have four chambers!) to determine crux anatomy, atrio-ventricular connections and function of the atrioventricular valvular apparatus, chordal attachments, ventricular septal anatomy, and ventricular morphology and function. In the horizontal plane, an anterior pulmonary artery and its bifurcation can be visualized by withdrawing the transducer and tilting superiorly, thereby establishing the great arterial positional relationships. The vertical plane is then used to reexamine atrioventricular valvular function and anatomy, ventricular function, the subarterial and membranous ventricular septum, relationships between ventricular inflow and outflow, the subvalvular areas of both great arteries, as well as conotruncal connections and the alignment of the great arteries relative to one another. Subsequently, transgastric horizontal and vertical views assess systemic venous connections and flow

TABLE 10-2   Biplane TEE in Adult Congenital Heart Disease

Imaging Plane	Native and Surgical Anatomy
Horizontal > vertical	Anomalous pulmonary venous connection
	Cor triatriatum
	Fontan RA-RV connection
	Fontan adjustable ASD
	Tricuspid and mitral atresia
	Cardiac crux anatomy
	Cushion (inlet) ASD or VSD
	Coronary anomalies
	Branch pulmonary arteries
	Great arterial positional relationships
Vertical > horizontal	Anomalous systemic venous connections
	Atrial situs
	Atrial septal defects
	Patent foramen ovale
	Atrial baffle anatomy (Mustard, Senning)
	Fontan RA-PA anastomosis
	Anomalous chordal insertions
	Outlet and membranous ventricular septum
	Left ventricular outflow and ascending aorta
	Complex right ventricular outflow lesions
	Ventriculoarterial alignment
	Aortic coarctation
	Glenn and Blalock-Taussig shunts

Source   Used by permission and modified from Marelli AJ et al, *Cardiol Clin*, in press.[6]

Key: ASD = atrial septal defect; RA-PA = right atrial–pulmonary artery; RA-RV = right atrial–right ventricle; VSD = ventricular septal defect.

patterns, ventricular morphology and function, and anatomy of the atrioventricular valves (with subvalvar apparatus, including chordal attachments and location of papillary muscles). The probe is then rotated to examine the descending thoracic aorta, then withdrawn to the isthmic level where it is examined in both horizontal and vertical planes for narrowing. The probe is further withdrawn and rotated to examine the dimensions of the arch, the ascending aorta, the right and left pulmonary artery, and any central systemic arterial shunts and systemic venous shunts. The origins of the carotid and subclavian vessels are assessed.

Advantages and Limitations of the Technique

Single-plane TEE adds important additional information with respect to systemic and pulmonary venous connections, atrial situs, atrial baffle integrity, atrioventricular anatomy and

function, left ventricular outflow tract lesions, central pulmonary arteries, and the Fontan circulation compared with standard transthoracic echocardiography.[5,6,14,19,26–28] The horizontal TEE plane is limited in the 2DE imaging and hemodynamic assessment of the more anterior cardiac structures such as an anterior right ventricular outflow tract, anterior sites of Fontan anastomosis, and the anteroapical septum.[5,6,14,19] The number of studies where additional information is gained from TEE depends closely on the available transthoracic window. Although in infants and children, in whom acoustic windows are more uniformly excellent than in adults, much information can be obtained by transthorac imaging; the gain can be as high as 55 percent in adolescents and adults.[5] In children and adolescents the combined use of the vertical and horizontal plane can provide additional diagnostic information in 75 percent of cases studied perioperatively.[29] Similar advantages of the vertical plane have been reported in adult acquired and congenital cardiac disease.[5,6,30,31] In the application of biplane TEE, the two planes are a continuum by virtue of skilled manipulation of the tip of the probe laterally and medially with simultaneous flexion or extension, rotation, and withdrawal or insertion. As such, the two planes are complementary, and both are desirable for complete assessment of congenital cardiac malformations. The vertical plane is generally superior to the horizontal plane examination for complex anomalies of the right ventricular outflow tract, origin and alignment of malposed great arteries, aortic coarctation, and assessment of atrial septal anatomy.[6] Table 10-2 summarizes our experience, highlighting the anatomy for which we generally find the horizontal plane to be more effective than the vertical plane (horizontal > vertical) and the vertical plane to be more effective than the horizontal plane (vertical > horizontal).

Intraoperative Transesophageal Echocardiography

TEE during congenital heart surgery is being increasingly used in the operating theater before cardiopulmonary bypass to refine anatomic diagnosis and detect previously unsuspected lesions (each of which may require modification of the operative approach) and, after going off cardiopulmonary bypass but prior to chest closure, to evaluate adequacy of repair and direct additional repair when the initial attempt is unsatisfactory, and finally to document surgical residua and sequelae (Table 10-3). Perioperative TEE has been found useful in anatomic diagnosis, in detection of wall motion abnormalities, and in intraoperative and perioperative management.[6–8,15,17,19,20,29,32–34] In the largest of these series,[29] 31 percent of the studies performed preoperatively provided diagnostic enhancement compared with the preoperative transthoracic echocardiogram, 10 percent of the studies performed after cardiopulmonary bypass revealed important hemodynamic or anatomic sequelae, and 15 percent of studies performed in the intensive care unit early postoperatively revealed findings relevant to the patient's management. As such, otherwise undiagnosed

TABLE 10-3   Objectives of Intraoperative TEE

Define cardiac malformation:
    Refine assessment of known lesions
    Detect unsuspected lesions
    Revise operative plan
Evaluate adequacy of repair:
    Examine surgical result in evolution
    Assist in surgical revision of unsatisfactory results
Establish postoperative residua and sequelae:
    Valvular regurgitation
    Residual atrial or ventricular septal shunts
    Prosthetic conduit obstruction
    Outflow tract obstruction or aneurysm
    Myocardial function

Source   Used by permission and modified from Marelli AJ et al, *Cardiol Clin*, in press.[6]

information was provided by TEE in 56 percent of the patients reported.[29] These observations are consistent with our data in adults with congenital heart disease undergoing surgical repair where the intraoperative TEE made a unique contribution to preoperative anatomy, intraoperative management, or postoperative residua in 50 percent of patients who had the procedure (Figs. 10-1, 10-2).[6] In addition, TEE can be of therapeutic assistance by directing a blade or balloon septostomy in the operating room or intensive care unit (Fig. 10-3).[6,12]

Echocardiography and Interventional Catheterization

The combination of invasive and noninvasive imaging procedures allows creative therapeutics. An example is the landmark balloon atrial septostomy of the newborn with transposition of the great arteries, first described by Rashkind in the setting of the catheterization laboratory[35] and now performed at the bedside under echocardiographic imaging.[36] The growing use of the cardiac catheterization laboratory as a site for percutaneous catheter intervention in congenital heart disease has given TEE a unique opportunity to complement classic fluoroscopic imaging. The usefulness of TEE in this regard is twofold: (1) to assist catheter and device manipulation and (2) to provide ongoing assessment of procedural residua, sequelae, and complications. TEE has been used

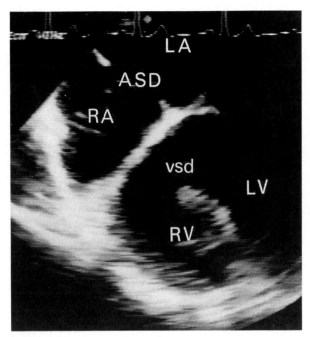

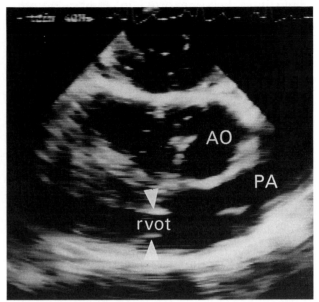

A.   B.

Figure 10-1
Intraoperative transesophageal echocardiogram (TEE) in a 35-year-old man with tricuspid atresia selected to undergo a Fontan procedure. *A.* Horizontal-plane TEE shows the band of tissue of the atretic tricuspid valve between the right atrium (RA) and right ventricle (RV). The large secundum atrial septal defect (ASD) allowed flow from RA into the left atrium (LA), left ventricle (LV), and then into the RV via a large ventricular septal defect (vsd). *B.* Preoperative angiograms and transthoracic echocardiograms suggested that his pulmonic stenosis was at the pulmonary valve level. This vertical-plane TEE view clearly demonstrated that there was a discrete subvalvar fibrous collar. This modified the surgical approach for the relief of the pulmonic stenosis. AO = aorta; PA = pulmonary artery; RVOT = right ventricular outflow tract.

effectively during pulmonary and aortic valvuloplasty, aortic coarctation dilatation, dilatation of atrial baffle obstruction, and device closure of patent ductus arteriosus and atrial septal defects.[7,11,12,16,37] The most important contributions of the TEE examination were in monitoring catheter and device position, in affording direct visualization of atrial septal tissue, in ongoing evaluation of aortic valvuloplasty, and in assessing postcoarctoplasty complications. Immediately following aortic coarctation dilatation, TEE appears to be more sensitive than angiography in detecting intimal flaps; at six months after the procedure, TEE seems more accurate in visualizing iatrogenic aortic dissection, undiagnosed with computed tomographic scanning.[37] Limitations of horizontal-plane TEE imaging that at times preclude adequate assessment of the right ventricular outflow tract, precise anatomy of the

aortic isthmus, and ductus arteriosus are overcome with the use of biplane TEE.[6,19]

Segmental Anatomic Examination

Examination at the Atrial Level

Systemic and Pulmonary Venous Connections and Flow Patterns
In the horizontal plane, at the base of the heart, a normal right-sided superior vena cava (RSVC) can be seen at several tomographic levels as it enters the right atrium. Anteflexion at the level of the lower pulmonary veins will display the RSVC entering the right atrium between the right upper pulmonary vein and the right atrial appendage. Using this plane,

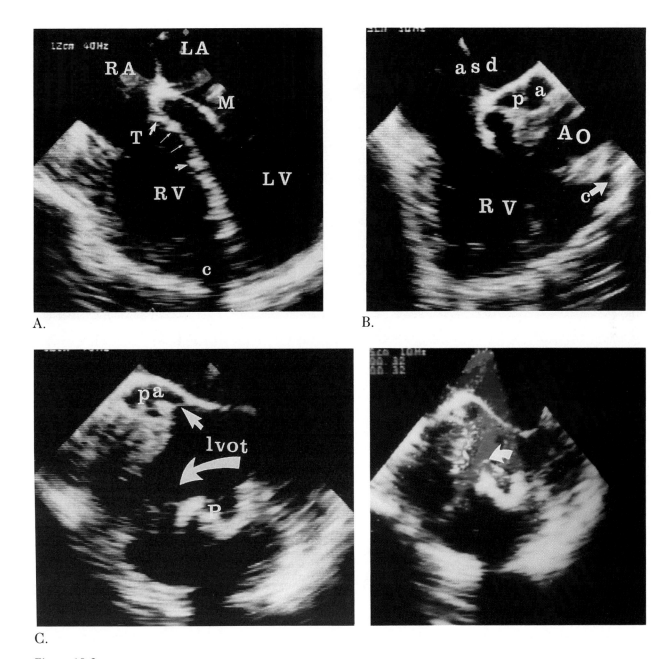

Figure 10-2

Preoperative transesophageal echocardiogram performed in the operating room in a 21-year-old man referred from an outside hospital for re-repair of D-transposition of the great arteries with a prior Rastelli repair in whom there was obstruction of conduit from right ventricle to pulmonary artery and a residual leak via the ventricular septal defect patch that also baffled flow from left ventricle to aorta. *A.* Basic "four-chamber" horizontal-plane view shows normal crux anatomy with an apical tricuspid (T) valve between the right atrium (RA) and right ventricle (RV) and the more superior plane of the mitral (M) valve between the left atrium (LA) and left ventricle (LV). The large arrows show the margins of the ventricular septal patch; the small arrows show the body of the patch that bows into the LV owing to increased RV pressure. The conduit exited the RV apex (c) but was not well seen in the horizontal plane. *B.* The vertical plane demonstrated the area of extracardiac conduit (c) obstruction after its exit from RV. The aorta (AO) no longer exits the RV though in this view the dropout of echo might suggest that it did. The pulmonary artery (pa) is small and posterior to the anterior aorta; the pulmonary valve had previously been oversewn. The atrial septal defect (asd) was a new finding, having been missed on the previous transthoracic echocardiograms and catheterizations at the referring hospital. *C* and *D.* A modified short-axis basal horizontal-plane view shows the echo and color flow images of the left ventricular outflow tract (lvot) and the septal patch (P); the color flow identified the patch leak at the margin of the patch (curved arrow).

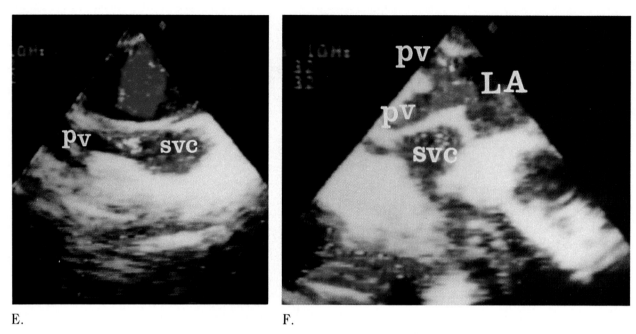

E.   F.

Figure 10-2
E. Also found was an unexpected anomalous pulmonary vein (pv) connecting to the superior vena cava (svc). *F.* The patch repair baffling the anomalous pulmonary vein into the left atrium (LA) instead of the svc is shown after coming off cardiopulmonary bypass.

the inferior vena caval drainage to the right atrium can be scanned by advancing the transducer to the "four-chamber view" and angling posteriorly and inferiorly. In the vertical plane both vena cava can be easily seen to enter the right atrium with sequential insertion of the TEE probe from a superior to inferior location in the esophagus.[6,13,21–23]

A persistent left superior vena cava (LSVC) is the most common anomaly of the superior caval system. It usually occurs as part of a bilateral superior caval system and is connected to the right atrium via the coronary sinus in over 90 percent of cases, thereby resulting in normal physiology. Hence its importance lies in the higher prevalence of associated cardiac defects and in the modifications that cavopulmonary anastomotic procedures will necessarily take into account. A persistent LSVC that joins the roof of the left atrium and communicates with the coronary sinus can be seen with the horizontal plane as an oval structure between the left atrial appendage and the left superior pulmonary vein. In the "four-chamber view," gradually angling the transducer inferiorly will track the LSVC into a

dilated coronary sinus. The vertical plane most directly shows the LSVC traversing superiorly toward the head (thus vertically) from its connection with the left side of the coronary sinus.[6,13,21–23]

Because of the proximity of the esophageal transducer to the four pulmonary veins, TEE is superior to transthoracic echocardiography in assessing venous connections and flow patterns.[38] In adults, even careful transthoracic imaging cannot uniformly determine connections of left and right inferior pulmonary veins. The normally connected superior pulmonary veins course anteroposteriorly at the level of the right and left atrial appendages.[22] The lower pulmonary veins have a variably postero-anterior course or course almost parallel to the frontal plane and enter the left atrium more laterally, posteriorly, and inferiorly than the upper veins.[22] Sweeping the vertical-plane TEE transducer to the far left, using the left atrial appendage as a landmark, and to the far right using the right pulmonary artery and right superior vena cava as landmarks allows identification of the superior pulmonary venous connections; advancing the probe slightly with

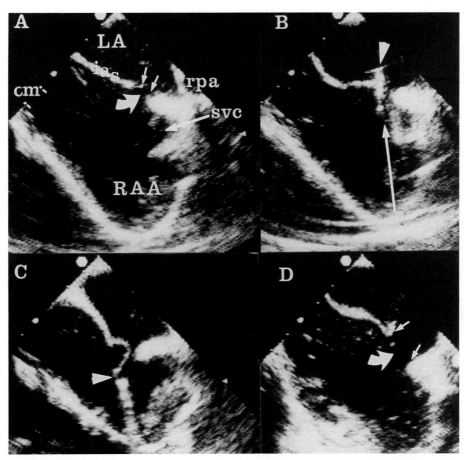

Figure 10-3
Intraoperative TEE-guided blade atrial septostomy. Patient with tricuspid atresia and a restrictive atrial septal defect had a Glenn shunt and an atrial septostomy without cardiopulmonary bypass; intraoperative TEE guidance allowed insertion of a scalpel through a small stab incision in the hypertrophied right atrial appendage (RAA) into the small atrial septal defect for septostomy enlargement. *A.* Small defect in the interatrial septum (ias) (small arrows) was seen only in the vertical plane; large arrow shows the direction of flow across the atrial septal defect into the left atrium (LA). (cm = centimeter, rpa = right pulmonary artery, svc = superior vena cava entrance to right atrium.) *B.* Scalpel handle passed into the right atrium (long arrow) with the tip of the scalpel (arrowhead) inserted across the defect. *C.* The interatrial septal tissue is now distorted because of a firm downward stroke of the scalpel tip (arrowhead). *D.* Surgically enlarged defect (two small arrows) with a tissue flap; large arrow depicts direction of flow. (With permission, Marelli AJ et al, *Cardiol Clin,* in press.[6])

further lateral rotation rightward or leftward allows visualization of the inferior right or left pulmonary veins, respectively. The horizontal or vertical planes vary in their display of the pulmonary veins depending on the individual's anatomic orientation. Our experience concurs with that of others in that complete and consistent interrogation of all four pulmonary venous connections and drainage sites is achieved best by the combined use of both planes.[6,19,21–23]

In the adult with congenital heart disease, the most commonly encountered variety of anomalous pulmonary venous connection is anomalous connection of the right upper pulmonary vein to the right atrium or superior vena cava (Fig. 10-2E), usually in association with a sinus venosus atrial septal defect (Fig. 10-4). There are few TEE reports on total anomalous pulmonary venous connection.[39] A coexisting ASD is the rule; the right atrium is dilated together with the superior vena cava if it receives the total anomalous pulmonary venous return via an innominate bridge. The malformation may coexist with more complex

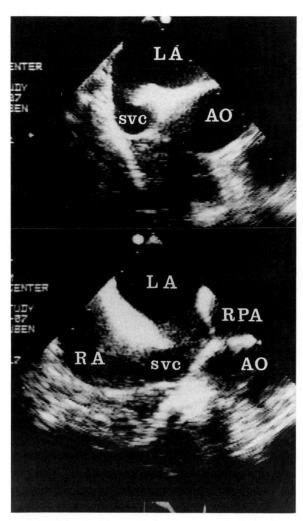

Figure 10-4
Sinus venosus atrial septal defect. The horizontal-plane basal view (top) and the rightward vertical plane (bottom) show a defect between left atrium (LA) and the superior vena cava (svc) at a level above the right atrium (RA). AO = aorta; RPA = right pulmonary artery. (With permission, Marelli AJ et al, *Cardiol Clin,* in press.[6])

anomalies. Identification of the entrance of the pulmonary veins into a retrocardiac venous confluence with subsequent connection to the superior vena cava or right atrium is possible because of the proximity of the TEE probe to the posterior cardiac structures. The patient with complete anomalous pulmonary venous connection who has been repaired requires careful Doppler interrogation of the anastomotic sites to ensure the absence of residual or acquired obstruction.

Atrial Situs and Anatomy

Transesophageal echocardiography is the procedure of choice to accurately determine atrial situs. In 132 patients, most of whom were adolescents, abnormal atrial situs was missed with transthoracic imaging but correctly identified in 5 patients using single-plane TEE.[40,41] The right atrial appendage can be identified in the basal short-axis view to the right of the aortic root. Typically, it is short and blunt with a broad junction to the right atrium. The left atrial appendage can be easily visualized with leftward rotation of the transducer. It is seated above the left atrioventricular valve anterior to the left upper pulmonary vein. Its identifying features include its long and fingerlike shape with a narrow junction to the left atrium. Additional structures between the left atrial appendage and left upper pulmonary vein can be an extra left atrial appendage, left juxtaposed atrial appendages, or a left superior vena cava. These can be differentiated on the basis of atrial septal orientation and by following the course of the structure with 2D and Doppler interrogation.[41]

Cor triatriatum represents the persistence of the dilated pulmonary vein of the embryo that fails to become incorporated into the left atrium; a fibromuscular diaphragm partitions the left atrium into a proximal chamber that receives the pulmonary veins and a distal or true left atrial chamber, which almost always contains the left atrial appendage and fossa ovalis. The two atrial partitions communicate through openings across the diaphragm, the number and degree of which determine the hemodynamic obstruction. This diagnosis is easily made with TEE because of the proximity of the probe to the left atrium. Several cases have been reported,[42–44] including acquired cor triatriatum after orthotopic heart transplantation.[45] Examination includes hemodynamic assessment of inflow obstruction using Doppler interrogation at the level of the intraatrial membrane and pulmonary veins.[42]

Atrial Septal Defect

In order of decreasing frequency, atrial septal defect (ASD) is likely to be of the secundum (Figs. 10-1*A*, *B*, 10-2*B*, 10-3), primum (Fig.

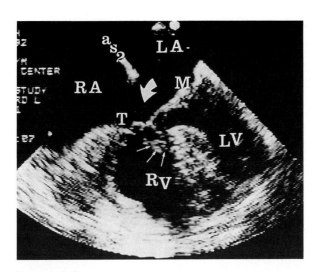

Figure 10-5
Endocardial cushion defect in 76-year-old woman undergoing repair. Intraoperative TEE demonstrates the large primum atrial septal defect (curved arrow) with a persistent left-to-right shunt from left atrium (LA) to right atrium (RA). The secundum atrial septum (as2) is intact. The cleft anterior mitral valve (M) was better seen in transgastric views. The tricuspid valve (T) had redundant tissue of its medial or septal portion (small arrows) which had effectively closed a small inlet ventricular septal defect. The right ventricle (RV) is dilated. LV = left ventricle.

10-5), or sinus venosus type (Fig. 10-4). The least common variety is the coronary sinus ASD. The echocardiographic examination is aimed at the diagnosis and localization of the defect, the precise definition of atrial septal anatomy in order to guide the therapeutic approach, the diagnosis of associated anomalies, and quantification of shunt size.

In adults, TEE is more sensitive than transthoracic echocardiography in the detection of atrial septal defect.[46–52] It is useful to supplement color Doppler examination of the atrial septum with peripheral venous contrast injection to detect both right-to-left and left-to-right shunting (right atrial negative contrast shadowing). Direct transthoracic echocardiographic visualization of the atrial septum, even in the subcostal view, is reliable in only 60 percent of adults studied with transthoracic imaging.[47] Up to 20 percent of atrial septal defects diagnosed with TEE have been missed by transthoracic studies.[48] The majority of defects undiagnosed by transthoracic echocar-

diography adequately detected by TEE are of the sinus venosus variety.[6,13,49,52] These occur high in the atrial septum close to the entry of the superior vena cava or rarely at the inferior vena caval junction. As mentioned above, both vena cava can be easily seen to enter the right atrium with superior and inferior scanning, particularly with the vertical plane. In our experience, the vertical plane is superior to the horizontal plane in the diagnosis of sinus venosus atrial septal defect.[6]

Recently, attention has been drawn to a possible association between a patent foramen ovale (PFO) or atrial septal aneurysms or both with otherwise unexplained neurologic events in adults.[53–55] Right-to-left shunting at the atrial level can be demonstrated with contrast echocardiography at rest or with the Valsalva maneuver in up to 23 percent of healthy volunteers.[56] In the detection of PFO, even with agitated saline echo-contrast injection, transthoracic imaging can lead to falsely negative studies.[57] Detection rates for PFO by TEE are three times higher than by transthoracic imaging and correspond more closely with the reported incidence of PFO in pathologic series.[57] Transesophageal echocardiographic detection and characterization of aneurysms of the atrial septum is superior to transthoracic imaging.[54,55] Criteria proposed for the definition of atrial septal aneurysm include a base width of 1.5 cm and an excursion ≥ 1.5 cm beyond the plane of the atrial septum or phasic excursion during the cardiorespiratory cycle >1.5 cm.[58]

The size of the septal defect, its location, the presence of tissue in the rim of the defect, and the presence or absence of an associated aneurysm will need to be determined prior to choosing an interventional or surgical therapeutic option. Equally important is the detection and quantitation of associated lesions. The secundum ASD can occur with a variable degree of mitral valve prolapse and mitral regurgitation, both of which can be well assessed with the horizontal and vertical imaging planes. An ostium primum defect is the most common form of partial atrioventricular canal defect and usually consists of a primum ASD and a cleft anterior mitral valve leaflet with a variable degree of mitral regurgitation (Fig. 10-5). The mitral valve cleft can best be visualized from the transgastric horizontal plane in a view similar to that seen from the parasternal short-axis view (Fig. 10-6).[6] Subaortic stenosis has been described and should be sought in patients with primum ASD.[59–61] The abnormal chordal attachments in the left ventricular outflow tract to the ventricular septum are best visualized in the vertical plane (Fig. 10-7).[6] The sinus venosus ASD is commonly associated with anomalous connection of the right pulmonary veins to the right atrium or superior vena cava. Because transthoracic imaging is inconsistently reliable in assessing pulmonary venous drainage, we recommend TEE if a sinus venosus ASD is suspected. The coronary sinus ASD usually occurs in the context of complex heart disease and can be associated with a persistent left LSVC that communicates with a dilated coronary sinus.

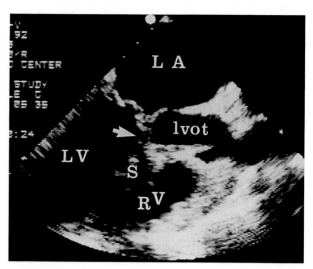

Figure 10-7
Abnormal ventricular septal (S) attachments (arrow) of cleft left anterior mitral leaflet partially obstructing the left ventricular outflow tract (lvot) are well shown in the vertical-plane TEE view with mild lateral tilting of the transducer head to best refine the anatomy. LA = left atrium; LV = left ventricle; RV = right ventricle.

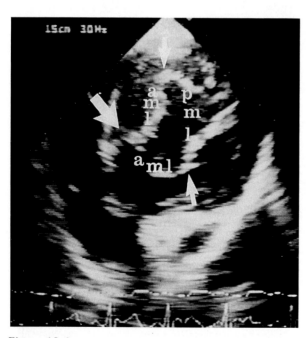

Figure 10-6
Cleft anterior mitral leaflet in conjunction with a primum atrial septal defect (partial endocardial cushion defect). This transgastric horizontal plane view shows a short-axis view of the mitral leaflets with two portions of the cleft anterior mitral leaflet (aml) shown. The large arrow shows the abnormal attachment to the ventricular septum. The posterior mitral leaflet (pml) and its junction with the aml is shown by the two smaller arrows.

The magnitude of left-to-right shunting across an ASD is inferred from the secondary increase in right atrial and right ventricular size as well as from direct assessment of ASD size using 2D and color Doppler imaging.[4] In the horizontal plane, combining direct measurement of the ASD in the horizontal plane with measurement of the width of the color flow jet in late systole and early diastole has shown good correlation with surgical measurements in adults.[46] Both methods tended to underestimate the ASD size as determined by surgical inspection. Quantitative assessment of shunt volumes using horizontal-plane TEE area measurements of the defect, and either time-velocity-integral or mean velocity of shunt flow have yielded correlation coefficients above 0.80 when compared with Qp/Qs ratios or Qp-Qs volumes obtained by cardiac catheterization.[50,51]

Atrial Baffles

Mustard and Senning atrial switch repairs for complete transposition of the great arteries are the most commonly encountered atrial baffles in the adult congenital population. A combination of atrial tissue, pericardium, or synthetic material is used to fashion a baffle that reroutes systemic venous return to the subpulmonary morphologic left ventricle and pulmonary venous return to the subaortic morphologic right ventricle. The atrial cavity is therefore divided into two portions: an anterior chamber receiving the systemic venous return and a posterior chamber receiving the pulmonary venous return (Fig. 10-8). Complications include baffle leaks, vena caval obstruction, and pulmonary venous obstruction.[62]

Precordial imaging with appropriate suprasternal, parasternal, apical, and subxiphoid views are routinely used to image the intraatrial pulmonary venous and systemic venous portions of the atrial baffles. Indirect evidence of inferior caval patency can be obtained by documenting flow reversal with atrial contraction in the hepatic venous confluence. Precordial imaging is limited and inconsistent in detection of baffle leaks, interrogation of the four pulmonary veins, and imaging of the caval junctions, particularly at the level of the inferior systemic venous baffle limb.[62]

In the appropriate clinical context, indications for TEE in this group of patients include the suspicion of a baffle leak otherwise undiag-

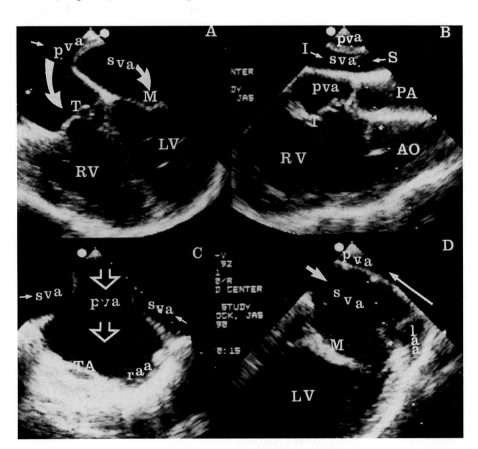

Figure 10-8

D-transposition of great arteries with ventricular septal defect, pulmonary vascular disease, and a palliative Mustard procedure. *A.* Horizontal-plane "four-chamber view" shows course of pulmonary venous atrium (pva) posterior to the systemic venous atrium (sva) with entrance to the right ventricle (RV) via the tricuspid valve (T). The sva is anterior to the pva and enters the left ventricle (LV) via the mitral valve (M). The plane of the TEE is inferior to the ventricular septal defect. *B.* Vertical-plane TEE approximately through the midline of frame *A* with aorta (AO) exiting RV anterior to the pulmonary artery (PA). Posterior and anterior portions of the pva are seen on each side of the sva. The connections with the superior (S) and inferior (I) vena cavae were open. *C.* Vertical-plane view with rotation rightward follows the body of the pva wrapping around the sva; direction of flow shown by arrows. (raa = right atrial appendage, TA = edge of tricuspid annulus.) *D.* Rotation of the vertical plane leftward from *B* shows the body of the sva, the entrance of the inferior vena cava (short arrow), and the entrance of the left superior pulmonary vein into the pva (long arrow). (laa = left atrial appendage.) (With permission, Marelli AJ et al, *Cardiol Clin,* in press.[6])

nosed with precordial imaging, or an abnormal flow pattern detected within the intraatrial portions of either systemic or pulmonary venous baffles suggestive of obstruction. Using the horizontal plane and withdrawing the probe from a high transgastric view to the basal short-axis view, baffle anatomy can be consistently assessed, including the caval junctions and pulmonary veins.[6,19,62] The vertical plane effectively visualizes the midportion of the baffles, the caval connections, and the entrance of the pulmonary veins (Fig. 10-8).[6] Peripheral venous contrast injections assist in the diagnosis of baffle leaks. Baffle obstruction is diagnosed with a combination of 2D color flow imaging and Doppler interrogation. Sites of narrowing, thrombus formation, and flaplike structures thought to represent folds within the baffle membrane can all cause various degrees of obstruction.[62] With TEE, obstructed caval-baffle junction sites can show areas of turbulent flow, although diastolic flow disturbances can occur within the posterior portions

of the pulmonary venous atrium without this necessarily implying baffle obstruction.[19,62] An increased peak velocity of continuous systolic and diastolic flow in combination with documented turbulence indicate baffle obstruction.[62]

Fontan Repair

There are several variants of the Fontan repair, all of which result in the complete or nearly complete (hemi-Fontan) separation of the pulmonary and systemic circulations in patients not eligible for biventricular repair.[3,63] The right atrium, an integral part of the Fontan anatomy, is anastomosed directly to the pulmonary artery, to the small right ventricle, or baffled to both vena cava in the total cavopulmonary connection.[3] The most commonly encountered complications in the atrial portion of the Fontan circulation include cavoatrial shunting, atrial septal shunting, thrombus (Fig. 10-9), and right atrial to pulmonary artery obstruction.[19,25–28] Surgical sequelae purposely

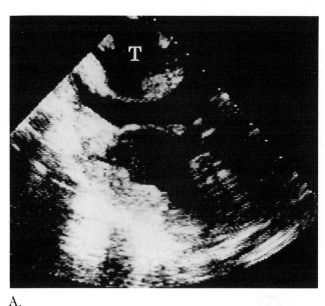

A.

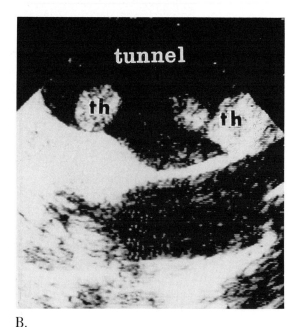

B.

Figure 10-9
Transesophageal echocardiogram performed in the surgical intensive care unit postoperatively in a 28-year-old woman with modified Fontan (total cavopulmonary anastomosis with a lateral tunnel) who has become hypotensive. A shows the two ventricles with the large ventricular septal defect and a bridging common atrioventricular valve that precluded biventricular repair. The ventricular function was normal and there was only mild valvular regurgitation. The lateral tunnel (T), better shown in the magnified view in B, has filling defects due to thrombus (th) formation, which caused pulmonary embolization and an increase in pulmonary artery pressures that caused the Fontan circulation to fail.

left behind in high-risk patients include atrial fenestrations and adjustable ASDs.[63]

Precordial echocardiographic scanning of the Fontan circulation is limited by incomplete imaging of the Fontan anastomosis and of complications of atrial function.[6,19,27] In a series of 18 patients (mean age of 13 years), the success rate of visualization of various forms of Fontan anastomoses was 86 percent with single-plane TEE versus 48 percent with transthoracic echocardiography.[27] In the same series, precordial imaging diagnosed 31 percent of the complications diagnosed with TEE. Right atrial to right ventricular conduits can sometimes be assessed with appropriate precordial examination whereas right atrial to pulmonary anastomotic sites are infrequently completely visualized. Using biplane TEE, we have consistently imaged the anatomy of the Fontan anastomosis, though not always with the necessary alignment to allow accurate spectral Doppler assessment of peak velocity profiles. In 15 adult patients, we have found that the right atrial to

pulmonary anastomosis is better seen with the vertical plane, particularly to a posterior pulmonary artery, while the right atrial to right ventricular anastomosis is better seen with the horizontal plane (Figs. 10-10 to 10-12).[6]

In following the Fontan patient, an important determinant of outcome is the function of the systemic ventricle and its atrioventricular valve both of which are usually readily interrogated by the precordial echo transducer and should be assessed at regular intervals. Patency of the Fontan anastomosis need not be routinely examined unless clinical deterioration points to obstruction or shunting within the Fontan atrium. Transesophageal echocardiography is most useful when directed at the detection and management of suspected complications or known residua of the Fontan atrial anatomy. It is known that the patient with a Glenn anastomosis (right superior vena cava end-to-side to right pulmonary artery) has a small but definite incidence of the development of right lower lobe pulmonary arteriovenous fistulas,

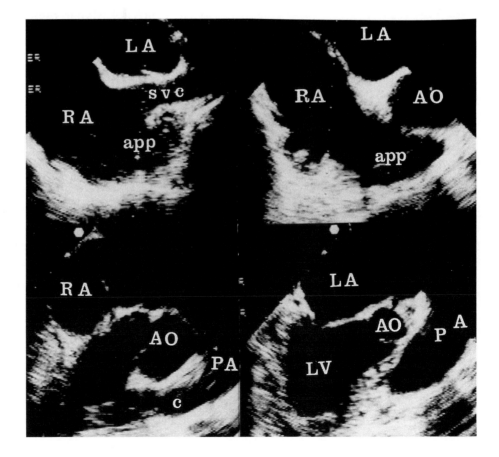

Figure 10-10
Fontan anatomy (right atrial appendage connection to pulmonary artery) in tricuspid atresia and normally related great arteries. Vertical-plane TEE shows sequential rotation from rightward in *A* to more leftward in *D* to follow the right atrium (RA) to anterior and leftward pulmonary artery (PA) connection using the right atrial appendage (app) and a pericardial conduit (c). (AO = aorta; LA = left atrium; LV = left ventricle; svc = superior vena cava.) (With permission, Marelli AJ et al, *Cardiol Clin,* in press.[6])

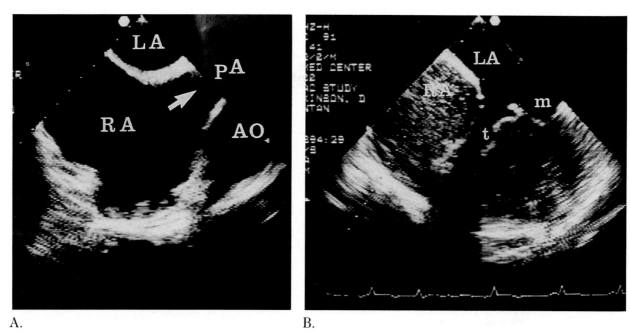

A.   B.

Figure 10-11
Fontan anastomosis from right atrium to pulmonary artery in a 25-year-old man with single ventricle and pulmonic stenosis. *A.* Fontan anastomosis (arrow) of right atrium (RA) to posterior and rightward pulmonary artery (PA) well seen in only the vertical TEE plane. *B.* Horizontal TEE plane shows both mitral (m) and tricuspid (t) valves entering the single ventricle with the right atrium (RA) baffled from the left atrium (LA). Echocontrast is seen in the RA; no baffle leaks were seen.

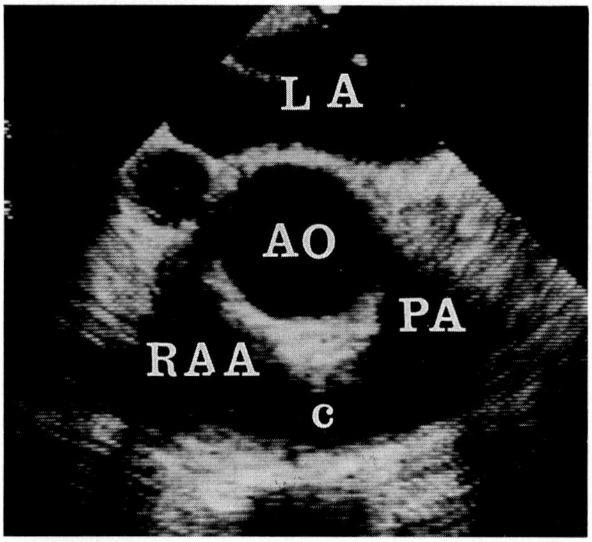

Figure 10-12
Horizontal TEE plane image of a Fontan right atrial appendage (RAA) connection (c) to pulmonary artery (PA) in a patient with tricuspid atresia. AO = aorta; LA = left atrium.

possibly due to nonpulsatile flow.[64] These fistulas are detectable by noting late appearance of echocontrast in the left atrium after intravenous echocontrast injection into a right arm vein. It has been postulated that similar right lower lobe pulmonary hemodynamics are present in the Fontan circulation. We have so far seen two patients where, by TEE only, we could see the reappearance of the echocontrast in the left atrium via the right inferior pulmonary vein that implicates pulmonary arteriovenous fistulas.

Examination of the Atrioventricular Junction and Ventricular Anatomy

Accurate morphologic assessment of the atrioventricular (AV) junction requires defining whether the AV valves are concordant (normal, D-ventricular loop), discordant (L-ventricular loop), imperforate, or absent (right- or left-sided atresia). In crisscross AV relations the

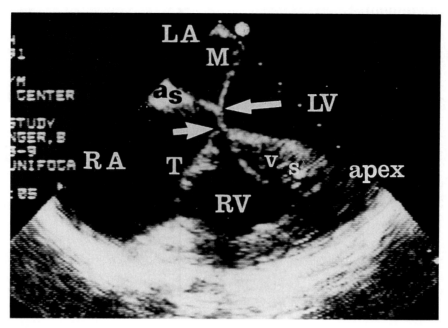

Figure 10-13
Normal crux anatomy on horizontal-plane TEE in a patient with tetralogy of Fallot. The tricuspid valve (T) is more apical than the mitral valve (M), which is more superior. The two large arrows highlight this offsetting of the two atrioventricular valves and also show the atrioventricular septum which is a potential site for connection from the left ventricle (LV) to the right atrium (RA). Not well shown in this still frame are the attachments of the septal tricuspid leaflet to the ventricular septum (vs). (as = secundum atrial septum; LA = left atrium; RV = right ventricle.)

tricuspid inflow may lie anterior to the mitral inflow either to its right or to its left. The typical offsetting of the right and left AV valves with respect to the crux with resulting apical displacement of the septal tricuspid leaflet should be defined (Fig. 10-13). In the presence of a defect in the inlet portion of the ventricular septum, offsetting of the AV valves cannot be used to determine atrioventricular concordance (Fig. 10-14). Right ventricular morphology can be determined using the septal attachment of the tricuspid medial chordal apparatus entering a coarse trabeculated endocardium with an apical moderator band. Left ventricular morphology is identified by a bileaflet atrioventricular valve whose chordal apparatus is attached to two discrete anteromedial and posterolateral papillary muscles seated in a smooth-walled ventricular chamber. Straddling chordal attachments precluding biventricular repair must be identified (Fig. 10-9). Atrioventricular valvular function also includes assessment of annular dimensions, the number and size of the leaflets, and points of poor coaptation

or deformity, all of which influence surgical management and outcome of valvuloplasty.

The above findings are used in the accurate diagnosis of mitral or tricuspid atresia (Fig. 10-1), atrioventricular septal defects (Figs. 10-5, 10-14), Ebstein deformity of the tricuspid valve (Fig. 10-15), double-inlet single ventricle (Fig. 10-11), and congenitally corrected transposition of the great arteries (S,L,L segmental anatomy). In adults, precordial imaging usually permits the accurate diagnosis of tricuspid or mitral atresia, of atrioventricular valve concordance in the presence of an intact ventricular septum,[65] and of Ebstein deformity of the tricuspid valve.[4] Single-plane TEE is reported to be superior to precordial imaging in the diagnosis of AV discordance with inlet ventricular septal defect and imperforate AV valve.[65] If chordal straddling is suspected from the precordial scan, TEE can be used to secure the diagnosis.[65] Using biplane TEE imaging, the horizontal plane more readily images atresia of the right-sided AV valve. The vertical transgastric views are useful in examining the mitral

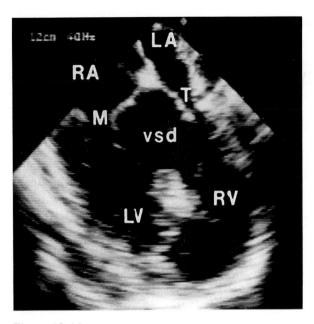

Figure 10-14
Large inlet ventricular septal defect (vsd) in patient with congenitally corrected transposition and pulmonic stenosis; preoperative TEE prior to Rastelli repair. The two atrioventricular valves arise from the crux at the same level. In other views, the left ventricle (LV) was identified by noting a bileaflet (mitral) valve (M) entering a smooth-chambered ventricle with two discrete papillary muscles; the right ventricle was identified by noting a trileaflet (tricuspid) valve (T) entering a coarse ventricle with an L-shaped configuration leading to the outflow tract. (LA = left atrium; RA = right atrium.)

papillary muscle anatomy and straddling of the right AV valve. Precise definition of the right-sided AV valve is occasionally difficult even using both horizontal- and vertical-plane imaging, but the size and mobility of the anterior tricuspid leaflet in Ebstein's anomaly can be assessed and the tricuspid valve anatomy in congenital tricuspid stenosis to ascertain eligibility for and the results of valvular reconstruction or commissurotomy.[6,66]

Ventricular Septal Defect

Ventricular septation occurs as a result of growth of the ventricles, the endocardial cushions, and the conal septum. Therefore, the ventricular septum in its entirety shows a complex longitudinal twist that does not lie in any single plane. Longitudinally, it extends from base to apex, assuming the shape of a crescent bulging from left to right. Horizontally, its outflow portion follows conotruncal anatomy and lies anterior and leftward while its inflow portion lies posterior and rightward. The ventricular septum itself is composed of a large muscular and small membranous portion. The membranous septum is divided into an interventricular portion and an atrioventricular portion by the insertion of the septal tricuspid leaflet (Fig. 10-13). The membranous ventricular septal defect (VSD) lies beneath the aortic valve and can have inlet, outlet, or muscular extension (Fig. 10-16). Muscular defects are commonly central or apical. Inlet defects lie on the ventricular base of the crux between the mitral and tricuspid leaflets posterior and inferior to membranous defects (Figs. 10-5, 10–14). Outlet defects that are roofed by the conjoined leaflets of the aortic and pulmonary valves are also termed doubly committed, subarterial, supracristal, conal, or infundibular VSDs. Malalignment of the ventricular septum occurs with more complex anomalies and results in the malaligned ventricular septal defect with aortic override that is seen, for example, in tetralogy of Fallot and at times D-transposition of the great arteries (Figs. 10-17, 10-18).

Precordial examination can usually accurately identify the presence of single ventricular septal defects owing to its liberal use of transducer positions to interrogate the septum in numerous planes, though muscular defects may occasionally be missed.[4] Transesophageal horizontal-plane imaging alone (single-plane TEE) is reliable in the assessment of the membranous and inlet portions of the ventricular septum.[19,20,31] Single-plane imaging has shown limitations in delineating doubly committed and muscular septal defects when compared with epicardial intraoperative echocardiography.[15,19,32] Visualization of the entire ventricular septum is successful with biplane TEE, the vertical plane being ideal for examination of the anterior subarterial, membranous, and muscular septum.[6,19] Intraoperative epicardial imaging is still required occasionally when prostheses or patches interfere with imaging

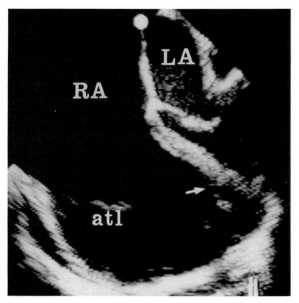

A.

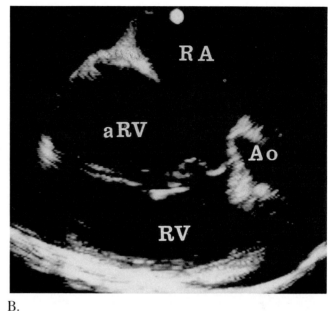

B.

Figure 10-15
Ebstein anomaly. *A* shows the horizontal-plane "four-chamber" view with a markedly dilated right atrium (RA) and right ventricle. The elongated anterior tricuspid leaflet (atl) is shown. The arrows points to the site of attachment of the septal tricuspid leaflet indicating excessive displacement from the crux of the heart. LA = left atrium. *B* shows the vertical-plane image aligned to best reveal the right inflow tract; the RV is dilated owing to severe long-standing tricuspid regurgitation. The right-sided atrioventricular groove is seen to separate the atrialized right ventricle (aRV) from the RA. Ao = aorta.

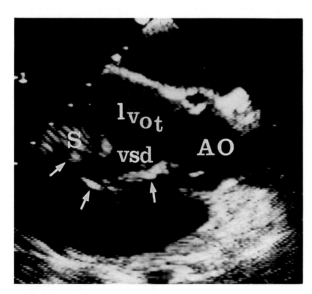

Figure 10-16
Membranous ventricular septal defect. The vertical plane is laterally aligned to show the aorta (AO) and left ventricular outflow tract (lvot) which best demonstrates an anatomically large membranous ventricular septal defect (vsd) that has undergone spontaneous closure owing to aneurysmal overlay (arrows) of septal tricuspid tissue adherent to the septum (S).

on the far-field side of the septum. Septal patch leaks can usually be detected by TEE with careful scanning of the margins of the VSD patch (Fig. 10-2).[6,19,20]

Defect size is best defined hemodynamically as nonrestrictive (left and right ventricular systolic pressures equalize) or restrictive (systolic gradient from left to right ventricle).[4] In VSD with Eisenmenger's reaction right ventricular function and pulmonary pressures should be determined.[4] Depending on the size and location of the VSD, secondary changes in the right- and left-sided cardiac chambers and valves should be sought. Spontaneous closure of VSD, most common with membranous defects, is due to aneurysm formation, often because of overlay of septal tricuspid valve tissue (Fig. 10-16).[67] Damage to the aortic valve, most frequently associated with defects in the outlet septum, occurs as a result of poor developmental tissue support of the cusps compounded by the effects of the underlying high-velocity jet.

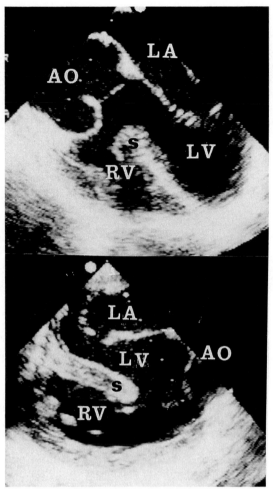

Figure 10-17
Malaligned ventricular septal defect in pulmonary atresia tetralogy of Fallot. Better appreciated in the horizontal plane (top) but well seen in the vertical plane (bottom), the aorta (AO) overrides the malaligned ventricular septal defect. The mitral valve is in continuity with the aorta. No right ventricular outflow tract was seen because of pulmonary atresia but the "blind pouch" (arrow) of the right ventricle (RV) was better seen in the vertical plane. (LA = left atrium; LV = left ventricle; s = septum.) (With permission, Marelli AJ et al, *Cardiol Clin*, in press.[6])

Examination of Conotruncal Anatomy

Accurate echocardiographic definition of conotruncal anatomy includes the determination of ventriculoarterial concordance or discordance, the relation of the great arteries to one another, and the details of subvalvular, valvar, and supravalvar anatomy for each of the outflow tracts.

Ventriculoarterial Alignment and Positional Relations of the Great Arteries

Integral to the determination of the ventriculoarterial alignment or the origins of the great arteries is the examination of the infundibulum. The distal infundibulum or conus connects the ventricle(s) below to the artery or arteries above. The infundibulum can be subpulmonary, subaortic, bilateral, or absent. The normal conus persists between the right ventricle and the pulmonary artery, thereby preventing continuity between the pulmonary valve and the atrioventricular valves. Conversely, the normal resorption of the subaortic conus enables fibrous continuity between the aortic annulus and anterior mitral valve. In simple transposition, the aorta is aligned with the right ventricle and the conus is therefore subaortic instead of subpulmonic, with resulting left-sided continuity between the pulmonary and mitral valves (Fig. 10-18). In double-outlet right ventricle, there are bilateral conuses and there is no semilunar atrioventricular continuity. Fallot's tetralogy with significant aortic override is differentiated from double-outlet right ventricle by the presence of mitral aortic continuity and the absence of subaortic conus (Fig. 10-17). To complete the determination of ventriculoarterial alignment or connection, the great artery should be followed from its ventricle of origin to determine if it branches (pulmonary artery) or if it can be identified as giving rise to the coronary arteries and brachiocephalic vessels (aorta) (Fig. 10-18).[4]

Examining the positional relationships of the great arteries relative to one another as they course out of their respective ventricles will determine if they are malposed or transposed, that is, with the aorta being anterior and to the right (D-transposition or malposition) (Fig. 10-18), or anterior and to the left (L-transposition or malposition) or side by side, with respect to the pulmonary artery.

In 15 adults with abnormally related great arteries, we consistently found the vertical plane to be useful in determining right- and

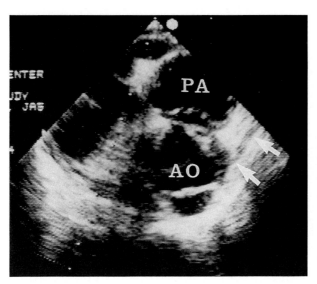

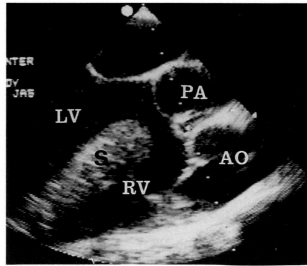

A.   B.

Figure 10-18
D-transposition of great arteries with ventricular septal defect and pulmonary vascular disease. *A.* Horizontal plane shows relative positional relationship of great arteries with aorta (AO) anterior and slightly rightward of the pulmonary artery (PA); the orifice of a left-sided coronary artery is seen (arrows) arising from the left posterior coronary cusp; the right-sided coronary artery was shadowed by PA-AO tissue. *B.* The vertical plane shows the AO anterior to the PA with the AO aligned with right ventricle (RV) and the PA aligned with left ventricle (LV) with an intervening ventricular septal defect (arrow) with the ventricular septum (S) mildly malaligned toward the PA. Note that the mitral valve is in continuity with the PA.

left-sided ventriculoarterial connections and showing the course of the great arteries while the horizontal plane more readily showed the positional relationship of the two great vessels. The use of both horizontal and vertical imaging planes is necessary for complete TEE assessment of conotruncal anatomy.[6] Once the ventriculoarterial connections and great arterial positional relations have been established, examination of both right and left ventricular outflow tract is pursued separately and in greater detail.[6]

Lesions of the Right Ventricular Outflow Tract

Right ventricular outflow tract (RVOT) malformations between a morphologic right subpulmonary ventricle and pulmonary trunk are an important and common group of congenital heart anomalies. In the native RVOT, the pulmonic valve, which normally has right, left, and anterior cusps, can be dysplastic or atretic (Figs. 10-17, 10-19) or functionally stenotic

but patent or regurgitant. Subvalvar stenosis can be fixed or dynamic, with or without the involvement of atrioventricular valvular tissue. Narrowing above the valve can occur within the main pulmonary artery, either as a primary lesion or secondary to previous surgical banding. Sizing the main pulmonary artery and its branches is important in the patient with Fallot's tetralogy with and without pulmonary atresia (Fig. 10-19) and in determining candidacy for procedures such as Fontan's operation. Branch pulmonary artery anatomy can vary from stenosis to atresia, the former being either primary or secondary (e.g., secondary to aortopulmonary surgical shunts). The reconstructed RVOT can have aneurysmal dilatation, as in Fallot's tetralogy with a pericardial transannular patch, or can consist of a valved or nonvalved conduit or homograft, as in the Rastelli procedure (Fig. 10-2).

Published transesophageal experience has clearly shown the limitations of the horizontal plane to adequately interrogate the proximal

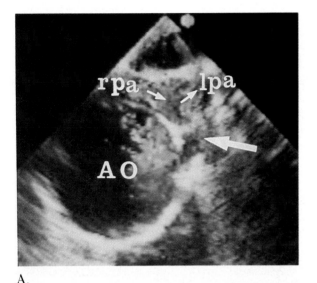

A.

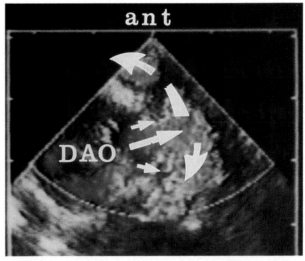

B.

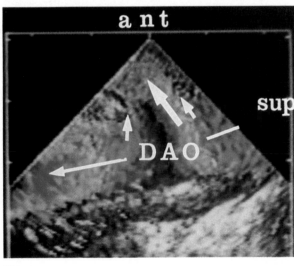

C.

Figure 10-19
Aortic-to-pulmonary arterial collaterals in pulmonary atresia with malaligned ventricular septal defect (tetralogy of Fallot). *A* shows pulmonary atresia and confluent small pulmonary arteries in the basal horizontal plane view of the ascending aorta (AO) above the level of the aortic valve. The arrow points to the atretic segment of the pulmonary artery. Flow from aortic-to-pulmonary artery collaterals entered the right pulmonary artery (rpa) and then fed the left lung via the left pulmonary artery (lpa). *B* and *C*. Aortic-to-pulmonary artery collaterals in the horizontal and vertical plane, respectively. The descending aorta (DAO) was imaged at the level of the carina where a conglomerate of collaterals exited (large arrows); the two smaller arrows point to the orifice of the collaterals.

RVOT.[6,14,15,19] The horizontal plane can be used to adequately assess the distal main pulmonary artery, the pulmonary artery bifurcation, and the main branch pulmonary artery (right more easily than the left) (Fig. 10-19). In our adults with repaired tetralogy of Fallot, RVOT conduits, pulmonary atresia with unifocalization of pulmonary blood flow, and valvar or subvalvular pulmonic stenosis, we consistently achieved complete imaging of the RVOT in its entirety using the vertical plane.[6] The vertical (longitudinal) plane is better able to assess the surgical patching of malaligned ventricular septal defects.[6,19] The vertical plane is essential for precise assessment of the valvar,

subvalvular, and proximal supravalvar RVOT lesions and ventricular-to-pulmonary arterial conduits (Fig. 10-20).[6]

Lesions of the Left Ventricular Outflow Tract

Lesions of the left ventricular outflow tract (LVOT) are here defined as those that occur between a morphologic left systemic ventricle and the aorta. Subvalvular aortic stenosis can be dynamic with or without involvement of atrioventricular valve tissue or can occur in the form of discrete membranous or tunnel fibromuscular obstruction (Fig. 10-21). Complete assessment of the aortic valve requires

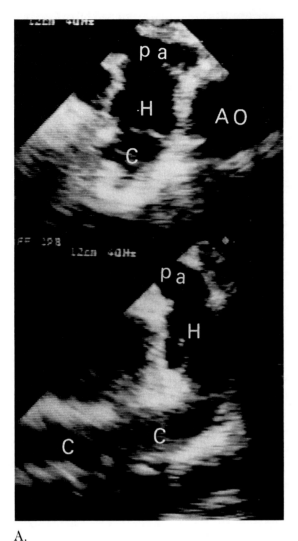

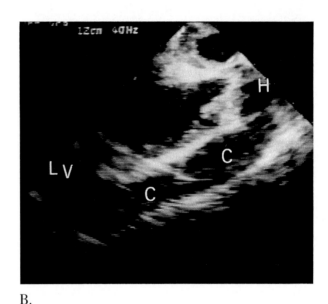

A.

B.

Figure 10-20

Extracardiac conduit from apex of left ventricle to pulmonary artery in patient with congenitally corrected transposition of arteries (patient from Fig. 10-4); intraoperative TEE. Because of the position of the pulmonary artery (pa) posterior and rightward to the aorta (AO) and the left ventricular apical position, the conduit was long and was placed along the right side of the heart so as to avoid kinking or compression by the sternum. *A.* The horizontal plane (top) and vertical plane (bottom) TEE views were performed intraoperatively to verify that the dacron conduit (C) and homograft (H) were unobstructed in their course. In addition, the homograft–to–pulmonary artery anastomosis was widely patent. The homograft is well seen in both planes but the vertical plane was required for full visualization of the conduit. *B.* The vertical plane is used to verify patency of the anastomosis of the conduit to the apex of the left ventricle (LV), a feat that was not possible with the horizontal plane.

anatomic definition of the sinuses of Valsalva, the number of aortic cusps (Fig. 10-22), the origins of the coronary arteries, and hemodynamic determination of regurgitation or stenosis. TEE has, in limited experience, proved to be useful in the detection of unruptured and ruptured sinus of Valsalva aneurysms.[68,69] Beyond the valve, obstruction can be supravalvar or can occur in the form of coarctation of the aorta. Complete assessment of aortic coarctation requires examination of the aortic isthmus, sizing of the transverse aorta, and study of the aortic valve.

Transesophageal echocardiography has established its contribution in the imaging of the valvar and subvalvar aortic areas.[6,13–15,19] The

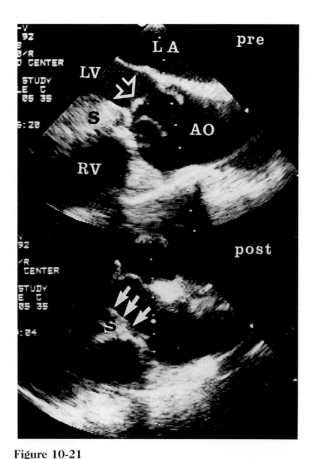

Figure 10-21
Discrete subaortic stenosis; intraoperative TEE pre- and postsurgical resection. Top: Vertical plane view of the discrete fibromembranous obstruction (arrow) situated immediately beneath the aorta (AO), on the septum (S) in the left ventricular outflow tract (LA = left atrium; LV = left ventricle; RV = right ventricle). Bottom: The three arrows show the site of surgical resection without evidence of perforation of the septum. Color flow imaging of the aortic valve (not shown) demonstrated mild residual aortic regurgitation.

horizontal-plane, short-axis and long-axis basal views (lateral and medial tip deflection, respectively) elucidate the aortic valve as well as the subvalvar area and proximal ascending aorta. Using the horizontal plane, the proximal ascending aorta can also be imaged by angling anteriorly and superiorly at the transgastric level. Nonetheless, biplane TEE imaging is essential to complete assessment of the LVOT and entire aorta.[6,19,21,24,25] In our TEE experience with malformations of the LVOT and aorta (including subaortic stenosis, bicuspid aortic valve, lesions of the sinus of Valsalva,

aortic coarctation, and Marfan's syndrome), we have found the vertical plane to be particularly useful for subaortic stenosis and aortic coarctation (Figs. 10-21, 10-23).[6]

In subaortic stenosis, the combination of the two planes affords a more complete definition of discrete membranes and allows intraoperative assessment of the adequacy of resection (Fig. 10-21) as well as competence of the aortic valve and the immediate detection of complications (e.g., perforation of the anterior mitral leaflet, iatrogenic VSD). In aortic coarctation, the vertical plane facilitates the diagnosis of discrete coarctation (Fig. 10-23), particularly recurrent postoperative coarctations, whereas combining the two planes enables more reliable sizing of all aortic segments. During balloon coarctation dilatation, TEE allows assistance in balloon placement across the defect and provides immediate detection of intimal flaps. In assessing the anatomy of a bicuspid aortic valve, we have found both planes equally useful, with either one of the two planes showing better resolution in the individual patient using careful medial-lateral manipulation of the transducer head. As with balloon dilatation of coarctation, TEE in the catheterization laboratory provides ongoing feedback as to balloon position across the valve and detection of valvular tears, as well as a semiquantitative estimate of the degree of residual aortic regurgitation.

Coronary Anomalies

Anomalous origin of a coronary artery can occur as a result of an ectopic ostium within or above the aortic sinuses or as a result of a coronary artery originating in the pulmonary trunk. An interesting group of patients who will become of long-term interest to adult congenital cardiologists are those with transposition of the great arteries in whom close to 40 percent have anomalous origins of the coronary arteries.[70] These variations in coronary anatomy are preserved after the transfer of coronary buttons to the neoaorta during the arterial switch operation.[70] Though possible, transthoracic scanning of the aortic sinuses and proximal coronary arteries is inconsistent in adults. Both single-plane and biplane TEE have been

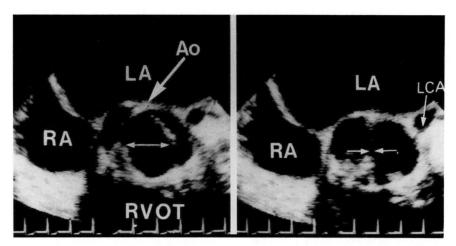

Figure 10-22
Horizontal-plane view of bicuspid aortic valve. Left: Systolic frame showing the oval opening of two leaflets within the aortic sinuses. Right: Diastolic frame shows the central closure line from 12 to 6 o'clock with mild focal thickening of the anterior rightward portion of the valve which may represent part of a false raphe. (Ao = aorta; LA = left atrium; LCA = left circumflex artery; RA = right atrium; RVOT = right ventricular outflow tract.)

used to diagnose anomalous coronary origins with a higher success rate than transthoracic echocardiography.[70–75]

Coronary fistulas occur most commonly between the right coronary artery and the right ventricle, right atrium, or pulmonary trunk. The fistulous connection may be so large as to allow a significant left-to-right shunt. A pulsed and color Doppler continuous-flow pattern with diastolic predominance can be detected in the low-pressure receiving chamber.[4] When the pulmonary trunk is the receiving chamber, this flow must be differentiated from PDA flow. Single-plane and biplane TEE have been used successfully to delineate the course and size of coronary fistulas.[71–74]

Figure 10-23
Coarctation of the aorta, recurrent postoperatively. The vertical-plane TEE image reveals the discrete membranelike narrowing (two large arrows) of the descending aorta (DA). The orifice was best found by tracking the color flow imaging to the flow acceleration into the narrowed orifice (two small arrows). Other views not shown revealed the coarctation to be just below a dilated left subclavian artery. TrAO = transverse aorta.

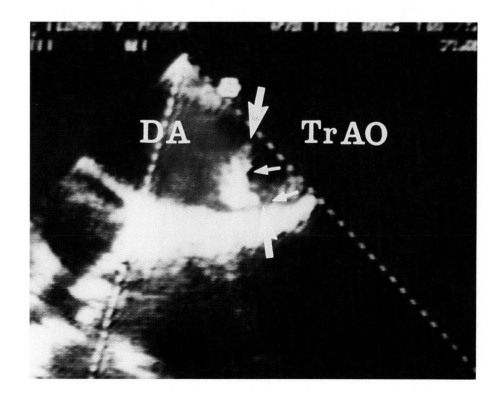

Systemic to Pulmonary Arterial Shunts

Reported experience is insufficient to cite definitive data on the use of TEE in this group of lesions; however, some general relevant remarks are possible.[6,80,81] For all systemic to pulmonary artery shunts, either native (PDA) or palliative (e.g., Blalock-Taussig subclavian to pulmonary artery branch anastomosis or Pott's anastomosis of the anterior wall of the descending aorta to the posterior wall of the left pulmonary artery), spectral and color Doppler examination is essential for detection and assessment of patency. TEE appears to be more accurate than standard transthoracic echocardiography in the detection of PDA, with the vertical plane being superior to the horizontal plane.[80,81] Flow through palliative systemic venous shunts and arterial shunt can usually be achieved with meticulous transthoracic scanning using appropriate suprasternal views. Single-plane TEE assessment of Glenn shunts is superior to transthoracic scanning but as would be expected of a vertical structure, the vertical TEE plane is more reliable than the horizontal plane in assessing flow through a Glenn or Blalock-Taussig shunt (Fig. 10-24).[6] In the absence of distal pulmonic stenosis, we have also found the vertical plane to be particularly helpful in aligning a continuous-wave Doppler beam to determine the gradient across a Pott's anastomosis, thus reflecting the pulmonary artery pressure in a potential Fontan candidate.[6]

Summary

Dramatic progress in diagnostic and surgical management of infants and children born with congenital heart disease over the last three decades has resulted in the frequent survival of this population into adulthood. The complexity of the underlying malformations with superimposed surgical intervention make accurate diagnostic imaging essential for adequate follow-up. Currently, much of the reported information on the utility of TEE in congenital heart disease is obtained from studies in children. The potential informational gain with TEE is higher in older adolescents and adults in whom transthoracic acoustic windows are at times poorer. The scope of information obtainable from high-quality transesophageal echocardiography makes this technique ideal for following both operated and unoperated adult patients as well as for assisting surgical

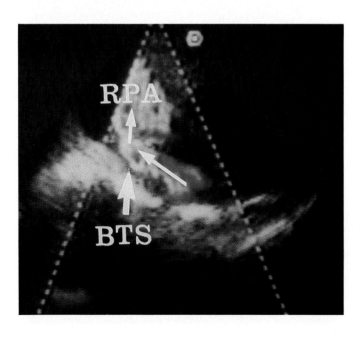

Figure 10-24
Blalock-Taussig shunt, right subclavian artery to right pulmonary artery branch anastomosis in patient with complex cyanotic heart disease. The vertical plane was used to image the patent Blalock-Taussig shunt (BTS) connection, with the right pulmonary artery using color flow imaging as an aid to track the continuous flow and localize the anastomosis.

and interventional procedures, though careful transthoracic imaging using the standardized segmental approach to diagnosis remains the cornerstone for assessment. Horizontal-plane TEE imaging provides important additional information with regard to pulmonary venous return, atrial situs, atrial baffle function, atrioventricular anatomy and function, lesions of the left ventricular outflow tract, central pulmonary arteries, and positional relationships of malposed great vessels. The vertical TEE plane enhances imaging of systemic and pulmonary venous connections, atrial situs, venosus atrial septal defects, right-sided atrioventricular anatomy, the ventricular septum, and the ventricular outflow tracts. Vertical-plane imaging is essential for complete assessment of complex right ventricular outflow tract anatomy, ventriculoarterial alignment, and coarctation of the aorta.

References

1. Perloff JK: 22nd Bethesda conference: Congenital heart disease after childhood: An expanding patient population. *J Am Coll Cardiol* 18:311, 1991.

2. Perloff JK: Congenital heart disease in adults: A new cardiovascular subspecialty. *Circulation* 84:1881, 1991.

3. Perloff JK, Child JS: *Congenital Heart Disease in Adults*. Philadelphia, Saunders, 1991.

4. Child JS: Echo-Doppler and color flow imaging in congenital heart disease. *Cardiol Clin* 8:289, 1990.

5. Sreeram N, Sutherland GR, Geuskens R, et al: The role of transesophageal echocardiography in adolescents and adults with congenital heart defects. *Eur Heart J* 12:231, 1991.

6. Marelli AJ, Child JS, Perloff JK: Transesophageal echocardiography in adult congenital heart disease. *Cardiol Clin*, in press.

7. Cyran SE, Kimball TR, Meyer RA, et al: Efficacy of intraoperative transesophageal echocardiography in children with congenital heart disease. *Am J Cardiol* 63:594, 1989.

8. Dan M, Bonato R, Mazzucco A, et al: Value of transesophageal echocardiography during repair of congenital heart defects. *Ann Thorac Surg* 50:637, 1990.

9. Feltes TF: Advances in transesophageal echocardiography: Impact of a changing technology on children with congenital heart disease. *J Am Coll Cardiol* 18:1515, 1991.

10. Fyfe DA, Kline CH: Transesophageal echocardiography for congenital heart disease. *Echocardiography* 8:573, 1991.

11. Hellenbrand WE, Fahey JT, McGowen FX, et al: Transesophageal echocardiographic guidance of transcatheter closure of atrial septal defect. *Am J Cardiol* 66:207, 1990.

12. Kipel G, Arnon R, Ritter SB: Transesophageal echocardiographic guidance of balloon atrial septostomy. *J Am Soc Echocardiogr* 4:631, 1991.

13. Seward JB, Tajik AJ: Transesophageal echocardiography in congenital heart disease. *Am J Cardiac Imag* 4:215, 1990.

14. Stumper O, Kaulitz R, Elzenga NJ, et al: The value of transesophageal echocardiography in children with congenital heart disease. *J Am Soc Echocardiogr* 4:164, 1991.

15. Stumper O, Kaulitz R, Sreeram N, et al: Intraoperative transesophageal versus epicardial ultrasound in surgery for congenital heart disease. *J Am Soc Echocardiogr* 3:392, 1990.

16. Stumper O, Witsenburg M, Sutherland GR, et al: Transesophageal echocardiographic monitoring of interventional cardiac catheterization in children. *J Am Coll Cardiol* 18:1506, 1991.

17. Ungerleider RM, Kisslo JA, Greeley WJ, et al: Intraoperative prebypass and postbypass epicardial color flow imaging in the repair of atrioventricular septal defects. *J Thorac Cardiovasc Surg* 98:90, 1989.

18. Van Der Velde ME, Perry SB, Sanders SP: Transesophageal echocardiography with color Doppler during interventional catheterization. *Echocardiography* 8:721, 1991.

19. Weintraub R, Shiota T, Elkadi T, et al: Transesophageal echocardiography in infants and children with congenital heart disease. *Circulation* 86:711, 1992.

20. Wienecke M, Fyfe DA, Kline CH, et al: Comparison of intraoperative transesophageal echocardiography to epicardial imaging in children undergoing ventricular septal defect repair. *J Am Soc Echocardiogr* 4:607, 1991.

21. Nanda NC, Pinheiro L, Sanyal RS, et al: Transesophageal biplane echocardiographic imaging: Technique, planes, and clinical usefulness. *Echocardiography* 7:771, 1990.

22. Pinheiro L, Nanda NC, Jain H, et al: Transesophageal echocardiographic imaging of the

pulmonary veins. *Echocardiography* 8:741, 1991.

23. Nanda NC, Pinheiro L, Sanyal R, et al: Transesophageal echocardiographic examination of left-sided superior vena cava and azygos and hemiazygos veins. *Echocardiography* 8:731, 1991.

24. Bansal RC, Shakudo M, Shah PM, et al: Biplane transesophageal echocardiography: Technique, image orientation, and preliminary experience in 131 patients. *J Am Soc Echocardiogr* 3:348, 1990.

25. Seward JB, Khandheria BK, Edwards WD, et al: Biplanar transesophageal echocardiography: Anatomic correlations, image orientation, and clinical applications. *Mayo Clin Proc* 65:1193, 1990.

26. Fyfe DA, Kline CH, Sade RM, et al: Transesophageal echocardiography detects thrombus formation not identified by transthoracic echocardiography after the Fontan operation. *J Am Coll Cardiol* 18:1733, 1991.

27. Fyfe DA, Kline CH, Sade RM, et al: The utility of transesophageal echocardiography during and after Fontan operations in small children. *Am Heart J* 122:1403, 1991.

28. Stumper O, Sutherland GR, Geuskens R, et al: Transesophageal echocardiography in evaluation and management after a Fontan procedure. *J Am Coll Cardiol* 17:1152, 1991.

29. Ritter SB: Transesophageal real-time echocardiography in infants and children with congenital heart disease. *J Am Coll Cardiol* 18:569, 1991.

30. Cohen GI, Chan KL: Biplane transesophageal echocardiography: Clinical applications of the long-axis plane. *J Am Soc Echocardiogr* 4:155, 1991.

31. Omoto R, Kyo S, Matsumura M, et al: Evaluation of biplane color Doppler transesophageal echocardiography in 200 consecutive patients. *Circulation* 85:1237, 1992.

32. Muhiudeen IA, Roberson DA, Silverman NH, et al: Intraoperative echocardiography for evaluation of congenital heart defects in infants and children. *Anesthesiology* 76:165, 1992.

33. Muhiudeen IA, Roberson DA, Silverman NH, et al: Intraoperative echocardiography in infants and children with congenital cardiac shunt lesions: Transesophageal versus epicardial echocardiography. *J Am Coll Cardiol* 16:1687, 1990.

34. Roberson DA, Muhiudeen IA, Silverman NH,

et al: Intraoperative transesophageal echocardiography of atrioventricular septal defect. *J Am Coll Cardiol* 18:537, 1991.

35. Rashkind W: Creation of an atrial septal defect without thoracotomy. *JAMA* 196:173, 1966.

36. Steeg C, Bierman FZ, Hardoff: Bedside balloon septostomy in infants with transposition of the great arteries: New concepts using two-dimensional echocardiographic techniques. *J Pediatr* 107:904, 1985.

37. Erbel R, Bednarczyk I, Pop T, et al: Detection of dissection of the aorta intima and media after angioplasty of coarctation of the aorta. An angiographic, computer tomographic, and echocardiographic comparative study. *Circulation* 81:805, 1990.

38. Castello R, Pearson AC, Lenzen P, et al: Evaluation of pulmonary venous flow by transesophageal echocardiography in subjects with a normal heart: Comparison with transthoracic echocardiography. *J Am Coll Cardiol* 18:65, 1991.

39. Romero-Cardenas A, Vargass-Barron J, Stumper O, et al: Total anomalous pulmonary venous return: Diagnosis by transesophageal echocardiography. *Am Heart J* 121:1831, 1991.

40. Stumper OF, Sreeram N, Elzenga NJ, et al: Diagnosis of atrial situs by transesophageal echocardiography. *J Am Coll Cardiol* 16:442, 1990.

41. Stumper O, Rijlaarsdam M, Vargas-Barron J, et al: The assessment of juxtaposed atrial appendages by transesophageal echocardiography. *Int J Cardiol* 29:365, 1990.

42. Patt MV, Obeid AI: Cor triatriatum with isolated pulmonary venous stenosis in an adult: Diagnosis with transesophageal two-dimensional echocardiography. *J Am Soc Echocardiogr* 4:185, 1991.

43. Schlüter M, Langenstein BA, Thier W, et al: Transesophageal two-dimensional echocardiography in the diagnosis of cor triatriatum in the adult. *J Am Coll Cardiol* 2:1011, 1983.

44. Ludomirsky A, Erickson C, Vick GW 3d, et al: Transesophageal color flow Doppler evaluation of cor triatriatum in an adult. *Am Heart J* 120:451, 1990.

45. Fagan LF Jr, Penick DR, Williams GA, et al: Two-dimensional, spectral Doppler, and color flow imaging in adults with acquired and congenital cor triatriatum. *J Am Soc Echocardiogr* 4:177, 1991.

46. Faletra F, Scarpini S, Moreo A, et al: Color

Doppler echocardiographic assessment of atrial septal defect size: Correlation with surgical measurements. *J Am Soc Echocardiogr* 4:429, 1991.

47. Hanrath P, Schlüter M, Langenstein BA, et al: Detection of ostium secundum atrial septal defects by transesophageal cross-sectional echocardiography. *Br Heart J* 49:350, 1983.

48. Lin SL, Ting CT, Hsu TL, et al: Transesophageal echocardiography detection of atrial septal defect in adults. *Am J Cardiol* 69:280, 1992.

49. Kronzon I, Tunick PA, Freedberg RS, et al: Transesophageal echocardiography is superior to transthoracic echocardiography in the diagnosis of sinus venosus atrial septal defect. *J Am Coll Cardiol* 17:537, 1991.

50. Mehta RH, Helmcke F, Nanda NC, et al: Transesophageal Doppler color flow mapping assessment of atrial septal defect. *J Am Cardiol* 16:1010, 1990.

51. Morimoto K, Matsuzaki M, Tohma Y, et al: Diagnosis and quantitative evaluation of secundum-type atrial septal defect by transesophageal Doppler echocardiography. *Am J Cardiol* 66:85, 1990.

52. Oh JK, Seward JB, Khanderia BK, et al: Visualization of sinus venosus atrial septal defect by transesophageal echocardiography. *J Am Soc Echocardiogr* 1:275, 1988.

53. Pearson AC, Labovitz AJ, Tatineni S, et al: Superiority of transesophageal echocardiography in detecting cardiac source of embolism in patients with cerebral ischemia of uncertain etiology. *J Am Coll Cardiol* 17:66, 1991.

54. Pearson AC, Nagelhout D, Castello R, et al: Atrial septal aneurysm and stroke: A transesophageal echocardiac study. *J Am Coll Cardiol* 18:1223, 1991.

55. Schneider B, Hanrath P, Vogel P, et al: Improved morphologic characterization of atrial septal aneurysm by transesophageal echocardiography: Relation to cerebrovascular events. *J Am Coll Cardiol* 16:1000, 1990.

56. Lynch JJ, Schuchard GH, Gross CM, et al: Prevalence of right-to-left atrial shunting in a healthy population: Detection by Valsalva maneuver contrast echocardiography. *Am J Cardiol* 53:1478, 1984.

57. Siostrzonek P, Zangeneh M, Gossinger H, et al: Comparison of transesophageal and transthoracic contrast echocardiography for detection of a patent foramen ovale. *Am J Cardiol* 68:1247, 1991.

58. Hanley PC, Tajik AJ, Hynes JK, et al: Diagnosis and classification of atrial septal aneurysm by two-dimensional echocardiography: Report of 80 consecutive cases. *J Am Coll Cardiol* 6:1370, 1985.

59. Lappen RS, Muster AJ, Idriss FS, et al: Masked subaortic stenosis in ostium primum atrial septal defect: Recognition and treatment. *Am J Cardiol* 52:336, 1983.

60. Reeder GS, Danielson GK, Seward JB, et al: Fixed subaortic stenosis in atrioventricular canal defect: A Doppler echocardiographic study. *J Am Coll Cardiol* 20:386, 1992.

61. Taylor NC, Samerville J: Fixed subaortic stenosis after repair of ostium primum defects. *Br Heart J* 45:689, 1989.

62. Kaulitz R, Stumper OF, Geuskens R, et al: Comparative values of the precordial and transesophageal approaches in the echocardiographic evaluation of atrial baffle function after an atrial correction procedure. *J Am Coll Cardiol* 16:686, 1990.

63. Laks H: The partial Fontan procedure: A new clinical concept and its clinical application. *Circulation* 82:1866, 1990.

64. Cloutier A, Ash JM, Smallhorn JF, et al: Abnormal distribution of pulmonary blood flow after the Glenn shunt or Fontan procedure: Risk of development of arteriovenous fistulae. *Circulation* 72:471, 1985.

65. Sreeram N, Stumper OF, Kaulitz R, et al: Comparative value of transthoracic and transesophageal echocardiography in the assessment of congenital abnormalities of the atrioventricular junction. *J Am Coll Cardiol* 16:1205, 1990.

66. Fram DB, Missri J, Therrien ML, et al: Assessment of Ebstein's anomaly and its surgical repair using transesophageal two-dimensional echocardiography and Doppler color flow mapping. *Echocardiography* 8:367, 1991.

67. Hornberger LK, Sahn DJ, Krabill KA, et al: Elucidation of the natural history of ventricular septal defects by serial color flow mapping studies. *J Am Coll Cardiol* 13:1111, 1989.

68. Blackshear JL, Stafford RE, Lane GE, et al: Unruptured noncoronary sinus of Valsalva aneurysm: Preoperative characterization by transesophageal echocardiography. *J Am Soc Echocardiogr* 4:485, 1991.

69. McKenney PA, Shemin RJ, Wiegers SE: Role of transesophageal echocardiography in sinus of Valsalva aneurysm. *Am Heart J* 128:228, 1992.

70. Mayer JE Jr, Sanders SP, Jonas RA, et al: Coronary artery pattern and outcome of arterial switch operation for transposition of the great arteries. *Circulation* 82(suppl IV):139, 1990.

71. Gaither NS, Rogan KM, Stajduhar K, et al: Anomalous origin and course of coronary arteries in adults: Identification and improved imaging utilizing transesophageal echocardiography. *Am Heart J* 122:69, 1991.

72. Smolin MR, Gorman PD, Gaither NS, et al: Origin of the right coronary artery from the left main coronary artery identified by transesophageal echocardiography. *Am Heart J* 123:1062, 1992.

73. Samdarshi TE, Hill DL, Nanda NC: Transesophageal color Doppler diagnosis of anomalous origin of left circumflex coronary artery. *Am Heart J* 122:571, 1991.

74. Boogaerts J, Samdarshi TE, Nanda NC, et al: Anomalous separate origin of left circumflex coronary from a separate ostium in the left coronary sinus: Identification by transesophageal color Doppler echocardiography. *Echocardiography* 7:165, 1990.

75. Koh KK: Confirmation of anomalous origin of the right coronary artery from the left sinus of Valsalva by means of transesophageal echocardiography. *Am Heart J* 122:851, 1991.

76. Calafiore PA, Raymond R, Schiavone WA, Rosenkranz ER: Precise evaluation of a complex coronary arteriovenous fistula: The utility of transesophageal color Doppler. *J Am Soc Echocardiogr* 2:337, 1989.

77. Samdarshi TE, Mahan EF 3d, Nanda NC, et al: Transesophageal echocardiography assessment of congenital coronary artery to coronary sinus fistulas in adults. *Am J Cardiol* 68:263, 1991.

78. Sunuga Y, Taniichi Y, Okubo N, et al: Biplane transesophageal echocardiographic study of left coronary artery to right atrium fistula. *Am Heart J* 123:1058, 1992.

79. Arazoza EA, Bowser M, Obeid AI: Coronary artery fistula: Diagnosis by biplane transesophageal echocardiography. *J Am Soc Echocardiogr* 5:277, 1991.

80. Mügge A, Daniel WG, Lichtlen PR: Imaging of patent ductus arteriosus by transesophageal color-coded Doppler echocardiography. *J Clin Ultrasound* 19:128, 1991.

81. Takenaka K, Sakamoto T, Shiota T, et al: Diagnosis of patent ductus arteriosus in adults by biplane transesophageal color Doppler flow mapping. *Am J Cardiol* 68:691, 1991.

11

The Evaluation of Aortic Dissection and Aortic Atheromatosis

Siva Arunasalam
Gerald Maurer
Robert J. Siegel

Aortic Dissection

Each year more than 2000 new cases of aortic dissection are diagnosed in the United States.[1] It is by far the most catastrophic disease of the aorta, with an early mortality as high as 1 percent per hour and over 90 percent mortality within 1 year if left untreated.[2] Aortic dissection is characterized by an accumulation of blood dissecting the media from the intima and adventitia. The majority of the cases are associated with an intimal flap (96 percent), and about 70 percent of the intimal tear occurs in the ascending aorta, 1 to 3 cm above the right or left sinus of Valsalva.[3–5] In the remaining 20 to 25 percent of cases, the intimal flap is located distal to the origin of the left subclavian artery near the attachment of the ligamentum arteriosum.[6–8] The tear is often transverse secondary to the pulsatile shearing force that is the underlying mechanism for the development of the intimal flap. The intimal tear often initiates the process of dissection; however, in a small percentage of dissections, subintimal hemorrhage of the vasa vasorum may precede

the tear, as illustrated by Fig. 11-1. Risk factors often associated with the development of aortic dissection are (1) systemic hypertension and (2) intrinsic aortic pathology. Systemic hypertension is present in 80 percent of patients diagnosed with aortic dissection. Aortic pathology includes elastic degeneration of the media, connective tissue disease (such as Marfan's syndrome, Ehlers-Danlos syndrome, and giant cell arteritis), and severe atherosclerosis.[9,10] Other risk factors associated with the development of aortic dissection include age greater than 50 years, male gender, pregnancy,[11,12] aortic coarctation, congenital bicuspid aortic valve,[13] iatrogenic causes during intravascular procedures, trauma,[14,15] and the use of intranasal or intravenous cocaine.[16,17]

Classification of Aortic Dissection

Three schemes have been proposed for the classification of aortic dissection. The DeBakey

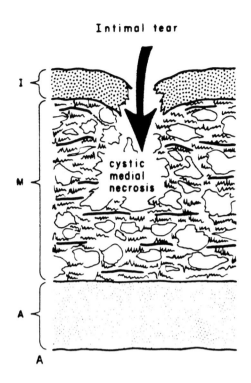

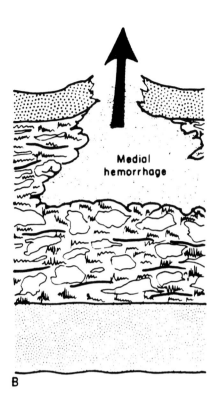

Intimal tear

cystic medial necrosis

Medial hemorrhage

A

B

Figure 11-1
Mechanisms of aortic dissection. (*A*) Intimal tear from lumen into the aortic wall, initiating an aortic dissection. (*B*) Subintimal hemorrhage of the vasa vasorum into the media, leading to rupture of intima into the lumen. (From Roberts WC: Aortic dissection: Anatomy, consequences and causes. *Am Heart J* 101:195, 1981, with permission.)

classification divides aortic dissection into three types (Fig. 11-2). Type I dissection involves the aortic root and extends into the descending aorta, type II is limited to the ascending aorta, and type III is confined distal to the origin of the left subclavian artery. The Stanford classification divides aortic dissection into proximal (type A) and distal (type B) aortic dissections.[18,19] Proximal dissection is inclusive of types I and II in the DeBakey classification while distal dissection is the equivalent of type III. Recently, Erbel et al. have proposed a new classification for aortic dissection based on TEE findings. They have divided aortic dissection into (a) aortic dissection with intimal tear and (b) without intimal tear. Aortic dissections with intimal tear are further categorized according to the amount of thrombus in the false lumen: (1) false lumen completely filled with thrombus, (2) false lumen partially filled with thrombus, and (3) no thrombus in the false lumen. Aortic dissection is further differentiated according to whether there is retrograde or antegrade dissection from the site of the most proximal intimal tear. Mediastinal hematoma defined as blood outside the pericardial sac is considered a special

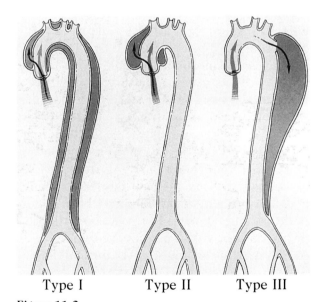

Type I   Type II   Type III

Figure 11-2
De Bakey classification of aortic dissection. **Type I:** Involves the ascending aorta and extends into the descending aorta. **Type II:** Limited to the ascending aorta. **Type III:** Limited to the descending aorta. (From DeBakey ME et al: Surgical management of dissecting of the aorta. *J Thorac Cardiovasc Surg* 49:130, 1965, with permission.)

TABLE 11-1a   TEE Classification for Aortic Dissection and Associated Mortalities (70 Patients)

	No Intimal Tear	Intimal Tear with Antegrade Dissection	Intimal Tear with Retrograde Dissection	Mediastinal Hematoma
No thrombus		20		
Partial thrombosis	5	13	11	
Complete thrombosis	11		10	9
% mortality	13	40	36	89

From Erbel R et al: *Circulation* 84 (suppl II) II:23, 1989, with permission.

TABLE 11-1b   Comparative Mortalities of Aortic Dissection by Stanford and DeBakey Classification

	Stanford Classification		DeBakey Classification		
	Proximal $n = 116$	Distal $n = 489$	I $n = 54$	II $n = 62$	III $n = 489$
% mortality	88	12	90	88	12

Source   Refs. 23, 24, 65.

group. Their follow-up of 70 patients demonstrated that mediastinal hematoma was associated with the highest mortality of 89 percent, while patients without an intimal tear had an overall mortality of 13 percent (Table 11-1a, 1b).[20] Proximal aortic dissection requires emergent surgical intervention since it carries a high mortality of 10 to 15 percent within the first 6 h of presentation, 30 to 35 percent within the first 24 h, 60 percent within the first 3 days, and almost 80 percent within the first 3 weeks.[21,22] However, distal aortic dissections have a 15 to 20 percent mortality in asymptomatic patients who are medically managed over a period of 24 to 36 months and a high initial surgical mortality that approaches 50 percent. Thus the latter group of patients are managed medically until they become symptomatic or there is significant dilation of the aorta (>6 cm).[23]

Clinical Manifestations

Aortic dissection generally presents with a history of sudden onset of severe chest and/or back pain, followed by a variety of complications, including congestive heart failure from acute aortic regurgitation, myocardial infarction secondary to acute dissection and/or occlusion of a coronary artery, organ ischemia from involvement of the major branches of the aorta, hemorrhagic shock, and cardiac tamponade.[24,25] In a small number of patients, aortic dissection may be painless. Thus there is a wide spectrum to the presentation of this entity. Although several studies have identified a number of clinical signs and symptoms associated with aortic dissection, they are often nonspecific and cannot be used reliably to make a definitive diagnosis in patients suspected of dissection (Table 11-2).[26–28]

TABLE 11-2   Clinical Presentations in Patients with Suspected Aortic Dissection

Clinical Features	Confirmed Dissection n = 18	No Dissection n = 22
Age (years)	59 ± 11.3	61 ± 16.6
Male : female	11 : 7	13 : 9
History of hypertension	10	8
Duration of symptoms < 24 h	8	11
Sudden chest or back pain	14	17
Migration of pain	7	8
Presence of neurologic or cardiac event	3	5
Enlarged aorta or widened mediastinum, on chest x-ray	17	13
Presence of aortic regurgitation	4	1
Left ventricular hyertrophy on ECG	1	5

From Chan KL: *Am Heart J*, 122:495, 1991, with permission.

Imaging of the Thoracic Aorta

Hanrath et al. first described the use of TEE for imaging the aorta as well as detecting aortic dissection.[29] Since their description in 1981, TEE as a diagnostic modality has gained widespread acceptance and application. The TEE probe is introduced (see Chap. 3) into the esophagus in the neutral position. By systematically examining the aorta, moving the TEE probe up and down the length of the esophagus, in both the horizontal (short-axis) and the longitudinal (long-axis) planes the aortic root, supravalvular aorta, transverse aortic arch, and left carotid and left subclavian arteries can be imaged. By rotating the probe posteriorly, the descending aorta and upper abdominal aorta can be imaged as well. Color Doppler further enhances the diagnostic utility of TEE by visualizing blood flow during various phases of the cardiac cycle in the true and false lumen in both the long and horizontal axes of the aorta (Fig. 11-3A–D). Longitudinal imaging is superior to horizontal views for imaging the aortic cusps and the proximal and distal sections of the ascending aorta. The blind spot due to trachea interference, which occurs in the upper (ascending) aorta, is almost elimi-

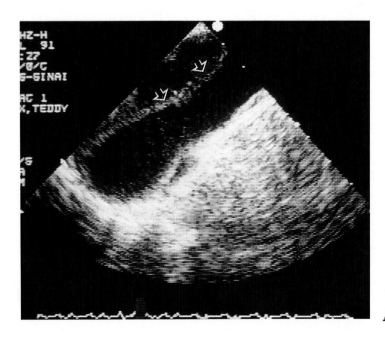

A.

Figure 11-3
TEE images of aortic dissection. (A) Dissection of the transverse aorta (long-axis view). Arrows identify intimal flap.

Figure 11-3
(*B*) Color Doppler identifies flow in the perfusing lumen (true lumen) and absence of flow in the false lumen.

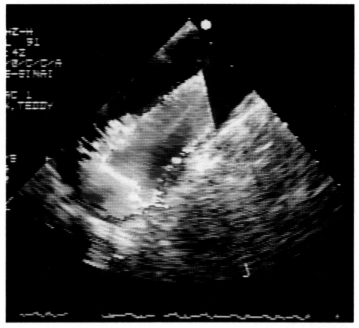

B.

Figure 11-3
(*C*) Dissection of the transverse aorta (short-axis view). Arrow identifies intimal flap.

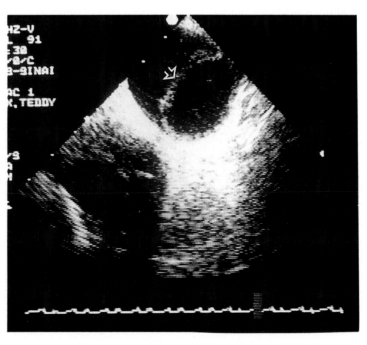

C.

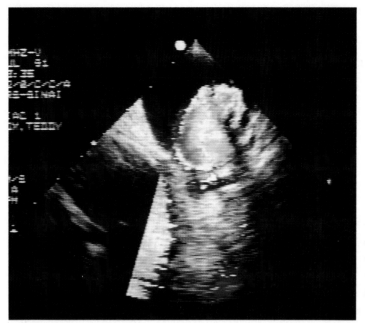

Figure 11-3
(*D*) Color Doppler in the
short axis identifies flow
in the perfusing lumen
(true lumen).

D.

nated with biplane imaging.[30] Use of the omniplane probe further enhances the ability and ease of imaging the ascending and transverse aorta.

Technique of TEE in Patients with Aortic Dissection

Control of blood pressure in patients with aortic dissection is essential in preventing aortic rupture. During the examination with TEE the systemic blood pressure should be carefully controlled by the use of sodium nitroprusside and beta blockers such as esmolol or labetalol. Blood pressure tends to increase with the insertion of the TEE probe if the local anesthesia of the posterior pharynx and throat is not adequate. A TEE examination of patients with acute aortic dissection should ideally be performed by an experienced examiner. With appropriate technical expertise and adequate analgesia insertion of the TEE probe causes minimal elevation of systemic arterial pressure.[31,32]

Safety of TEE in Aortic Dissection

The use of TEE in patients with aortic dissection has been safe in the over 450 patients reported (Table 11-3). Complications such as aspiration and various forms of arrhythmias are infrequent and without significant clinical sequelae.[37] However, there have been reports of rupture of the adventitia of the aortic dissection during TEE.[38] While the relation between the

TABLE 11-3 Literature review:[28,33,34,38,99] Reasons for Interruption of TEE Study before Completion in a Total of 450 Patients (1.1 percent) with Aortic Dissection

Aortic rupture	1
Inability to successfully intubate esophagus with probe	1
Major bleeding complication	1
Hemodynamic instability for interruption	1
Malignant arrhythmia	1

aortic aneurysm rupture and TEE in these cases could be circumstantial, the need for control of blood pressure and heart rate in this setting and during TEE needs to be recognized.

Transthoracic Echocardiography in Aortic Dissection

In any TEE study, including the use of TEE in patients with diseases of the aorta, transthoracic echocardiography (TTE) should be used to complement the study. TTE is especially useful in assessing ventricular wall motion, measurement of chamber sizes, wall thickness, and aortic regurgitation.[39] Furthermore, the suprasternal window augments the assessment of the transverse aorta. However, TTE alone in the diagnosis of aortic dissection has a sensitivity of only about 30 percent[40,41] and in approximately 33 percent of patients undergoing TTE examination, the aorta is inadequately imaged, especially in patients who are obese, those with chest wall abnormalities, Chronic obstructive pulmonary disease (COPD), and in patients who are on a respirator or unable to be still during the TTE examination.[42–44]

Diagnostic Criteria in Aortic Dissection by TEE

With TEE, a diagnosis of aortic dissection is made if two lumens separated by an intimal flap are seen within the aorta (Fig. 11-4). If a false lumen is completely thrombosed, central displacement of intimal calcification with bright echo densities within the aorta or separation of the intimal layers from the thrombus are regarded as positive findings. Figure 11-5A and B demonstrates thrombosis in the nonperfusing lumen. The site of an intimal tear is defined as a disruption in the continuity of the flap, often seen best by color Doppler (Fig. 11-6). The perfusing or true aortic lumen is often differentiated from the false or nonperfusing lumen by the identification of systolic bulging of the dissection flap toward the nonperfusing lumen. Figure 11-7 identifies this motion by two-dimensional and M-mode TEE tracings. Figure 11-8 demonstrates a case of dissection at the site of an atherosclerotic plaque. There is no systolic or diastolic motion of the flap but the presence of flow by Doppler is recorded with flow signals moving from the perfusing into the nonperfusing lumen during systole. The dissection flap can also move inward during systole owing to the suction

Figure 11-4
Short-axis view of the descending aorta. An intimal flap separates the true lumen (L) and false lumen.

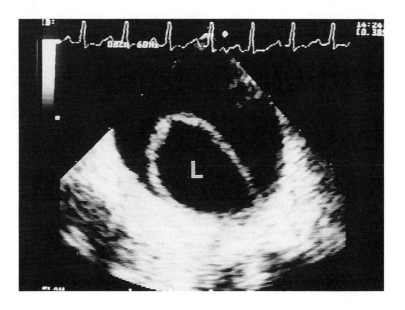

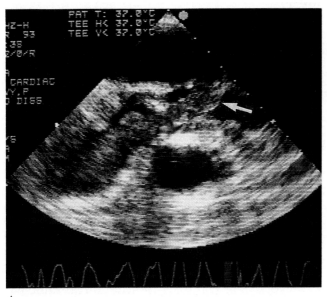
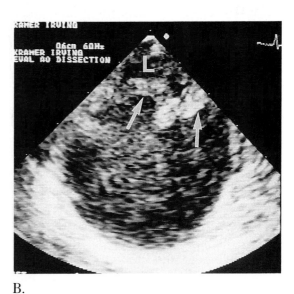

A.

B.

Figure 11-5
Thrombosis in aortic dissection. (*A*) Thrombus extending from false lumen into the aorta and LV outflow tract. Arrow identifies thrombus in LV outflow tract. (*B*) Short-axis view of descending thoracic aortic dissection. **L** identifies the compromised true lumen. The false lumen is filled with specular echoes due to slow blood flow and thrombus. Arrows identify intimal flap.

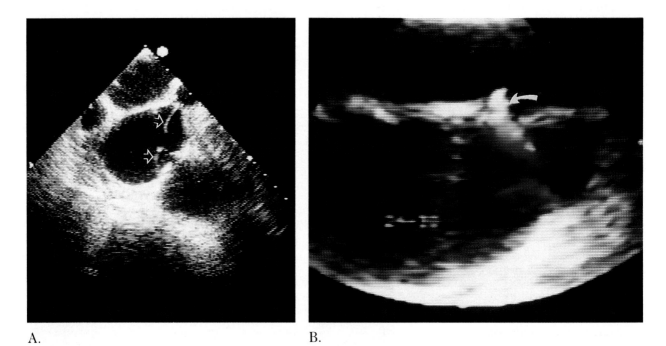

A.

B.

Figure 11-6
Identification of intimal tears. (*A*) Ascending aorta. An intimal flap is seen (arrows). The discontinuity in the midportion represents the site of the intimal tear ("entry site"). (*B*) Descending aorta. Color Doppler in the longitudinal axis demonstrates entry site of dissection (arrow).

Figure 11-7
Short-axis view of dissection in the descending thoracic aorta. M-mode echocardiography demonstrates motion of the intimal flap throughout the cardiac cycle.

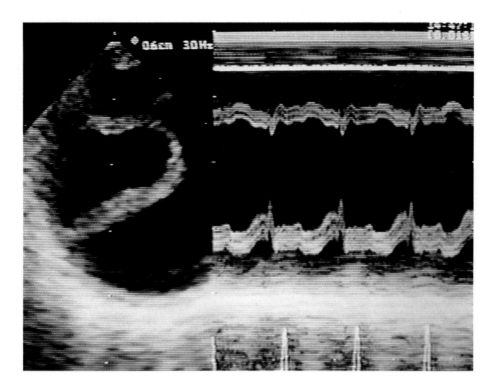

caused by high-velocity flow (Venturi effect), as shown in Fig. 11-9. Communications between the false and true lumen can be identified with pulsed and color Doppler. With color Doppler, smaller intimal tears can be identified, which are not visualized by two-dimensional echocardiography. A turbulent jet is depicted as a bright mosaic color flow when seen traversing from the true to the false lumen.[45–48] As demonstrated by Fig. 11-8 the pressure differential between the true and false lumens may be assessed by pulsed or continuous-wave Doppler assessment.

Sensitivity and Specificity of TEE in Aortic Dissection

Using the standard TEE images described earlier, the ascending, transverse, and descending thoracic aorta can be visualized clearly. Intimal flaps can be detected in 96 percent of patients and the type of aortic dissection diagnosed accurately (Table 11-4).[33–36] The initial studies with single-plane TEE probes failed to recog-

nize dissection in the transverse aorta in about 7 percent of cases, decreasing the overall sensitivity to 92 percent. Studies using biplane probes, however, have increased the sensitivity of TEE in the diagnosis of thoracic aortic dissection to 96 percent, close to the 98 percent sensitivity reported with MRI (Table 11-5).[28,33,99] The reported specificity of TEE in the detection of aortic dissection is 96 percent. Adachi et al. detected intimal flaps in 96 percent of proximal and 100 percent of distal dissections, while the site of entry of the tear was seen in 89 percent of cases (Table 11-6). TEE is sensitive and specific for the diagnosis of aortic dissection. In addition it provides accurate information on ventricular function, the presence and extent of pericardial effusion, as well as the assessment of other vital organ involvement which is required for optimal medical and surgical management of patients with aortic dissection.[49–53] Comprehensive evaluation of aortic regurgitation and involvement of coronary arteries with aortic dissection are also critical considerations when surgical intervention is being assessed. Increasingly, cardiovascular surgeons operate on patients with type A dissections based on TEE without adjunctive

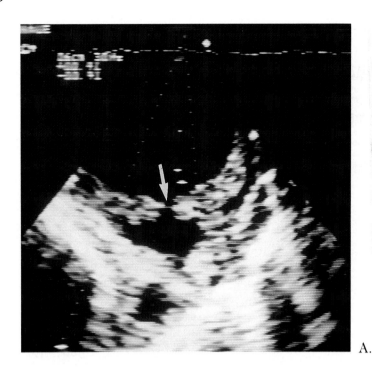

A.

Figure 11-8
Aortic dissection of the descending thoracic aorta secondary to ruptured atherosclerotic plaque. (*A*) Intimal flap is not mobile and separation in the plaque is clearly seen (arrow).

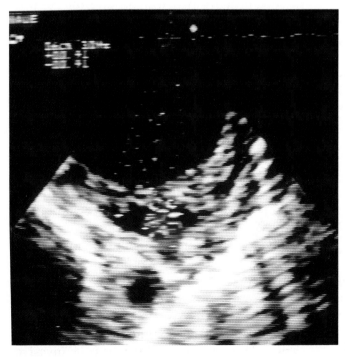

B.

Figure 11-8
(*B*) Color Doppler demonstrates flow from the true lumen to the false lumen (blue).

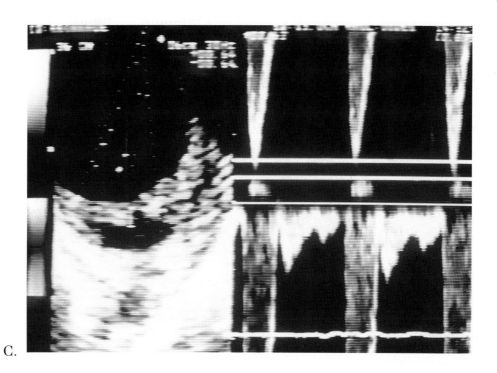

Figure 11-8
(C) Pulsed Doppler at the same site demonstrates gradient and flow from the true lumen into the false lumen at the entry site. (Courtesy of Dr. Richard Wright, Pacific Heart Institute, Santa Monica, California.)

C.

studies such as angiography, MRI, or CT scans.[55,56]

The specificity of TEE has been reported to be lower in the ascending aorta. False-positive interpretation of an intimal flap has been associated with ectatic aortas as well as with the presence of extensive plaquing—both of which may result in echo reverberations. Use of pulsed and color Doppler as well as biplane interrogation of a "possible" site of an intimal flap may improve specificity.

Advantages of TEE in Aortic Dissection (Tables 11-7 and 11-8)

TEE is useful in defining and detecting proximal coronary anatomy and stenoses.[57] Atherosclerotic plaques are easily visualized and appear as highly reflective discrete echoes. In 88 percent of patients, the left main coronary artery can be visualized from its origin to the bifurcation by TEE. In 50 to 60 percent of patients the proximal left anterior descending

and circumflex coronary arteries are also successfully imaged and discrete stenoses identified.[58–60] The proximal right coronary artery can also be imaged and the anatomy defined in 50 percent of patients. In about 21 percent of patients with type A aortic dissection there is involvement of the coronary arteries. In all 21 percent of patients with coronary artery involvement the right coronary artery was dissected. In 9 percent of acute aortic dissections both the right and left coronary arteries were involved. Ballal et al. found that with TEE they successfully identified coronary artery involvement in 86 percent of patients (Table 11-7).[57] CT and standard MRI do not provide information about coronary anatomy. Thus evaluation of patients with aortic dissection by these methods may require further diagnostic investigation before appropriate interventions may be initiated. While angiography provides greater details regarding coronary anatomy, coronary arteriography is often unnecessary in patients with aortic dissection. The utility of obtaining a coronary angiogram has to be counterbalanced against the time delay to surgery and potential complications from invasive

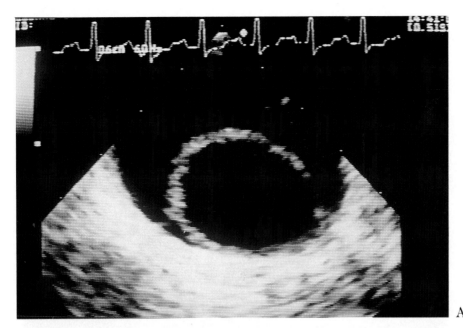

A.

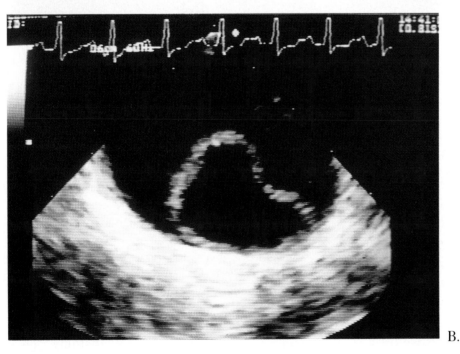

B.

Figure 11-9
Motion of the intimal flap on TEE cross-sectional view of a descending thoracic aortic dissection. In diastole the true lumen appears circular (*A*). During systole, the dissection flap moves inward (distorting the circular lumen) owing to Venturi effect caused by high-velocity systolic flow (*B*).

angiography. While at present there are no data to show that coronary artery bypass grafting affects the ultimate outcome in patients with dissection of the aorta,[61,62] coronary artery involvement in patients with proximal aortic dissection is an indication for urgent surgery.[63,64] TEE, which enables rapid diagnosis and relatively sensitive assessment of the proxi-

mal coronary arteries, is thought by many to be the test of choice for defining the coronary anatomy in the setting of aortic dissection.[65] The outcome of aortic dissection is highly dependent on the extent of the aortic dissection, the rapidity with which the diagnosis is made, and on left ventricular function (Table 11-8). Thus TEE has a clear advantage over

TABLE 11-4   Sensitivity and Specificity of TEE in the Diagnosis of Proximal and Distal Aortic Dissection

	Proximal	Distal	Sensitivity, %	Specificity, %
Nienaber et al.,[99] $n = 110$	31	28	98	77
Erbel et al.,[33] $n = 28$	9	12	100	100
Adachi et al.,[34] $n = 57$	24	21	100	100
Chan et al.,[28] $n = 18$	9	9	100	100
European Cooperative study,[33] $n = 164$	47	35	99	98
Overall			96	87

TABLE 11-5   Sensitivity and Specificity of TEE, MRI, Aortography, and Chest CT in the Diagnosis of Aortic Dissection[28,33,39,55,56,75,79,80,82]

$n = 225$	Sensitivity, %	Specificity, %
Type A ($n = 120$):		
XCT	90	100
TEE	95	84
MRI	100	98
Aortography	91	100
Type B ($n = 105$):		
XCT	96	96
TEE	96	100
MRI	96	100
Aortography	93	100

TABLE 11-7   TEE Findings in 33 Patients with Proximal Aortic Dissections and Coronary Artery Involvement. Coronary Artery Involvement Proved by Angiogram, Surgery, or Autopsy

Coronary Artery(s) Involved in Aortic Dissection Diagnosed by TEE	No. of Patients
Left main coronary artery and right coronary artery	3
Right coronary artery alone	3
Right coronary artery dissection with false-negative result by TEE	1

From Ballal et al: *Circulation* 84:1903, 1991, with permission.

TABLE 11-6   Visualization of Intimal Flap and Site of Entry of Tear in Patients with Aortic Dissection by TEE[2,65,72-86]

	Site of Entry Tear, %	Visualization of Intimal Flap, %
Type A ($n = 24$)	88	96
Type B ($n = 21$)	91	100
Overall	89	98

other diagnostic modalities since it can be performed at the bedside even in critically ill patients. This further reduces the time between diagnosis and appropriate intervention. While it takes an average of 15 min to perform TEE, it takes generally 45 to 60 min to perform MRI, 35 to 40 min for completion of contrast CT, and 60 min to perform and complete an angiographic examination in most centers, including our institution.[69-72] In one series TEE was

TABLE 11-8   Advantages and Disadvantages of TEE over MRI, CT, Aortography in the Diagnosis of Aortic Dissection

	Aortography with Ventriculogram	CT	MRI	TEE
1. Need for contrast	+	+	–	–
2. Intraop evaluation	–	–	–	+
3. Diagnosis of				
a. Thrombus	+	+	+	+
b. Intimal flap	+	+	+	+
c. Tamponade	–	–	+	+
d. False lumen	+	+	+	+
e. Aortic regurgitation	+	–	+	+
f. Branch artery occlusion	+	–	+	–
g. Segmental wall motion abnormalities	+	–	+	+
4. Assessment of left ventricular function	+	–	+	+
5. Suitability in critically ill patients	–	–	–	+
6. Assessment of coronary artery disease	+	–	–	+/–

performed within 15 min of test request in patients with a possible aortic dissection (Table 11-9).[66] Kotler et al. found most patients with aortic dissection can successfully undergo TEE; those who were unable to undergo TEE examination were too unstable to undergo other diagnostic investigations as well. In this subgroup of patients mortality approached 100 percent. TEE yields information concerning wall motion, presence of pericardial effusion or tamponade, valvular disease, and the presence and extent of aortic regurgitation as well as the location of the entry site as shown in Fig. 11-6A and B. These advantages are summarized in Table 11-8. Aortic regurgitation is present in 50 percent of proximal and 10 percent of descending thoracic aortic dissections. The diagnosis and quantitation of the severity of aortic regurgitation is easily obtained with TEE using color Doppler (Fig., 11-12). TEE is more sensitive than aortography as it detects mild aortic regurgitation not evident by angiography.[67,68] TEE can also demonstrate the causes of aortic regurgitation which facilitates surgical repair. Possible etiologies of aortic regurgitation in patients with aortic dissection include (1) dilatation or aneurysm formation of the ascending aorta, (2) thickening of the aortic leaflets, (3) prolapse of one of the aortic cusps (Fig. 11-10A–C), and (4) prolapse of the dissection flap into the aortic valve orifice or the left ventricular outflow tract (Fig. 11-11A–C).

TABLE 11-9   Average Length of Time (in Minutes) Required to Complete Study in Patients Suspected of Aortic Dissection*

	Time, min
TEE	15
XCT	35
MRI	48
Aortography	60

*Cedars-Sinai Medical Center experience.

Figure 11-10
Dissection longitudinal
view originating at the sinuses of Valsalva. (*A*) A
systolic image shows a
"double-barrel" aortic lumen. (*B*) In diastole the
intimal flap prolapses,
creating a "triple-barrel"
aortic lumen. In addition
the right aortic valve
leaflet (arrow) prolapses
into the LV outflow
tract, resulting in severe
aortic regurgitation.

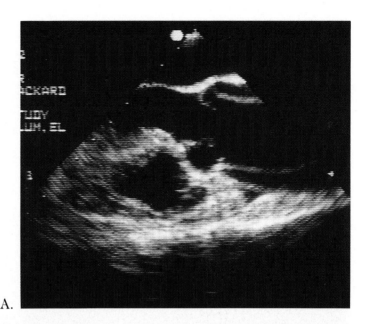

A.

B.

The Use of Other Imaging Modalities in the Diagnosis of Aortic Dissection

Aortography

Aortography has traditionally been considered the diagnostic test of choice in the detection of aortic dissection.[54] Although angiography can be used reliably to detect dissections, it can no longer be considered to be the "gold standard," owing to a sensitivity of only 92 percent.[71] With contrast aortography the detection of aortic dissection is primarily based on direct or indirect findings, with the demonstration of false lumen in 87 percent of cases, intimal flaps in 70 percent, and the site of the intimal tear in only 56 percent of patients.[2]

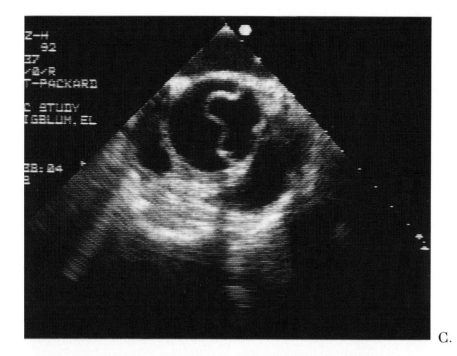

C.

Figure 11-10
(*Continued*)
(*C*) A short-axis view of
the aorta at this level
demonstrates the com-
plex three-dimensional
geometry of the flap.

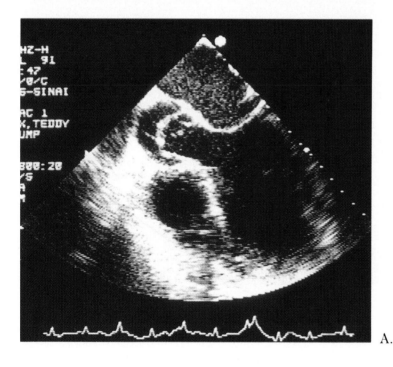

A.

Figure 11-11
Aortic insufficiency due
to prolapse of intimal
flap; five-chamber view.
(*A*) In systole the aortic
valve opens and the inti-
mal flap moves cepha-
lad.

Furthermore, angiography is associated with a significant potential risk of extending the dissection due to catheter placement in the false lumen. Angiography does not permit direct visualization of thrombus in the false lumen. When the false lumen is completely thrombosed, it cannot be opacified by contrast angiography. Angiography, however, can delineate arterial side branches and coronary arterial anatomy, the presence and extent of aortic insufficiency, as well as left ventricular function. However, a recent study by Kotler et al. found that almost 15 percent of patients with aortic dissection were unable to undergo angio-

Figure 11-11
(*Continued*)
(*B*) In diastole the intimal flap (arrow) prolapses through the aortic valve into the LV outflow tract and prevents leaflet closure. (*C*) Color Doppler demonstrates the severe aortic regurgitation resulting from prolapsing intimal flap into the aortic valve orifice.

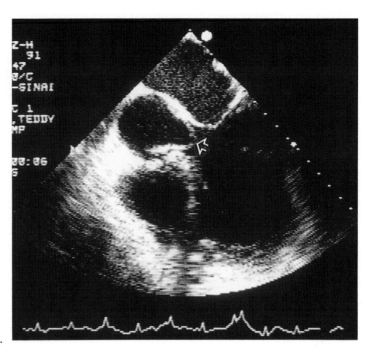

B.

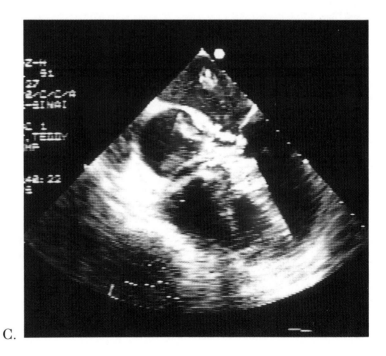

C.

graphy because of the inability to obtain arterial access or the clinical instability of the patient.[72–74]

Computerized Tomography

Computerized tomography (CT) yields descriptive information similar to that of angiography, but CT has the advantage of being noninvasive and offers additional information regarding mediastinal disease.[75–79] However, CT is not feasible in unstable patients who cannot be moved out of the intensive care unit. CT has limited resolution for identifying mobile structures such as intimal flaps, which are detected in

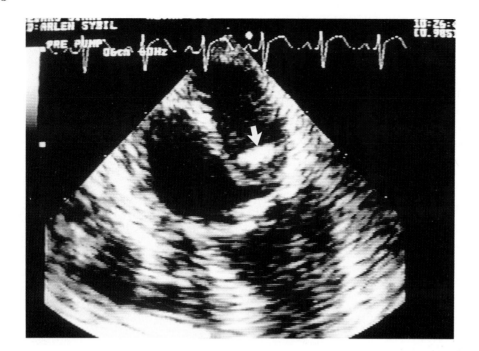

Figure 11-12
Iatrogenic aortic dissection caused by insertion of an intraaortic balloon pump. The distal tip (arrow) of the balloon counterpulsation catheter is shown by TEE in the false lumen.

only 65 to 70 percent of cases. CT does not usually provide information about the site of entry or intimal tear and does not identify the degree of aortic regurgitation. The European Cooperative Study on aortic dissection concluded that CT has a specificity of 100 percent and a sensitivity of only 83 percent. The study of Ballal et al. found CT to be only 90 percent sensitive. These studies indicate that in patients with a negative CT scan, other diagnostic tests should be performed if there is clinical suspicion of aortic dissection.[75–79] Recent advances in CT using ultrafast CT improve the spatial resolution of CT imaging. Thus ultrafast CT may have an improved sensitivity over standard CT for aortic dissection.

Magnetic Resonance Imaging

MRI has been reported to have a sensitivity of 98 percent and specificity of 99 percent in the diagnosis of aortic dissection.[80–82] MRI is useful for identifying the presence of an intimal flap, the false lumen, branch artery occlusion, the severity of aortic regurgitation, left ventricular function, and the presence of a pericardial effusion. MRI may be the imaging method of choice in patients with chronic, stable aortic dissection. However, unlike TEE, MRI is less suited for unstable or critically ill patients because of the difficulty in monitoring patients and the time it takes to perform the study. About 15 percent of patients with aortic dissection cannot undergo MRI testing owing to the requirement for mechanical ventilation, or the presence of prosthetic Bjork-Shiley valves, permanent pacemakers, or automatic implantable cardiac defibrillators (Table 11-10).[78–82]

TABLE 11-10   Contraindications to the Use of MRI[78–81]

Patients with:

1. Pacemakers

2. AICD

3. Bjork-Shiley and Starr Edwards cardiac valves

4. Aneurysm and hemostatic clips

5. Swan-Ganz catheter

6. Cochlear implants

7. Bullets or shrapnel

Other Advantages of TEE in Aortic Dissection

TEE holds an additional advantage over other diagnostic modalities, as it lends itself to be used in the intraoperative setting. TEE is now routinely used intra- and postoperatively to assess the integrity of the aortic graft and to detect residual flow signals in the false lumen. In addition, TEE may identify suspected aortic dissection as shown in Fig. 11-12 in a patient in whom dissection was iatrogenically produced during insertion of an intraaortic balloon pump. The absence of false lumen blood flow after surgery indicates successful closure of the true and false lumen communication, reducing the risk of aortic rupture, and thereby improving prognosis and a higher survival rate of 90 percent.[83–85] Figure 11-13 is a TEE image of an intramural hematoma that is not identifiable by angiography. This is an important diagnosis, as intramural hematoma has a high risk of rupture. With TEE the number of patients with aortic dissection who have also been found to have pericardial effusion has increased to 20 percent as compared with the 10 percent reported by TTE, probably because of the 10 percent higher resolution of TEE. Similarly because of the excellent resolution, wall motion abnormalities in patients with aortic dissection are readily identified.

Limitations of TEE

TEE is a minimally invasive procedure but has some potential risks which are described in Chap. 3. As with all procedures, results and interpretation are influenced by the technical adequacy of the study. Further visualization of cardiac structures can be suboptimal in patients with abnormal anatomic relationships of the esophagus and stomach with the aorta. In addition, the presence of esophagogastric disease limits the use of TEE for evaluation of the aorta.

TEE in Aortic Atheromatosis

Up to 40 percent of patients with stroke have no identifiable etiology.[86–89] Atherosclerotic

Figure 11-13
Rupture of the descending aorta into the pleural cavity: hematoma (arrow) is present in the aortic wall, which is approximately 1 cm thick. A hemorrhagic pleural effusion containing thrombus (asterisk) is present in the pleural space (A = aortic lumen).

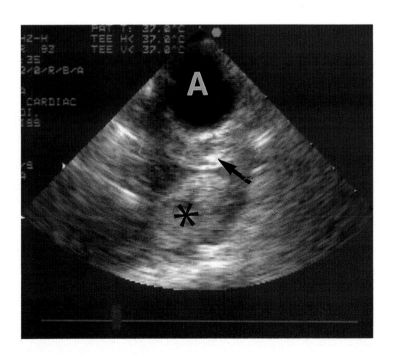

plaques protruding into the thoracic aorta have been reported to account for 1 percent of patients with otherwise unexplained strokes and 2 percent of arterial embolization.[86–89] Figure 11-14 demonstrates a dense plaque in the transverse aorta. Recently it has been found that ulcerated plaques in the aortic arch, as assessed by TEE, occur in up to 58 percent of patients with no known cause of stroke.[90] Thus ulcerated plaques in the aortic arch may play a more prominent role as a causative factor than previously thought. Furthermore, cerebral vascular accidents and peripheral emboli are significant and often devastating complications of cardiac surgery, with an incidence of 1 to 5 percent.[89,90] Gardner et al. found that the risk of stroke associated with cardiac surgery increased from 0.6 percent in 1979 to 2.4 percent in 1983.[91] This increase in the incidence of stroke is attributed to the increasing age of patients undergoing cardiac surgery. During cardiac surgery the ascending aorta is manipulated for cannulation, placement of the cross clamp, the anastomosis of bypass grafts to the aorta, and the infusion of cardioplegia. Such manipulations can result in the dislodgment of atheromatous material. Kouchoukos[93]

and others have shown that intraoperative TEE can be used to visualize and characterize the composition of the ascending aorta, thereby allowing the surgeon to identify potential sources of embolism.[92–94] Kouchoukos et al. performed TEE of the ascending aorta at the time of cardiac surgery in 100 consecutive patients.[95] They divided the ascending aorta into three segments. They graded the severity of atherosclerosis of the aorta as mild when intimal thickening was less than 3 mm and was localized to one segment, moderate when intimal thickening was greater than 3 mm and was present in one or two segments, and severe when intimal thickening was greater than 3 mm and was present throughout the entire circumference in all three segments. They found that 30 percent of the patients studied had normal aortic anatomy, 33 percent had mild atherosclerosis, 19 percent had moderate atherosclerosis, and 18 percent had severe atherosclerosis. By stepwise logistic regression analysis they showed age and the presence of diabetes to be significant independent predictors of the presence of atherosclerosis in the ascending aorta.[95] Kusukawa et al. studied 137 consecutive patients between the

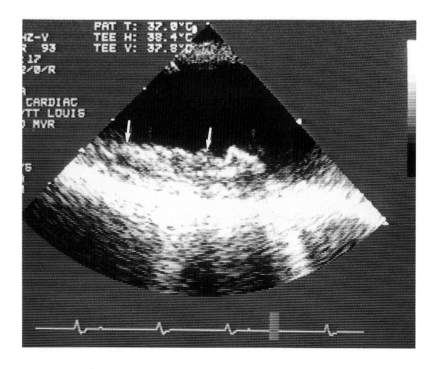

Figure 11-14
An extensive atheromatous plaque is present in the descending aorta.

ages of 49 and 69 with TEE of the thoracic aorta. They found a high incidence of atherosclerotic lesions in patients with hypertension (72 percent), hypercholesterolemia (57 percent), and coronary artery disease (57 percent). They concluded that hypertension, elevated cholesterol, and coronary artery disease are important risk factors for atherosclerosis in the thoracic aorta.[96] Since the aorta, especially the thoracic aorta, can be visualized with great detail, TEE is increasingly applied to evaluate the extent of aortic atherosclerosis. Aortic atherosclerosis has clinical implications in the development of strokes, TIA, and peripheral emboli. Spencer et al. have also developed a grading system for atheromatous disease of the aorta by TEE:[98]

Grade I = minimal intimal thickening
Grade II = extensive intimal thickening
Grade III = sessile atheroma
Grade IV = protruding atheroma
Grade V = mobile atheroma

Grade IV and V lesions carry an almost fourfold increase in risk of peripheral embolization. During coronary artery bypass grafting, these patients demonstrated a 23 to 25 percent incidence of stroke, with 15 percent early mortality. Figure 11-15 shows a mobile plaque in the aortic arch. This patient developed a cerebral vascular accident after aortocoronary bypass surgery. Thus TEE can be successfully used to evaluate the thoracic aorta for protruding atheromas and to assess patients with an unexplained source of embolic strokes, TIA, and peripheral emboli. Furthermore, TEE can be used to assess the risk of stroke from an aortic source in patients undergoing bypass surgery. Patients with grades IV and V protruding atheromas defined by TEE carry the highest risk,[97,98] and surgical resection of these atheromas or alterations in aortic manipulation and cannulation may reduce stroke risk.

Future Directions

With the advent of omniplane and higher-resolution biplane probes three-dimensional reconstruction of the aorta and cardiac structures will soon be possible. Three-dimensional reconstructed images may provide more accurate depiction of the aortic pathology for successful surgical or medical intervention.

Figure 11-15
A highly mobile protruding plaque (arrow) is shown in the aortic arch. Such plaques have a greater risk of embolization than nonmobile plaques.

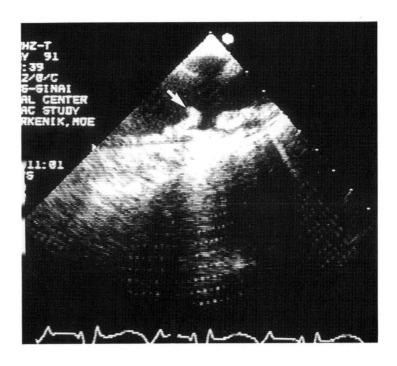

Conclusion

TEE is increasingly used as the procedure of choice for the diagnosis and assessment of aortic dissection as well as aortic atheromatosis. TEE is a safe procedure that can be performed in awake outpatients, in critically ill patients in an ICU or ER, as well as in an intraoperative setting. The outcome of aortic dissection is dependent on the rapidity and accuracy of diagnosis. Based on these factors, we believe TEE to be the initial diagnostic test of choice for aortic dissection. In the setting of aortic dissection TEE is useful for assessing the cause and severity of associated aortic insufficiency, proximal coronary artery involvement, detecting thrombi in the nonperfusing lumen, identifying communications between false and true lumen, assessing the presence and severity of pericardial fluid, and immediately evaluating the adequacy of surgical repair. At present TEE is the most definitive diagnostic modality for aortic atheromatosis. The identification of aortic atheromatosis is likely to reduce morbidity due to aortic manipulation and cannulation during cardiovascular surgery, as well as provide a definitive diagnosis in patients with embolization due to atherosclerotic disease of the aorta.

References

1. Wolfe WJ, Moran JF: The evolution of medical and surgical management of aortic dissection. *Circulation* 56:503, 1977.
2. Cigarroa JE, Isselbacher EM, DeSanctis RW, et al: Diagnostic imaging in the evaluation of suspected aortic dissection: Old standards and new directions. *N Engl J Med* 328:35, 1993.
3. Roberts WC: Aortic dissection: Anatomy, consequences and causes. *Am Heart J* 101:195, 1981.
4. Cooke JP, Safford RE: Progress in the diagnosis and management of aortic dissection. *Mayo Clin Proc* 61:147, 1986.
5. Yamada T, Tada S, Harada J: Aortic dissection without intimal rupture: Diagnosis with MR imaging and CT. *Radiology* 168:347, 1988.
6. Hasleton PS, Leonard JC: Dissecting aortic aneurysm: A clinicopathological study: II. Histopathology of the aorta. *Q J Med* 48:63, 1979.
7. Schlatman TJM, Becker AE: Pathogenesis of dissecting aneurysm of the aorta: Comparative histopathologic study of the significance of medical changes. *Am J Cardiol* 39:21, 1977.
8. Wheat MW Jr: Pathogenesis of aortic dissection, in Doroghazi RM, Slater EE (eds): *Aortic Dissection*, New York, McGraw-Hill, 1983, p 55.
9. Loeppky CB, Alpert MA, Hamel PC, et al: Extensive aortic dissection from combined-type cystic medial necrosis in a young man without predisposing factors. *Chest* 79:116, 1981.
10. McKusick VA, Logue RB, Bahnson HT: Association of aortic valvular disease and cystic medial necrosis of the ascending aorta; Report of four instances. *Circulation* 16:188, 1957.
11. Pumphrey CW, Fay T, Weir L: Aortic dissection during pregnancy. *Br Heart J* 55:106, 1986.
12. Williams GM, Gott VL, Brawley RK, et al: Aortic disease associated with pregnancy. *J Vasc Surg* 8:470, 1988.
13. Nicod P, Bloor C, Godfrey M, et al: Familial aortic dissecting aneurysm. *J Am Coll Cardiol* 13:811, 1989.
14. Lefemine AA, Kosowksy B, Madoff I, et al: Results and complications of intra-aortic balloon pumping in surgical and medical patients. *Am J Cardiol* 40:416, 1977.
15. Nicholson WJ, Crawley IS, Logue RB, et al: Aortic root dissection complicating coronary bypass surgery. *Am J Cardiol* 41:103, 1978.
16. Gadaleta D, Hall MH, Nelson RL: Cocaine induced acute aortic dissection. *Chest* 96:1203, 1989.
17. Barth CW III, Bray M, Roberts WC: Rupture of the ascending aorta during cocaine intoxication. *Am J Cardiol* 57:496, 1986.
18. DeBakey ME, Henly WS, Cooley DA, et al: Surgical management of dissecting aneurysm of the aorta. *J Thorac Cardiovasc Surg* 49:130, 1965.
19. Slater EE, DeSanctis RW: The clinical recognition of dissecting aortic aneurysm. *Am J Med* 60:625, 1976.
20. Erbel R, Oelert H, Meyer J, et al: New classification of aortic dissection by transesophageal echocardiography (abstract). *Circulation* 84 (suppl II):II-23, 1989.
21. Anagnostopoulos CE, Prabhakar MJS, Kittle

CF: Aortic dissections and dissecting aneurysm. *Am J Cardiol* 30:263, 1972.

22. Gurin D, Bulmer JW, Derby R: Dissecting aneurysms of the aorta. Diagnosis and operative relief of acute arterial obstructions due to this course. *NY State J Med* 35:1200, 1935.

23. Wheat MW Jr, Palmer RF, Barley TD, et al: Treatment of dissecting aneurysms of the aorta without surgery. *J Thorac Cardiovasc Surg* 50:364, 1965.

24. Slater EE: Aortic dissection: Presentation and diagnoses, in Doroghazi RM, Slater EE (eds): *Aortic Dissection*, New York, McGraw-Hill, 1983, p 61.

25. Slater EE, DeSanctis RW: The clinical recognition of dissecting aortic aneurysm. *Am J Med* 60:625, 1976.

26. Logue RB, Sikes C: New sign in dissecting aneurysm of the aorta: Pulsation of sternoclavicular joint. *JAMA* 148:1209, 1952.

27. Earnest F IV, Muhm JR, Sheedy PF: Roentgenographic findings in thoracic aortic dissection. *Mayo Clin Proc* 54:43, 1979.

28. Chan KL: Usefulness of transesophageal echocardiography in the conditions mimicking aortic dissection. *Am Heart J* 122:495, 1991.

29. Hanrath P, Schluter M, Langenstein BA, et al: Transesophageal horizontal and sagittal imaging of the heart with a phased array system: Initial clinical results, in Hanrath P, Bleifeld W, Souquet J (eds): *Cardiovascular Diagnosis by Ultrasound*, Boston, Martinus Nijhoff Publishers, 1982, pp 280–288.

30. Seward JB, Khandheria BK: Biplanar transesophageal echocardiography: Anatomic correlations, image orientation, and clinical applications. *Mayo Clin Proc* 65:1193, 1990.

31. Seward JB, Khanderia BK, Oh KJ, et al: Transesophageal echocardiography: Technique, anatomic correlations, implementation, and clinical applications. *Mayo Clin Proc* 63:649, 1988.

32. Ballal RS, Nanda NC, Gatewood RG, et al: Usefulness of transesophageal echocardiography in assessment of aortic dissection. *Circulation* 84:1903, 1991.

33. Erbel R, Engberding R, Daniel W, et al: Echocardiography in diagnosis of aortic dissection. *Lancet* 1:457, 1983.

34. Adachi H, Kyo S, Takamoto S, et al: Early diagnosis and surgical intervention of acute aortic dissection by transesophageal color flow mapping (abstract). *Circulation* 80 (suppl II): II-24, 1989.

35. Omoto R, Kyo S, Matsumura M, et al: Evaluation of biplane color doppler transesophageal echocardiography in 200 consecutive patients. *Circulation* 85:1237, 1992.

36. Mohr-Kahaly S, Erbel R, Steller D, et al: Aortic dissection detected by transesophageal echocardiography. *Int J Cardiac Imaging* 2:31, 1986.

37. Chan KL: Usefulness of transesophageal echocardiography in the diagnosis of conditions mimicking aortic dissection. *Am Heart J* 122:495, 1991.

38. Silvey S, Stoughton T, Pearl W, et al: Rupture of the outer partition of aortic dissection during transesophageal echocardiography. *Am J Cardiol* 68:286, 1991.

39. Iliceto S, Antonelli G, Biasco G, et al: Two-dimensional thoracic aorta. *Circulation* 5:1045, 1982.

40. Victor MF, Mintz GS, Kotler MN, et al: Two-dimensional echocardiographic diagnosis of aortic dissection. *Am J Cardiol* 48:1155, 1981.

41. Mathew T, Nanda NC: Two-dimensional and Doppler echocardiographic evaluation of aortic aneurysm and dissection. *Am J Cardiol* 54:379, 1984.

42. Iliceto S, Ettorre G, Francioso G, et al: Diagnosis of aneurysm of the thoracic aorta. Comparison between two noninvasive techniques: Two-dimensional echocardiography and computed tomography. *Eur Heart J* 5:545, 1988.

43. Kasper W, Meinertz T, Kersting F, et al: Diagnosis of dissecting aortic aneurysm with suprasternal echocardiography. *Am J Cardiol* 42:291, 1978.

44. Victor MF, Mintz GS, Kotler MN, et al: Two-dimensional echocardiographic diagnosis of aortic dissection. *Am J Cardiol* 48:1155, 1981.

45. Mathew T, Nanda NC: Two-dimensional and Doppler echocardiographic evaluation of aortic aneurysm and dissection. *Am J Cardiol* 54:379, 1984.

46. Dagli SV, Nanda NC, Roitman E, et al: Evaluation of aortic dissection by Doppler color flow mapping. *Am J Cardiol* 56:497, 1985.

47. Iliceto S, Nanda NC, Rizzon P, et al: Color Doppler evaluation of aortic dissection. *Circulation* 75:748, 1987.

48. Hashimoto S, Kumada T, Osakada G, et al: Assessment of transesophageal doppler echography in dissecting aortic aneurysm. *J Am Coll Cardiol* 14:1253, 1989.

49. Omoto R: *Color Atlas of Real-Time Two Di-*

mensional Doppler Echocardiography, 2d ed, Tokyo, Shindan-To-Chiryo, 1987, pp 80–112.

50. Takamoto S, Hojo H, Adachi H: Diagnosis of dissecting aortic aneurysm by transesophageal color flow mapping: Comparison with CT scanning, in Erbel R (ed): Transesophageal Echocardiography. Berlin, Springer-Verlag, 1989, pp 146–152.

51. Omoto R, Kyo S, Matsumura M: Recent technological progress in transesophageal color Doppler flow imaging with special reference to newly developed biplane and pediatric probe, in Erbel R (ed): Transesophageal Echocardiography, Berlin, Springer-Verlag, 1989, pp 21–26.

52. Miller DC, Mitchell RC, Oyer PE, et al: Independent determinants of operative mortality for patients with aortic dissections. Circulation 70 (suppl I):I-153, 1984.

53. Matuzaki M, Toma Y, Kusukawa R: Clinical applications of transesophageal echocardiography. Circulation 82:709, 1990.

54. Nanda NC, Gramiak R: Pericardial effusion, in Nanda NC, Gramiak R (eds): Clinical Echocardiography, St Louis, CV Mosby, 1978, p 268.

55. Miller DC, Stinson EB, Shumway NE: Realistic expectations of surgical treatment of aortic dissections: The Stanford experience. World J Surg 4:571, 1980.

56. Berga JJ, Yao JST: Aneurysms, Diagnosis and treatment, Newark, Grune and Stratton, 1982, p 105.

57. Ballal RS, Nanda NC, Gatewood R, et al: Usefulness of transesophageal echocardiography in assessment of aortic dissection. Circulation 84:1903, 1991.

58. Roberts WC: Aortic dissection: Anatomy, consequences and causes. Am Heart J 101:195, 1981.

59. Hirst AE, Johns VJ, Kime SW: Dissecting aneurysm of the aorta: A review of 505 cases. Medicine 37:217, 1958.

60. Oram S, Holt MC: Coronary involvement in dissecting aneurysm of the aorta. Br Heart J 12:10, 1950.

61. Debakey ME, McCollum CH, Crawford ES, et al: Dissection and dissecting aneurysms of the aorta: Twenty year follow-up of five hundred twenty seven patients treated surgically. Surgery 92:1118, 1982.

62. Jex RK, Schaff HV, Orszulak TA, et al: Repair of ascending aortic dissection: Influence of associated aortic valve insufficiency on early

and late results. J Thoraac Cardiovasc Surg 93:375, 1987.

63. Miller DC, Mitchell RC, Oyer PE, et al: Independent determinants of operative mortality for patients with aortic dissections. Circulation 70 (suppl I):I-153, 1984.

64. Svensson LG, Coselli JS, Safi HJ, et al: Aortic dissection: Improving surgical results (abstract). Circulation 80 (suppl):II-24, 1989.

65. Adachi H, Omoto R, Kyo S, et al: Emergency surgical intervention of acute dissection with the rapid diagnosis by transesophageal echocardiography. Circulation 84 (suppl III):III-14, 1991.

66. Kotler MN: Is transesophageal echocardiography the new standard for diagnosing dissecting aortic aneurysms? J Am Coll Cardiol 14:1263, 1989.

67. Ballal RS, Nanda NC, Gatewood R, et al: Usefulness of transesophageal echocardiography in assessment of aortic dissection. Circulation 84:1903, 1991.

68. Hunt D, Baxley WA, Kennedy JW, et al: Quantitative evaluation of cineaortography in the assessment of aortic regurgitation. Am J Cardiol 31:696, 1973.

69. Goldman AP, Kotler MN, Scanlon MH, et al: The complementary role of magnetic resonance imaging, Doppler echocardiography, and computed tomography in the diagnosis of dissecting thoracic aneurysms. Am Heart J 111:970, 1986.

70. Godwin JD, Breiman RS, Speckman JM: Problems and pitfalls in the evaluation of thoracic aortic dissection by computed tomography. J Comput Assist Tomogr 5:1045, 1982.

71. Wechsler RJ, Kotler MN, Steiner RM: Mutimodality approach to thoracic aortic dissection, in Kotler MN, Steiner RM (eds): Cardiac Imaging: New Technologies and Clinical Application. Cardiovascular Clinics, Philadelphia, FA Davis, 1986, p 385.

72. Goldman AP, Kotler MN, Scanlon M, et al: The role of non-invasive techniques in the diagnosis of dissecting thoracic aneurysms. Circulation 74 (suppl II):II-146, 1986.

73. Dinsmore RE, Rourke JA, DeSanctis RD, et al: Angiographic findings in dissecting aortic aneurysm. N Engl J Med 275:1152, 1966.

74. Soto B, Herman MA, Ceballos R, et al: Angiographic diagnosis of dissecting aneurysm of the aorta. Am J Roentgenol 116:146, 1972.

75. Moncada R, Salinas M, Churchill R: Diagnosis

of dissecting aortic aneurysms by computed tomography. *Lancet* I:238, 1981.

76. Thorsen MK, San Doetto MA, Lawson TL, et al: Dissecting aortic aneurysms: Accuracy of computed tomographic diagnosis. *Radiology* 148:773, 1983.

77. Larde D, Bellor C, Vasile N, et al: Computed tomography in dissection of the thoracic aorta. *Radiology* 136:147, 1980.

78. Heiberg E, Wolverson M, Sundaram M, et al: CT findings in aortic dissection. *AJR* 136:13-7, 1981.

79. Godwin JD, Herfkens Skioldebrand CG, Feder le MP, et al: Evaluation of dissection and aneurysms of the thoracic aorta by conventional and dynamic CT scanning. *Radiology* 136:125, 1980.

80. Amparo G, Higgins CB, Hricack H, et al: Aortic dissection: Magnetic resonance imaging. *Radiology* 155:399, 1985.

81. Geisinger MA, Risius B, O'Connel JA: Thoracic aortic dissections: Magnetic resonance imaging. *Radiology* 155:407, 1985.

82. Goldman AP, Kotler MN, Scanlon MH, et al: Magnetic resonance imaging and two dimensional echocardiography: Alternative approach to aortography in diagnosis of aortic dissecting aneurysm. *Am J Med* 80:1225, 1986.

83. Mohr-Kahaly S, Erbel R, Rennollet H, et al: Ambulatory follow-up of aortic dissection by transesophageal two-dimensional and color-coded Doppler echocardiography. *Circulation* 80:24, 1989.

84. Guthaner DF, Miller DC, Silverman JF, et al: Fate of the false lumen following surgical repair of aortic dissections: An angiographic study. *Radiology* 133:1, 1979.

85. Heinemann M, Laas J, Haverich A, et al: Fate of the descending aorta after operation for acute aortic dissection type A. Follow-up and indication for replacement (abstract). *J Thorac Cardiovasc Surg* 36(suppl 1):85, 1980.

86. Perez JE: Non invasive diagnosis, in Doroghazi RM, Slater EE (eds): *Aortic Dissection*, New York, McGraw-Hill, 1983, p 133.

87. Tunick PA, Kronzon I: Protruding atherosclerotic plaque in the aortic arch of patients with systemic embolization: A new finding seen by transesophageal echocardiography. *Am Heart J* 120:658, 1990.

88. Karalis DG, Chandrasekaran K, Victor MF, et al: The recognition and embolic potential of intra aortic atherosclerotic debris. *Circulation* 82 (suppl):III-246, 1990.

89. Simon AJ, Carlson R, Hare CL, et al: The use of transesophageal echocardiography in detecting aortic atherosclerosis in patients with embolic disease. *Am Heart J* 123:224, 1992.

90. Coy KM, Maurer G, Goodman D, et al: Transesophageal echocardiographic detection of aortic atheromatosis that provides clues to occult renal dysfunction in the elderly. *Am Heart J* 123:1684, 1992.

91. Gardner TJ, Horneffer PJ, Manolio TA, et al: Stroke following coronary artery bypass grafting: A ten year study. *Ann Thorac Surg* 48:574, 1985.

92. Barzilai B, Saffitz JE, Miller JG, et al: Quantitative ultrasonic characterization of the nature of atherosclerotic plaques in human aorta. *Cir Res* 659:459, 1987.

93. Marshall WG, Barzilai B, Kouchoukos NT, et al: Intraoperative ultrasonic imaging of the ascending aorta. *Ann Thorac Surg* 48:339, 1989.

94. Hosoda Y, Watanabe M, Hirooka Y, et al: Significance of atherosclerotic changes of the ascending aorta during coronary bypass surgery with intraoperative detection by echography. *J Cardiovasc Surg* 32:310, 1991.

95. Davila-Roman VG, Barzilai B, Wareing TH, et al: Intraoperative ultrasonographic evaluation of the ascending aorta in 100 consecutive patients undergoing cardiac surgery. *Circulation* 84(suppl III):III-47, 1991.

96. Ono S, Matsuzaki M, Michishige H, et al: Estimation of atherosclerotic lesions in the thoracic aorta by transesophageal echocardiography. *J Cardiology* (Japanese) suppl 26:57, 1991.

97. Ribakove GH, Katz ES, Galloway AC, et al: Surgical implications of transesophageal echocardiography to grade the atheromatous aortic arch. *Ann Thorac Surg* 53:758, 1992.

98. Katz ES, Tunick PA, Rusinek H, et al: Protruding aortic atheromas predict stroke in elderly patients undergoing cardiopulmonary bypass: Experience with intraoperative transesophageal echocardiography. *J Am Coll Cardiol* 20:70, 1992.

99. Nienaber CA, Von Kodolitsh Y, Nicolas V, et al: The diagnosis of thoracic aortic dissection by noninvasive imaging procedures. *N Engl J Med* 328:1, 1993.

12

Transesophageal Echocardiography during Catheter Interventions

Shunei Kyo
Ryozo Omoto
Takeshi Mototyama
Naomasa Miyamoto
Toshiki Kobayashi
Kazuyuki Koike
Jui-Sung Hung

Introduction

Transesophageal echocardiography (TEE)[1,2] has been increasingly applied in various clinical settings as a potent and rapid diagnostic tool for valvular, congenital, and ischemic heart disease[3–6] as well as cardiovascular disease including acute aortic dissection[7] and cerebral stroke due to intracardiac thrombus.[8] Its clinical utility was first recognized as an intraoperative monitoring method for cardiac function by anesthesiologists;[1] however, TEE has been accepted more widely by cardiologists and cardiac surgeons as an intraoperative diagnostic tool for mitral valvuloplasty[9] and a rapid diagnostic tool for acute aortic dissection in emergency[10] after color flow mapping was incorporated into TEE.

Transcatheter therapy for many different types of acquired and congenital heart disease has been well developed and established in the past three decades.[11–14] Almost all techniques employed for transcatheter therapy have been performed under fluoroscopic monitoring in the cardiac catheterization laboratory. However, in some specific situations, echocardiographic monitoring has been employed as a guiding tool instead of fluoroscopy for catheter interventions, usually in the intensive care unit in an emergency setting when fluoroscopic monitoring is not available.[15–17]

The effectiveness of echocardiographically assisted balloon atrial septostomy was first reported by Perry et al. in 1982,[15] and currently most of these procedures are performed in the neonatal ICU simply with transthoracic or

215

transesophageal echo guidance without fluoroscopic monitoring. In some other situations echocardiographic monitoring has been employed to make the procedure of catheter interventions easier and safer even when combined with fluoroscopic monitoring in the cardiac catheterization laboratory.[18,19]

Transseptal cardiac catheterization was developed in 1960 by Brockenbrough and Braunwald,[20] and complications associated with the transseptal puncture procedure have been reported as relatively rare in experienced hands; however, overall mortality of this procedure was reported as 1 case out of 1500 procedures.[21]

Kronzon and Glassman[19] reported clinical effectiveness of transthoracic echo monitoring during transseptal puncture, but also pointed out its limitation as a guiding tool. The poor quality of echocardiograms prevented demonstration of the relation between the needle tip and the interatrial septum in 15 to 27 percent of studied cases and did not allow definite identification of the needle tip position.

Percutaneous transvenous mitral commissurotomy (PTMC) is one of the alternative therapeutic procedures for mitral stenosis. Inoue[12] recommended performing PTMC using echocardiographic guidance for the selection of appropriate balloon size and for evaluation of the effect of balloon dilation on the mitral

valve area, therefore avoiding creation of severe mitral regurgitation (more than Sellers grade 3) using a step-by-step dilatation technique. However, it is not easy to examine mitral valve function in terms of measurement of mitral valve area and the evaluation of mitral regurgitation, because the patient is covered with sterile cloths, and is in a supine position that is unfavorable for the transthoracic echo. Moreover, echo image and Doppler flow signals obtained by the transthoracic approach cannot always provide adequate information for the evaluation of mitral valve area and regurgitation. Currently, after the development of color flow mapping technique[9], intraoperative echo monitoring is indispensable for the surgical mitral valvuloplasty.

After intraoperative direct scanning with color flow mapping (epicardial echo) was introduced to the operating room in 1984,[22] transesophageal color flow mapping has gradually taken over the role of intraoperative monitoring[3] because of the convenience for the surgeon and because of advances in TEE technology, such as development of biplane and pediatric TEE probes. As an extension of the intraoperative application, TEE monitoring during catheter interventions[23] started in 1990 in Saitama Medical School (Fig. 12-1) and also in the United States.[24] In this chapter the utility of

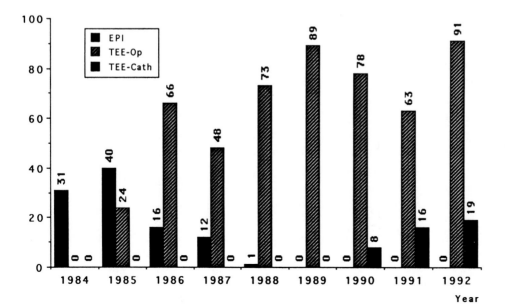

Figure 12-1
Intraoperative echo examinations from 1984 to 1992 in Saitama Medical School. Intraoperative application of epicardial echo (EPI) started in 1984, transesophageal echo during surgery (TEE-Op) in 1985, and during catheter interventions (TEE-Cath) in 1990.

clinical application of intraoperative TEE and its effects during catheter interventions are described.

Intraoperative TEE during Percutaneous Transvenous Mitral Commissurotomy (PTMC)

Inoue et al. developed a special balloon catheter for nonsurgical mitral commissurotomy, and reported the first clinical application of the technique as "transvenous mitral commissurotomy" in 1982;[25] later they renamed this technique "percutaneous transvenous mitral commissurotomy (PTMC)."[12] This technique has gained worldwide acceptance and prevails as an effective method for the treatment of mitral stenosis. However, an accompanying complication rate of 6 percent of development of severe mitral regurgitation greater than Sellers grade 3 has been reported.[26]

The National Heart, Lung, and Blood Institute balloon valvuloplasty registry[27] reported 12 percent serious complication, 1.6 percent procedure-related death, and 1.6 percent in-hospital death more than 24 h after the procedure in 738 patients. Although several valvuloplasty techniques were used in this study, transseptal puncture was performed on all 738 patients. Twenty-nine patients (4 percent) required emergency cardiac surgery including 27 patients (4 percent) with cardiac tamponade due to cardiac perforation. The transseptal puncture is usually performed with x-ray guidance, but this technique is not always easy and safe, because of the difficulty in achieving three-dimensional orientation of the anatomical structure of the cardiac cavities, especially for the less experienced operator. Mitral regurgitation relating to this method has been evaluated by transthoracic echocardiography in most institutes, but the supine position of the patients prevents good imaging in some cases, making effective echo examination difficult; moreover the echo examination itself may interfere with the sterile field.

TEE has been reported to be a very effective intraoperative monitoring method during surgical mitral valvuloplasty, because of the good echo penetration to the heart from the esophageal echo window that is just next to the left atrium (LA), and because of its ability to obtain a precise pathology of the mitral valve and mitral valve flow dynamics. Therefore, it seems reasonable to introduce the TEE technique as an intraoperative monitoring method during PTMC (Fig. 12-2). Orihashi et al.,[28] Inoue's coworkers, first reported the clinical use of TEE monitoring during PTMC, and observed all PTMC procedures with the exception of the Brockenbrough transseptal puncture. They found that an entire view of the catheter was rather difficult in a single picture since the plane of the scanning was not always identical to that of the catheter plane.

We first reported the use of biplane TEE as a guiding method for Brockenbrough transseptal puncture during PTMC,[23] and confirmed the effectiveness of the longitudinal plane guiding the Brockenbrough needle approaching the atrial septum since the plane of the scanning was easily adjustable to that of the catheter plane (Fig. 12-3). Also, at the time of transseptal puncture the needle tip position on the septum can be confirmed precisely using orthogonal biplane images of TEE. The confirmation technique is to push up the septum slightly with small force and to observe the so-called tent formation of the septum by biplane TEE. To observe the tent formation simultaneously in both orthogonal biplane images, the matrix-biplane TEE technology is preferable, because both images can be monitored simultaneously as a side-by-side image on the monitor (Fig. 12-4).

From March 1990 to November 1991, we performed PTMC on 23 patients with mitral stenosis (male = 8, female = 15, mean age = 50.3 ± 10.6 years old) with guidance of matrix-biplane TEE monitoring. PTMC was performed in patients without mitral regurgitation greater than Sellers grade 2 by angiography and without thrombus in the left atrium. Prior to PTMC patients were kept fasting for at least 6 h and premedication was performed with intravenous butylscopolamine (20 mg). Also, the throat was

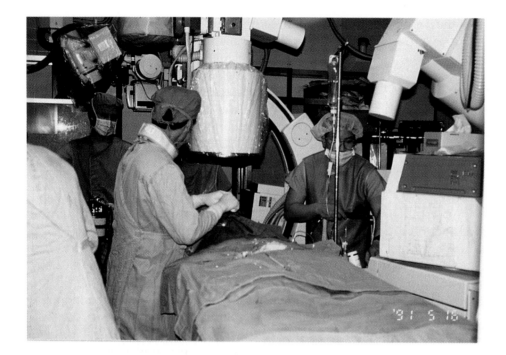

Figure 12-2
Intraoperative TEE monitoring during catheter intervention (PTMC). The TEE examiner and TEE system including the TEE probe do not interfere with the catheter operator in any step of the procedure during PTMC.

treated with local anesthesia (lidocaine viscous and aerosol) before the PTMC procedure. After the pre-PTMC angiographic and hemodynamic study was finished, the TEE probe was introduced, with cooperation of the supine patients, who were mildly sedated with intravenous diazepam (5 to 10 mg). During PTMC the sedation was maintained with intermittent IV diazepam (total 20 mg including the initial dose). A right atriogram was obtained in 2 patients prior to Brockenbrough transseptal puncture; however, in the latter 21 patients the right atriography was eliminated after we confirmed the utility of TEE as a guiding

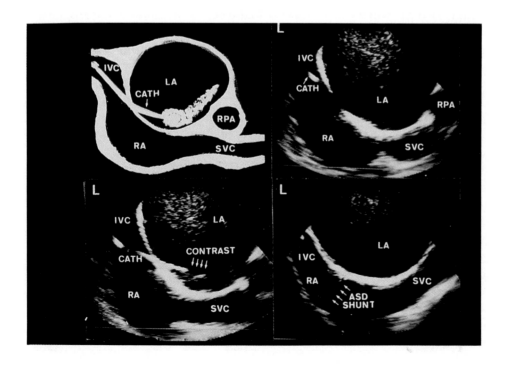

Figure 12-3
The longitudinal image plane of the Brockenbrough needle approaching the atrial septum. The right upper contrast echo is useful (left lower panel). Post-PTMC ASD shunt flow is seen in all patients (right lower panel).

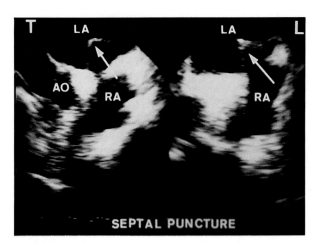

Figure 12-4
Matrix-biplane TEE images of the atrial septum where the Brockenbrough needle is positioned for transseptal puncture in both orthogonal planes. The side-by-side real-time image is a very effective guide for the safe transseptal puncture.

method for transseptal puncture. After introduction of a guidewire into the right atrium, a Brockenbrough needle was inserted into the right atrium. Almost the entire image of the needle tip and its excursion could be visualized clearly in the longitudinal image plane of TEE in 100 percent of the patients, but in only 3 patients (13 percent) in the transverse plane,

demonstrating the importance of the longitudinal plane for this procedure. In all 23 patients monitored by matrix-biplane TEE, the "tent formation of the septum" was clearly demonstrated in the side-by-side biplane image on the screen at the time of transseptal puncture.

Our policy for PTMC was a step-by-step dilatation method (Fig. 12-5), as recommended by Inoue, to avoid the creation of severe mitral regurgitation. The average dilation time was 2.4 ± 1.2 (1 to 5) times in this series. After each dilatation procedure the mitral valve orifice was measured and the grade of mitral regurgitation was evaluated by TEE. The mitral valve orifice was increased from 7.0 ± 2.7 to 11.2 ± 4.3 mm (longitudinal split) in the transverse image plane and from 9.8 ± 3.8 to 15.3 ± 5.2 mm in the longitudinal image plane (transverse split) (Fig. 12-6). The mitral valve area as obtained by pressure half-time method using high pulse-repetition-frequency interrogation of mitral valve flow was increased from 1.2 ± 0.4 to 2.0 ± 0.7 cm^2, and that obtained by the Gorlin formula was increased from 1.1 ± 0.3 to 2.3 ± 1.1 cm^2, respectively. In each balloon dilatation the grade of MR was accurately and promptly evaluated by TEE (Fig. 12-7). The grade of mitral regurgitation remained unchanged in 18 patients; however, in 5 patients

Figure 12-5
X-ray image of step-by-step dilatation of mitral valve using Inoue's balloon catheter; the balloon size was increased from 23 to 26 mm. In this case PTMC procedure was monitored using standard biplane TEE probe.

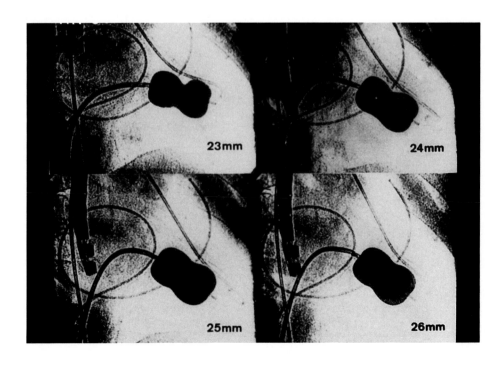

Length of Longitudinal Split

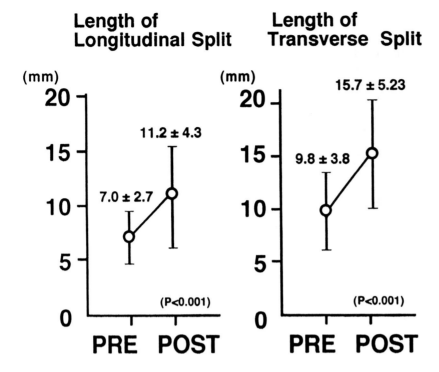

(mm)

11.2 ± 4.3

7.0 ± 2.7

(P<0.001)

PRE   POST

Length of Transverse Split

(mm)

15.7 ± 5.23

9.8 ± 3.8

(P<0.001)

PRE   POST

Figure 12-6
Intraoperative evaluation of longitudinal and transverse splits of mitral valve orifice by matrix-biplane TEE. Increase in mitral valve orifice in both image planes are significant after PTMC.

new mitral regurgitation or increase of mitral regurgitation was observed; MR increased to grade 2 in 3 patients and grade 1 in 2 patients (Fig. 12-8).

After PTMC, shunt flows through the interatrial septum were observed in all patients; one shunt flow was observed in 22 patients who had only one transseptal puncture by Brockenbrough needle, and two shunt flows were observed in 1 patient in whom transseptal puncture had been performed twice. Only in 3 patients was a significant shunt flow

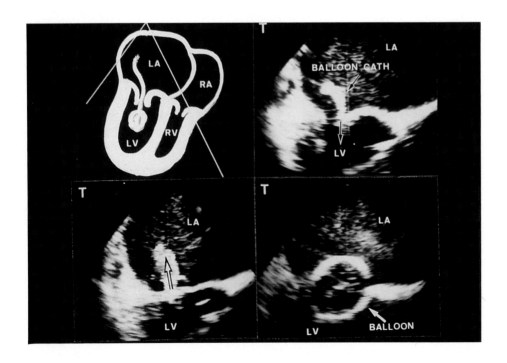

Figure 12-7
Intraoperative evaluation of transesophageal echocardiograms during PTMC. Inoue's balloon catheter was introduced into the left ventricle (right upper panel); then the balloon was dilated (right lower panel). After the first dilatation a small MR jet was detected, but it was judged as less than grade 1.

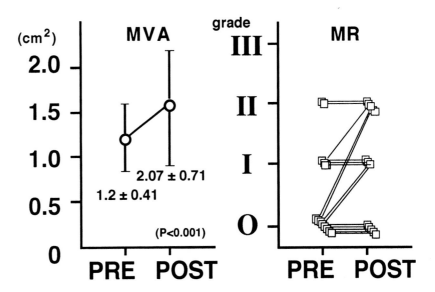

Figure 12-8
Intraoperative evaluation of mitral valve area (MVA) and mitral regurgitation (MR) by matrix-biplane TEE. For the evaluation of MVA, the pressure half-time method was used with high PRF Doppler.

(Qp/Qs > 1.2) observed hemodynamically. The endpoint of the PTMC procedure was to obtain an adequate mitral valve area or increase of the mitral regurgitation up to grade 2. Then the TEE probe was removed from the patients and post-PTMC angiography and hemodynamic study were performed. The usual duration of transesophageal intubation was 30 to 40 min.

The technical difficulty of the intraoperative TEE monitoring during PTMC is the main limitation, also the patient's throat discomfort due to the placement of the TEE probe for about 30 min. On the other hand, intraoperative TEE guidance and monitoring have definite advantages, such as safe introduction of the Inoue balloon catheter into the left atrium, the transseptal puncture, avoidance of creation of severe mitral regurgitation, and ability to evaluate the mitral valve orifice. Therefore, whether we can monitor the patients successfully by TEE depends on the technique of patient management during PTMC.

The effective local anesthesia of the throat and the repeated suction of the secretions from the oral cavity are most important. A deeply sedated condition does not seem favorable unless the patient is intubated, because of the high possibility of aspiration in the supine position. We kept the patients mildly sedated with intermittent low dose of intravenous diazepam during the procedure. All patients in this series had experienced TEE examinations several times prior to PTMC in the outpatient echo laboratory. They understood the TEE procedure and the clinical advantage of TEE monitoring during PTMC.

Another important point is the advancement of TEE technology. We can obtain orthogonal biplane images in real time with side-by-side display on the TV screen; therefore, there is no need to change the position of the TEE probe to observe both planes, which makes the examination time shorter and lessens patient discomfort. Moreover, we can easily obtain the three-dimensional orientation of the anatomy of the heart and intracardiac flow dynamics, which is quite advantageous as to guide the PTMC procedure. With a skillful TEE examiner and the most advanced technology, TEE can be a reasonable monitoring method during PTMC and we believe that it actually improves its clinical outcome.

Left Atrial Cannulation for Percutaneous Left-Heart Bypass with Biplane TEE Guiding

Percutaneous cardiopulmonary support (PCPS) is one recent advance of mechanical assist circulation systems[30] used for circulatory support of high-risk patients during coronary angioplasty and during cardiopulmonary resuscitation. Although the advantage of PCPS support is well understood, venoarterial bypass support by PCPS has a strong limitation for patients with severe left ventricular failure because of the limitation of the bypass flow rate and left ventricular unloading. Theoretically left-heart bypass support is considered more effective for left-heart failure, but percutaneous approach to the left heart is not easy nor safe, especially in the intensive care unit (ICU) without x-ray monitoring facility.

Dennis et al.[31] developed a percutaneous left-heart bypass system (AAB = left atrioarterial bypass), but their system never gained acceptance and did not have widespread clinical application until recently. We[23,29,32] and other researchers[24] demonstrated the usefulness of the TEE guidance for Brockenbrough transseptal puncture during PTMC, and the same transseptal puncture technique can be applied for the introduction of left atrial cannula for the percutaneous AAB. We have developed a special left atrial drainage cannula (Fig. 12-9) for AAB that can be easily introduced into the left atrium with the same technique used for the introduction of the Inoue PTMC catheter into the left atrium with biplane TEE guidance.[29,32]

In our first report three clinical cases supported by our system were described; in all three patients, the LA cannula was successfully introduced without any difficulty under TEE guidance. AAB was successfully weaned off in two patients after 94 h and 30 min of mechanical circulatory support. Figure 12-10 shows another cardiogenic shock patient supported by our AAB system. The patient had been supported by intraaortic balloon pumping for about 1 month and finally developed severe congestive heart failure and acute renal failure. Immediately after presentation to us, we introduced an 18 French left atrial cannula under TEE guidance and AAB support was started with 3.0 liters/min of bypass flow. Three days later congestive heart failure was no longer present and renal function recovered.

The major advantage of TEE guidance for the introduction of an LA cannula is that AAB support can be set up even without x-ray monitoring. In severe cases of cardiac failure the patients cannot be transferred to the catheterization laboratory for setup of AAB; therefore, it may be preferable to set up the AAB system under biplane TEE guidance in the ICU or the emergency room.

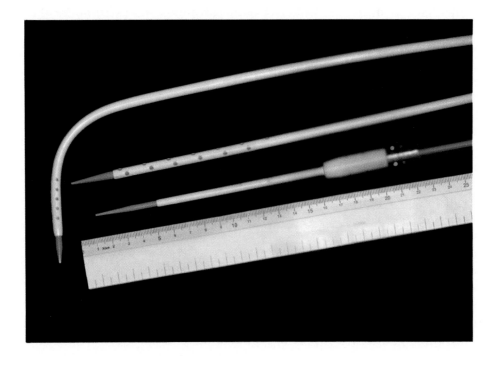

Figure 12-9
Cannulas used for percutaneous cardiopulmonary bypass (PCPS). The upper angulated cannula is a left atrial cannula (18 French), the middle straight cannula is a right atrial cannula (18 French), and the small straight cannula on the bottom is a femoral arterial cannula (14 French).

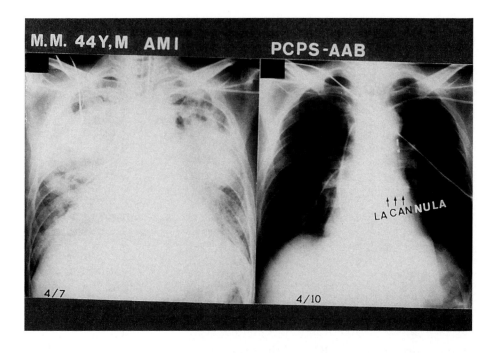

Transcatheter Therapy for Congenital Heart Disease with TEE Guidance

Balloon Atrial Septostomy

Transcatheter therapy for many different congenital heart defects has been performed by pediatric cardiologists. Almost all transcatheter techniques employ fluoroscopic image monitoring in the cardiac catheterization laboratory. However, in some specific situations echocardiographic monitoring has been used as a guiding tool for catheter interventions instead of fluoroscopy.[15–17] The effectiveness of echocardiographically assisted balloon atrial septostomy was first reported by Perry et al.[15] in 1982, and currently this procedure is performed most often in the neonatal ICU simply with transthoracic or transesophageal echocardiographic guidance without fluoroscopic monitoring.

Echocardiography is very effective to confirm the position of the balloon in the LA, for the selection of appropriate balloon size, and for evaluation of the size and flow dynamics of the enlarged ASD. Therefore, we can effectively avoid serious complications relating to the BAS procedure, such as rupture of chordae tendinae, rupture of tricuspid or mitral valve leaflet, or rupture of the inferior vena cava.[33] Usually transthoracic echocardiography is an adequate guiding tool for BAS; however, TEE can be the method of choice in some settings. For continuous monitoring of cardiac function during BAS, TEE is superior to transthoracic echo, and also for the operator of catheter intervention TEE is more preferable to transthoracic echo for maintaining sterility in the operating field. On the other hand, if the patient is not intubated, management of the patient's respiratory status during continuous TEE monitoring may be difficult, and the TEE examiner should always be very careful to avoid aspiration. Therefore, our policy is to use transthoracic echo when the patient is not intubated and to use TEE when the patient is intubated.

Figure 12-11 shows the transesophageal echocardiograms during BAS of a patient with transposition of the great arteries and coarctation. The patient underwent subclavian flap repair of the coarctation at first; however, 6 h after surgery severe hypoxemia developed. BAS was then performed under TEE guidance in the intensive care unit (Fig. 12-12). The size of the interatrial communication was increased from 2 by 4 to 6 by 8 mm by BAS, and an adequate shunt flow was obtained after BAS (Fig. 12-13).

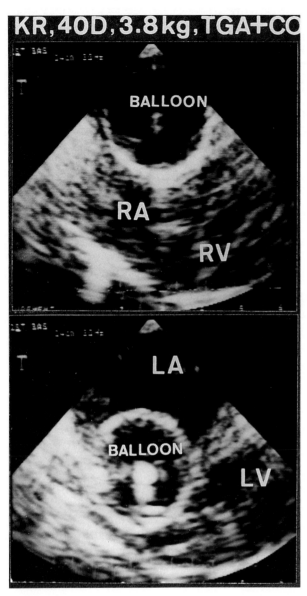

Figure 12-11
TEE images of balloon atrial septostomy in the case of transposition of great arteries (TGA) and coarctation (COA). The Miller balloon was located in the left atrium (LA) before BAS and in the right atrium (RA) after BAS.

Closure of Atrial Septal Defect

In some other scenarios of congenital heart disease, echocardiographic monitoring has been employed to make the procedure of catheter intervention easier and safer even with fluoroscopic monitoring. Hellenbrand et al.[18] first reported the utility of TEE for the guidance of transcatheter closure of atrial septal defects (Fig. 12-14). They examined the use of TEE for guidance of ASD closure in terms of evaluating defect size, position, and number of defects and ascertaining appropriate seating of the defect occluder within the ASD. They concluded that the concomitant use of TEE with fluoroscopic imaging provides information that may improve the efficacy and safety of the procedure. Patients who are treated by this technique are usually anesthetized with endotracheal intubation; therefore, management of TEE monitoring is very easy during the procedure.

Figure 12-15 shows the schematic presentation of the procedure, and all steps can be easily monitored by TEE as illustrated. We have tried to close ASDs by this technique in 7 patients, but since preprocedure TEE examination showed a maximum diameter of ASD of 22 mm in one patient, we performed clamshell closure in only 6. TEE measurement of ASD area estimated by ellipse approximation and the balloon stretched area directly measured by the balloon catheter have a very good correlation ($r = 0.93$) (Fig. 12-16); therefore, TEE is also effective for the selection of the device size. Postclosure TEE examination showed two cases of mild residual shunt (Fig. 12-17), but no case, significant shunt (Qp/Qs > 1.2) hemodynamically.

In high-risk patients for Fontan procedures the fenestrated Fontan operation is one option to overcome the early postoperative right ventricular failure, and the fenestrated atrial septal patch requires delayed closure with a clamshell device.[34] Usually closure of the fenestration on the prosthetic patch with a clamshell device is not difficult and does not require TEE guidance. However, we experienced one patient with extreme Ebstein's anomaly with severe right ventricular failure, who underwent tricuspid valve replacement and closure of the ASD with a fenestrated Gore-tex patch. The patient recovered from right ventricular failure 3 months after the closure of the ASD, and closure of the fenestration with a clamshell

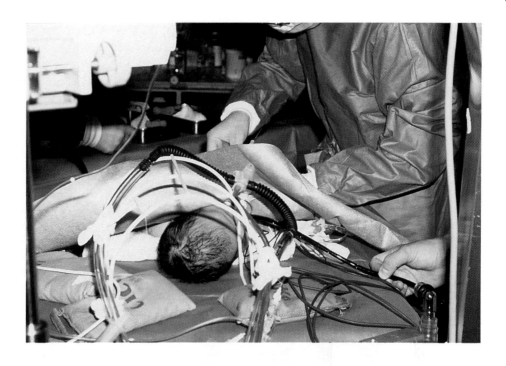

Figure 12-12
BAS under TEE guidance in the intensive care unit. TEE monitoring does not interfere with the BAS procedure; therefore, TEE guidance is much preferable with an intubated patient.

device was attempted. Unfortunately, both femoral veins of this patient were completely occluded by previous cardiac catheterizations, so the heart could be approached only from a jugular or subclavian vein. It was quite difficult to approach the fenestration through the superior vena cava by fluoroscopic guidance; however, a guidewire was very easily introduced into the LA through the fenestration under TEE guidance. The longitudinal image plane was particularly effective to observe the entire tip of the guidewire (Fig 12-18, right upper panel). In this case clamshell occlusion of the fenestrated ASD was performed easily and successfully with TEE guidance (Fig. 12-19) even with the approach from the right jugular vein.

Experience of TEE Monitoring of Other Congenital Defects

In two cases, transcatheter closure of a patent ductus arteriosus was performed with intraoperative TEE monitoring: in an adult patient with standard biplane probe of adult size and in a child with a pediatric probe. Both patients were anesthetized and endotracheally intu-

bated, and TEE monitoring was performed throughout the procedure. The PDA was completely closed with a Rashkind device in the adult patient (Fig. 12-20); however, a minor residual shunt was detected by TEE in the pediatric patient, which could not be seen by transthoracic echocardiography. Although the transthoracic echo is sensitive for the detection of residual leakage after device closure of PDA, we believe TEE is more sensitive to evaluate the position of the Rashkind device and minor leakage. In one patient (5-month-old female) balloon angioplasty was performed to correct restenosis of the coarctation. After several attempts of balloon dilatation, deterioration of the patient's condition was noticed with a sudden drop of blood pressure. Although angiography of the descending aorta indicated the creation of acute aortic dissection, an intimal flap could not be clearly demonstrated (Fig. 12-21). On the other hand, biplane TEE visualized the intimal flap very clearly in both the longitudinal and transverse image (Fig. 22-22). Based on the TEE findings, this patient was promptly operated and underwent subclavian flap repair of COA.

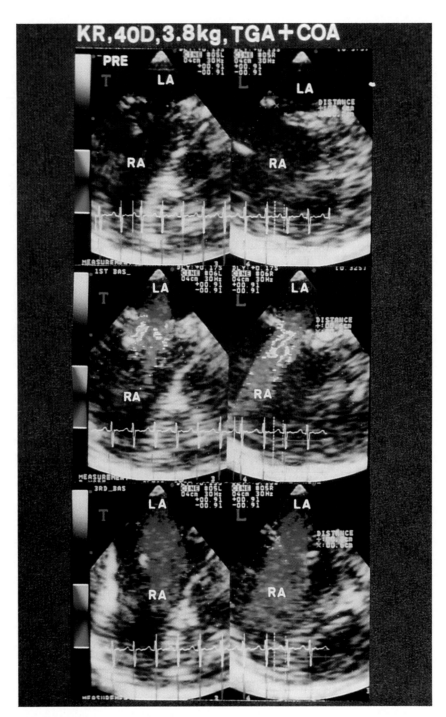

Figure 12-13
Biplane TEE images of the ASD in the patient with
TGA + COA before and after BAS.

Figure 12-14
Clamshell device for ASD closure.

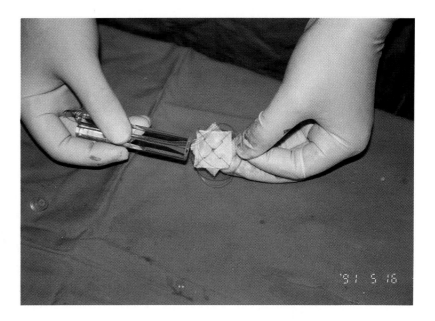

Figure 12-15
Schematic presentation of TEE images of clamshell device closure of ASD. Each step of the procedure can be monitored clearly by TEE as illustrated.

Chapter 12

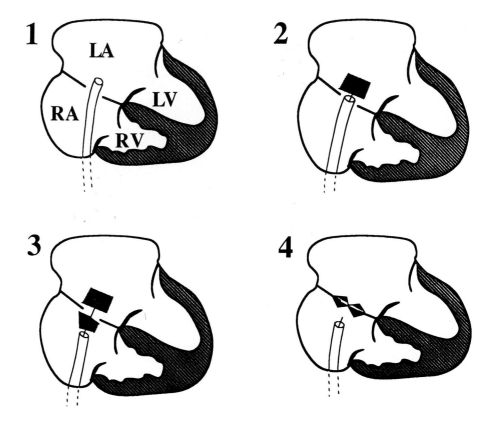

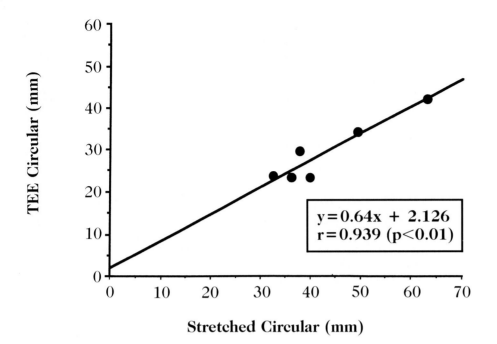

Figure 12-16
Correlation between the TEE measured circular by the ellipse approximation method and the balloon stretched circular. The correlation coefficient number (r) is 0.939.

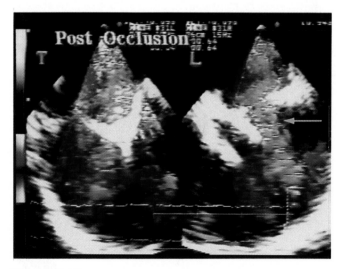

Figure 12-17
Matrix-biplane TEE images of clamshell closure of ASD in 4-year-old male patient. A small residual leakage is seen in both TEE image planes clearly.

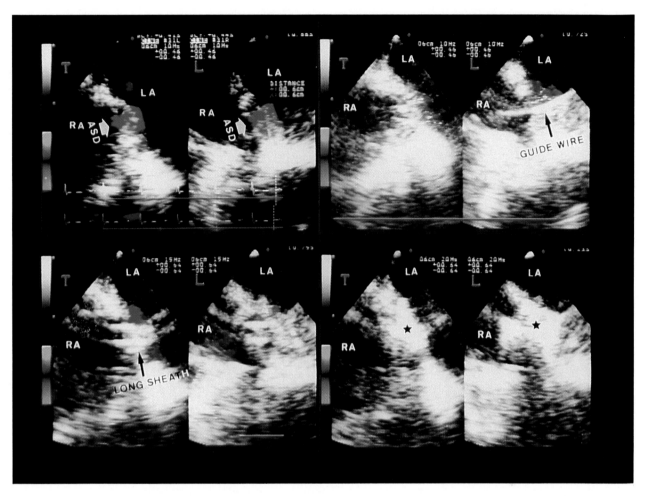

Figure 12-18
Biplane TEE images of clamshell closure of a fenestrated ASD in the patient with Ebstein's anomaly (13-year-old male). The fenestrated ASD with its shunt flow is seen in the left upper panel. The longitudinal image plane (L) is very useful for the introduction of a guidewire into LA (right upper panel). After introduction of the guidewire the long sheath for the delivery of the clamshell device could be easily inserted into LA (left lower panel). Finally the clamshell device (*) was securely placed on the fenestrated ASD (right lower panel).

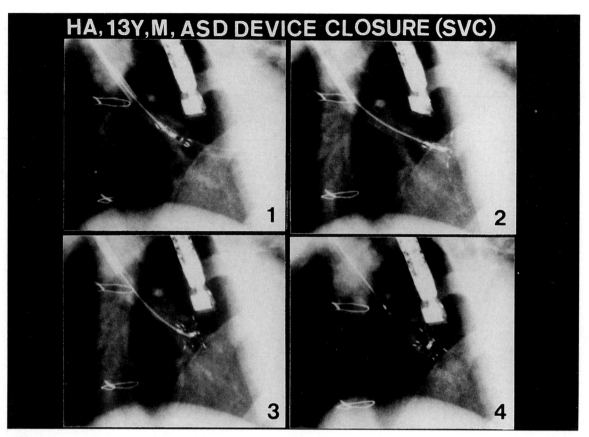

HA, 13Y, M, ASD DEVICE CLOSURE (SVC)

Figure 12-19
X-ray images of clamshell closure of a fenestrated ASD in the patient with Ebstein's anomaly (13-year-old male). 1. The clamshell device is introduced into the LA through a long sheath. 2. The distal umbrella of the device is opened and fixed on the left side of the fenestrated ASD. 3. Then the proximal umbrella of the device is opened on the right side of the fenestrated ASD. 4. The device is released from the delivery catheter.

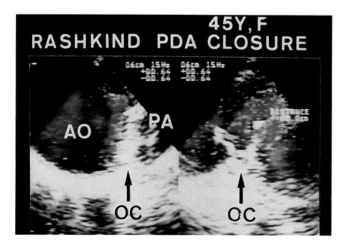

45Y, F
RASHKIND PDA CLOSURE

Figure 12-20
Biplane transesophageal echocardiogram showing the device closure of patent ductus arteriosus. After closure no leakage was detected.

Figure 12-21
Angiography and x-ray images of balloon angioplasty on a patient (5-month-old female) with restenosis of coarctation (COA). After several balloon dilatations severe aortic dissection was created; however, intimal flap (IF) was not clearly visualized by angiography.

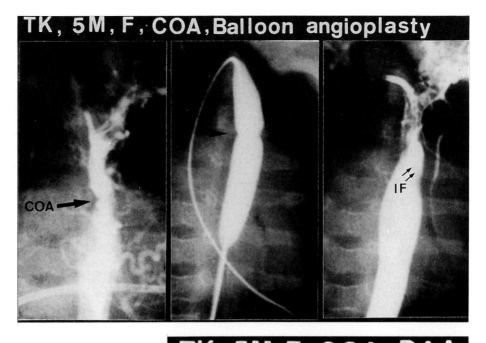

Figure 12-22
Intraoperative transesophageal echocardiograms of a patient (5-month-old female) with restenosis of coarctation (COA). The stenotic portion of coarctation (COA) and the intimal flap (IF) is clearly demonstrated in both the longitudinal plane (upper panel) and transverse plane (lower panel).

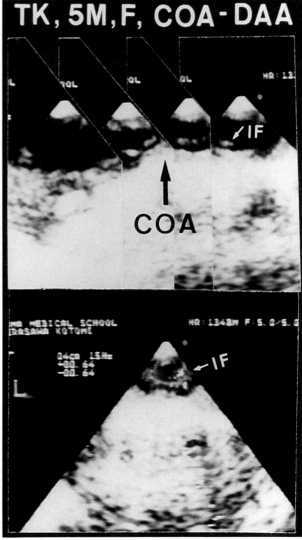

Future Aspect of TEE during Catheter Intervention

TEE is a very sensitive intraoperative monitoring method for various kinds of catheter interventions in adult and congenital heart diseases. Theoretically intraoperative TEE is considered to be effective to improve the results of many types of catheter interventions. Usually catheter interventions in adult patients are performed in the awake state in the supine position; therefore, management of the patient's discomfort relating to TEE can be properly controlled. Particular attention must be paid to suction secretions and to administer mild sedation, while closely monitoring respiration and vital signs. Also, proper selection of the TEE probe is very important in continous monitoring of cardiac function, since large probes may actually interfere with ventilation in very small patients. We have developed various types of TEE probes to be properly utilized in pediatric and adult patients.[35–38] However, for the purpose of intraoperative continuous monitoring in awake patients, highly flexible nasogastric-sized matrix-biplane TEE probes should be developed in the near future.

References

1. Matsumoto M, Oka Y, Strom J, et al: Application of transesophageal echocardiography to continuous intraoperative monitoring of left ventricular performance. *Am J Cardiol* 46:95, 1980.

2. Schlüter M, Langenstein BA, Hanrath P, et al: Assessment of transesophageal pulsed Doppler echocardiography in the detection of mitral regurgitation. *Circulation* 66:784, 1982.

3. Kyo S, Takamoto S, Matsumura M, et al: Immediate and early postoperative evaluation of cardiac surgery by transesophageal two-dimensional Doppler echocardiography. *Circulation* 76(suppl 5):113, 1987.

4. Yoshida K, Yoshikawa J, Yamaura Y, et al: Assessment of mitral regurgitation by biplane transesophageal color Doppler flow imaging. *Circulation* 82:1121, 1990.

5. Nellessen U, Schnittger I, Appleton CP, et al: Transesophageal two-dimensional echocardiography and color Doppler flow velocity mapping in the evaluation of cardiac valve prosthesis. *Circulation* 78:848, 1988.

6. Topol EJ, Weiss JL, Guzman PA, et al: Immediate improvement of dysfunctional myocardial segments after coronary revascularization: Detection by intraoperative transesophageal echocardiography. *J Am Coll Cardiol* 4:1123, 1984.

7. Takamoto S, Omoto R: Visualization of thoracic dissecting aortic aneurysm by transesophageal Doppler color flow mapping. *Herz* 12:187, 1987.

8. Aschenberg W, Schlüter M, Kremer P, et al: Transesophageal two-dimensional echocardiography for the detection of left atrial appendage thrombus. *J Am Coll Cardiol* 7:163, 1986.

9. Yoshikawa J, Yoshida K, Yamaura Y, et al: Intraoperative biplane transesophageal color Doppler echocardiography for assessment of valve repair for mitral regurgitation (abstract). *J Am Soc Echocardiogr* 3:220, 1990.

10. Adachi H, Kyo S, Takamoto S, et al: Early diagnosis and surgical intervention of acute aortic dissection by transesophageal color flow mapping. *Circulation* 82(suppl 5):19, 1990.

11. Rashkind WJ, Miller WW: Creation of an atrial septal defect without thoracotomy: A palliative approach to complete transposition of the great arteries. *JAMA* 196:991, 1966.

12. Inoue K, Owaki T, Nakamura T, et al: Clinical application of transvenous mitral commissurotomy by a new balloon catheter. *J Thorac Cardiovasc Surg* 87:394, 1984.

13. Rashkind WJ, Mullins CE, Hellenbrand WE, et al: Nonsurgical closure of patent ductus arteriosus: Clinical application of the Rashkind PDA Occluder system. *Circulation* 75:583, 1987.

14. King TD, Mills NL: Nonoperative closure of atrial septal defects. *Surgery* 75:383, 1974.

15. Perry LW, Ruckman RN, Galioto FM Jr., et al: Echocardiographically assisted balloon atrial septostomy. *Pediatrics* 70:403, 1982.

16. Bullboy CA, Jennings RB, Johnson DH, et al: Bedside balloon atrial septostomy using echocardiographic monitoring. *Am J Cardiol* 53:971, 1984.

17. Kyo S, Omoto R: Color flow Doppler guiding of atrial septostomy, in Cikes I (ed): *Echocar-*

diography in Cardiac Interventions. Netherlands, Kluwer Academic Publishers, 1989, p 45.

18. Hellenbrand WE, Fahey JT, McGowan FX, et al: Transesophageal echocardiographic guidance of transcatheter closure of atrial septal defect. *Am J Cardiol* 66:207, 1990.

19. Kronzon I, Glassman E: Echocardiography in transseptal cardiac catheterization, in Cikes I (ed): *Echocardiography in Cardiac Interventions.* Netherlands, Kluwer Academic Publishers, 1989, p 57.

20. Brockenbrough EC, Braunwald E: A new technique for left ventricular angiography and transseptal left heart catheterization. *Am J Cardiol* 6:1002, 1960.

21. Conti CR, Grossman W: Percutaneous approach and transseptal catheterization, in Grossman W (ed): *Cardiac Catheterization and Angiography.* Philadelphia, Lea & Febiger, 1974, p 59.

22. Takamoto S, Kyo S, Adachi H, et al: Intraoperative color flow mapping by real-time two-dimensional Doppler echocardiography for evaluation of valvular and congenital heart disease and vascular disease. *J Thorac Cardiovasc Surg* 90:802, 1985.

23. Kyo S, Hung JS, Omoto R, et al: Intraoperative monitoring of balloon percutaneous mitral valvuloplasty by biplane transesophageal echocardiography (abstract). *Circulation* 82(suppl III): III-80, 1990.

24. Ballal RS, Mahan III EF, Nanda NC, et al: Utility of transesophageal echocardiography in interatrial septal puncture during percutaneous mitral balloon commissurotomy. *Am J Cardiol* 66:230, 1990.

25. Inoue K, Nakamura T, Kitamura F, et al: Nonoperative mitral commissurotomy by a new balloon catheter (abstract). *Jpn Circ J* 46:877, 1982.

26. Hung J, Chern M, Wu J, et al: Short and long-term results of catheter balloon percutaneous transvenous mitral commissurotomy. *Am J Cardiol* 67:854, 1991.

27. NHLBI Balloon Valvuloplasty Registry Participants: Complications and mortality of percutaneous balloon mitral commissurotomy. A report from the National Heart, Lung, and Blood Institute Balloon Valvuloplasty Registry. *Circulation* 85:2014, 1992.

28. Orihashi K, Matsumura Y, Ishihara H, et al: Transvenous mitral commissurotomy examined with transesophageal echocardiography. *Heart Vessels* 3:209, 1987.

29. Kyo S, Noda H, Motoyama T, et al: Percutaneous introduction of left atrial cannula for left heart bypass: Effectiveness of transesophageal echo guidance for transseptal cannulation. *Jpn J Artif Organs* 21:347, 1992.

30. Phillips SJ, Ballentine B, Slonine D, et al: Percutaneous initiation of cardiopulmonary bypass. 36:223, 1983.

31. Dennis C, Carlens E, Senning A, et al: Clinical use of a cannula for the left heart bypass without thoracotomy. *Ann Surg* 156:623, 1962.

32. Kyo S, Motoyama T, Noda H, et al: Percutaneous introduction of left atrial cannula for left heart bypass: Utility of biplane transesophageal echo guidance for transseptal puncture. (abstract) *C Artif Organs* 15:312, 1991.

33. Rashkind WJ: The complication of balloon atrioseptostomy. *J Pediatr* 76:649, 1970.

34. Kopf GS, Kleinman CS, Hijazi ZM, et al: Fenestrated Fontan operation with delayed transcatheter closure of atrial septal defect. *J Thorac Cardiovasc Surg* 103:1039, 1992.

35. Omoto R, Kyo S, Matsumura M, et al: Recent advances in transesophageal echocardiography: Development of biplane and pediatric transesophageal probes. *Am J Cardiac Imag* 4:207, 1990.

36. Kyo S, Omoto R, Matsumura M, et al: Intraoperative transesophageal echocardiography in pediatric patients. *J Thorac Cardiovasc Surg* 99:373, 1990.

37. Omoto R, Kyo S, Matsumura M, et al: Biplane color Doppler transesophageal echocardiography: Its impact on cardiovascular surgery and further technological progress in the probe, a matrix phased-array biplane probe. *Echocardiography* 6:423, 1989.

38. Omoto R, Kyo S, Matsumura M, et al: Evaluation of biplane color Doppler transesophageal echocardiography in 200 consecutive patients. *Circulation* 85:1237, 1992.

13

Transesophageal Color Doppler Echocardiography in Surgical Repair of Valvular and Ischemic Heart Disease

Yuk Kong Lau
Lawrence S.C. Czer

Introduction

Surgical procedures that repair, reconstruct, or remodel cardiac structures are being performed with increasing frequency. Because these procedures are often complex and the results may be variable, a careful intraoperative assessment is essential before and after the procedure. Traditionally, this evaluation has been performed in the arrested heart by direct inspection of the affected structure. While helpful, this does not usually provide sufficient information about the adequacy of the repair procedure.[1-3]

Echocardiography with conventional and color Doppler flow mapping provides real-time tomographic imaging of intracardiac morphology and blood flow in the beating and ejecting heart. The examination can be performed under physiologic conditions in the operating room immediately before and after cardiopulmonary bypass with clinically available portable equipment. Because of these attributes, Doppler echocardiography has become the preferred method for the evaluation of patients undergoing reparative or reconstructive cardiac surgery.

Indications

Transesophageal imaging is very useful in suspected pathology of the atrial chambers (such as thrombi, tumors) or of the descending thoracic aorta (such as dissection), because of the proximity of these structures to the transducer. With suspected mitral prosthetic valve dysfunction, regurgitation into the left atrium is readily identified and is not subject to acoustical interference, which occurs with epicardial imaging. Furthermore, the effects of anesthesia, pressors, vasodilators, and other interventions on wall motion, blood flow, and valvular function can be monitored continuously. Imaging can be accomplished without interruption of the surgery, and contamination of the operative field is not a concern. Intracardiac air can be

235

watched for immediately after discontinuation of cardiopulmonary bypass.

Contraindications

Transesophageal imaging is contraindicated in patients with esophageal disease (such as stricture, web, diverticulum, erosion, or neoplasm), which places them at risk for esophageal rupture, patients who had a prior laryngectomy, and patients who are at extraordinary risk for mucosal bleeding (due to varices or a severe coagulopathy). When intraoperative echocardiographic imaging is required for these patients, the epicardial approach should be used.

Techniques

Transesophageal Approach

Transesophageal imaging utilizes a transducer mounted on the tip of an instrument similar to an endoscope. Induction of general anesthesia should be accomplished prior to insertion of the probe. Because bacteremia may occur, though infrequently,[4,5] antibiotic prophylaxis is recommended for patients with poor oral hygiene and history of endocarditis or prosthetic valves, according to the American Heart Association guidelines for upper gastrointestinal endoscopy.[6] However, as of today, there are no available data to support the use of antibiotic prophylaxis routinely.

With the patient in the supine position and the probe lubricated, an endoscopically mounted 5.0-MHz ultrasound transducer is inserted into the esophagus and is advanced at least 20 cm from the teeth (in adults) to the level of the structure of interest. Most cardiac structures are imaged at the level of the left atrium (Fig. 13-1). Transverse views are obtained at multiple levels by moving the transducer cephalad and caudad within the esophagus, and by angulating the tip of the transducer ventrally and dorsally. Longitudinal views may

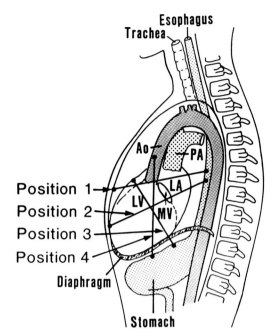

Figure 13-1
Transesophageal imaging positions (left lateral view). The superior portion of the left atrium, the aortic valve leaflets within the sinuses of Valsalva, and proximal coronaries are seen in the transverse plane at position 1. With clockwise rotation of the transducer, the interatrial septum, right atrium, and origin of the superior vena cava can be seen; with counterclockwise rotation, the left atrial appendage and the descending aorta are seen. With slight advancement and downward angulation of the transducer (position 2), a four-chamber transverse view is obtained, including the left and right atria, the mitral and tricuspid valves, and the left and right ventricles. The pulmonary veins may be visualized as they empty into the left atrium. If the left ventricular outflow tract, aortic valve, and aortic root are seen, a five-chamber view is obtained. With advancement of the probe, the mitral annulus and proximal left ventricle are seen. With the probe advanced past the gastroesophageal junction and reflected upward against the diaphragm to obtain a transgastric view (positions 3 and 4), the left and right ventricles are imaged in short axis (transverse plane) and long axis (longitudinal plane). Ao, aorta; PA, pulmonary artery; LA, left atrium; LV, left ventricle; MV, mitral valve. (From Czer, Siegel, Maurer, et al.,[40] with permission.)

also be obtained in multiple planes with the biplane probe by rotating clockwise or counterclockwise and by tilting the transducer tip from side to side with the manual controls. With the omniplane probe, cardiac structures may be visualized at an almost infinite number of views as desired. An example of an intraoperative biplane transesophageal color Doppler study is shown in Fig. 13-2.

Transgastric short- and long-axis views of the heart are obtained by advancing the probe through the gastroesophageal junction into the stomach and reflecting it upward against the diaphragm (Fig. 13-1). These views are especially useful in evaluation of ventricular function.

Figure 13-2
Biplane intraoperative transesophageal color Doppler study (systolic frames) before and after mitral valve repair with a Carpentier-Edwards ring. Before repair (A), severe mitral regurgitation can be seen, as represented by the jet in the left atrium (LA). The largest regurgitant jet area is obtained in the transverse plane (left part of panel A); however, the jet's inferior direction is best appreciated in the longitudinal plane (right part of panel A). After repair (B), there was no residual mitral regurgitation despite pressor challenge with phenylephrine and achievement of a comparable blood pressure. The diameter of the mitral annulus is decreased compared with that in the prerepair study. The left part of each panel represents the transverse plane, while the right part of each panel represents the longitudinal plane. Right (R), left (L), inferior (I), superior (S), left atrium (LA), left ventricle (LV). (From Maurer, Siegel, and Czer,[7] with permission.)

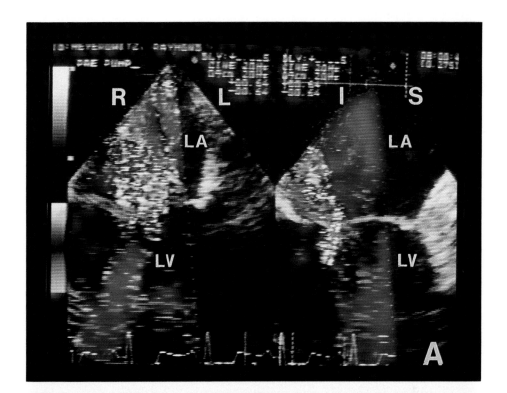

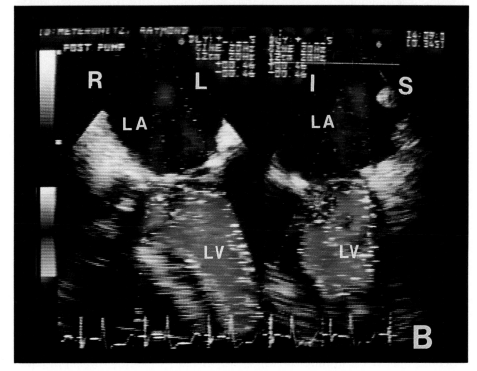

Image Acquisition

Imaging is performed immediately before and after cardiopulmonary bypass. Simultaneously, right atrial, pulmonary arterial, and systemic arterial pressures are recorded. If the systolic arterial pressure is more than 15 mmHg below a patient's baseline value or a fixed reference level (e.g., 140 mmHg), imaging and hemodynamics are repeated after an intravenous bolus of phenylephrine (50 to 500 μg). Color Doppler gain is adjusted to a level just below excessive random noise (5 percent of pixels). Studies are obtained at frame rates of 7.5 to 30 per second and are recorded on 1/2-in. videotape.

Safety Considerations

Electric current consumption ranges from 7 to 15 A for most color Doppler systems. To prevent potentially catastrophic power failure or circuit overload, the imaging system should be connected to an isolated electric circuit that does not supply other operating room equipment. Hospital-grade plugs with appropriate grounding must be employed. Leakage currents should be minimal. Caution is advised when using color Doppler systems in the presence of flammable gases.

For cleansing of the transesophageal probe, immersion in Cidex (or comparable bactericidal solution) for at least 15 to 30 min followed by copious rinsing with water is recommended.

Special Considerations

Valve Repair

Properly performed valve repair surgery is associated with greater survival, better ventricular function, and fewer thromboembolic complications than prosthetic valve replacement.[8–13] However, because of its greater complexity, valve repair requires careful intraoperative assessment before and after the procedure. Most commonly, valve repair is performed in patients with mitral or tricuspid valve disease, although reparative procedures have been described for all valve positions.

Echocardiography with Doppler color flow mapping has been applied intraoperatively in patients with mitral or tricuspid valve disease to determine the nature and severity of the valve disorder, the need for valve repair, and the feasibility of repair, and to aid planning of the surgical procedure. Other important issues such as the impact of physiologic interventions on regurgitation severity, the presence of associated lesions, and the state of ventricular function can also be addressed. In the patient who has undergone a valve repair, this technique can be used prior to chest closure to assess the adequacy of the repair procedure and to detect associated complications such as outflow tract obstruction.

Atrioventricular valve regurgitation is graded semiquantitatively on a scale of 0 to 4+ according to the maximal systolic length of the regurgitant jet in relation to the atrium: 1+ is assigned if the jet extends immediately behind the valve, 2+ if it extends up to one-third the length of the atrium, 3+ if up to two-thirds, and 4+ if more than two-thirds into the atrium.[1,2] Alternatively, a grading system modified from Helmcke's criteria[14] may be used, relating the jet area to the atrial area: 1+ if the jet extends just behind the valve, 2+ if up to 20 percent, 3+ if up to 40 percent, and 4+ if more than 40 percent of the left atrial area is occupied by the regurgitant jet.

Annulus

The need for an annulus-reducing procedure can be determined by echocardiographic measurement of annular size (Fig. 13-3). The normal mitral annulus has an elliptical shape in systole, and a nearly circular shape in diastole.[15] The maximal annular area occurs in late diastole, at the end of the P wave; if measured at this time, the area in normal adults ranges from 5.3 to 8.9 cm^2 (mean 7.1), the circumference from 8.0 to 10.5 cm (mean 9.3), and the diameter from 2.5 to 3.4 cm (mean 3.0). In systole, the area is reduced by 26 percent and the diameter by 13 percent.[15]

With chronic regurgitation, the annulus and atrium dilate and the annulus loses its elliptical shape, becoming more circular. Annular dilation, in turn, leads to poor coaptation of the valve leaflets and worsening of valve incompetence. Reestablishment of a normal annular

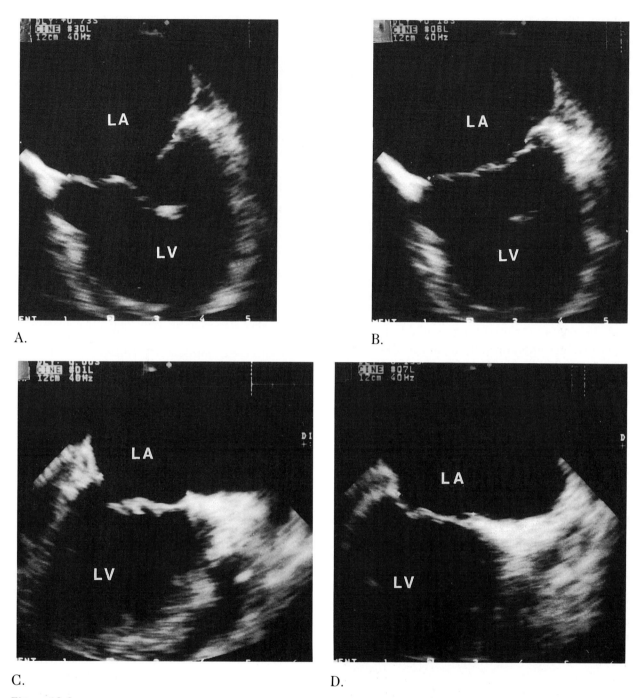

A.

B.

C.

D.

Figure 13-3
Dilation of mitral annulus and left atrium in patient with severe mitral regurgitation. Transesophageal transverse view at end diastole (A), and systole (B); longitudinal view at end diastole (C) and end systole (D). Note the larger annular diameter when measured during diastole (A, C).

size and shape can reduce or eliminate the regurgitation. Thus an annulus-reducing procedure is nearly always required when annular dilation is present. With acute regurgitation, annular and atrial size are usually normal and an annulus-reducing procedure is often not required; rather, other techniques of repair are indicated.

Annulus reduction can be achieved by two methods: suture annuloplasty and ring annuloplasty. Placement of sutures along portions of the annulus can effectively shrink the annulus; however, this shrinkage occurs only in areas where the sutures were placed. The most commonly used suture annuloplasty techniques are those described by Kay and Zubiate for the mitral valve[16] and DeVega for the tricuspid valve.[17] A more evenly spaced or circumferential reduction of the annulus can be accomplished by a ring annuloplasty,[18] whereby a prosthetic ring is attached to the annulus at numerous points along most or all of the circumference.[19,20] Several types of prosthetic rings are available, including the Carpentier-Edwards, Duran, Puig-Massana, and St. Jude BiFlex rings.

The ring can be imaged in transesophageal and transgastric views (Figs. 13-4 and 13-5), and the cross-sectional area available for flow can be determined directly from the short-axis view by planimetry of the internal orifice of the ring. Alternatively, pulsed or continuous-wave Doppler velocity measurements can be used to determine the pressure half-time of transvalvular flow; the valve area (A) can be calculated from the formula $A = 220/\text{pressure half-time}$ (in ms). In general, the orifice area

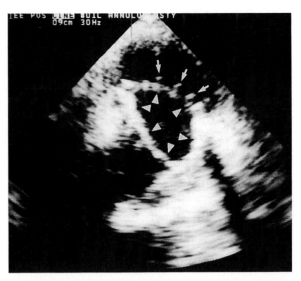

Figure 13-5
The elliptical shape of a prosthetic ring (arrows) is apparent when imaged in the plane of the ring following mitral annuloplasty with a Carpentier-Edwards prosthesis. Transgastric short-axis view at level of mitral annulus. Arrows indicate individual sutures placed around prosthetic ring by the surgeon.

should be greater than $1 \text{ cm}^2/\text{m}^2$ of body surface area. Overcorrection of regurgitation by insertion of a small ring can produce functional stenosis.

Leaflets and Chordae

The pathological changes in the leaflets or chords and the cause of the valve disease can often be identified by echocardiography prior to cardiopulmonary bypass. This information aids in determining the need for and feasibility of valve repair.

Myxomatous degeneration produces ballooning and scalloping of the valve leaflets as well as localized areas of thinning and thickening that can be seen echocardiographically. Elongated chords may produce prolapse of one or both attached leaflets; if only one leaflet is affected, leaflet malalignment may occur during systole. Excessively mobile structures near the leaflet tips during diastole may represent elongated chords or ruptured minor chords (Fig. 13-6). These structures do not prolapse into the atrium during systole.

Ruptured major chords are identified as thin structures with a fluttering appearance in the

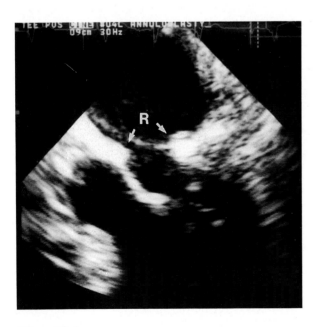

Figure 13-4
Carpentier-Edwards prosthetic ring (R) in cross section following mitral annuloplasty. Transesophageal transverse view during diastole.

Figure 13-6

Myxomatous mitral valve with prominent scalloping, especially of the posterior leaflet. An excessively mobile structure (arrow) is identified between the posterior leaflet and papillary muscle during diastole, representing an elongated chord attached to the posterior leaflet. This finding was confirmed at surgery. Such excessively mobile structures which do not prolapse into the left atrium can represent elongated chords or ruptured minor chords. The valve was successfully repaired. Transesophageal view obtained in the transverse plane at the level of the left atrium. (From Czer and Maurer,[39] with permission.)

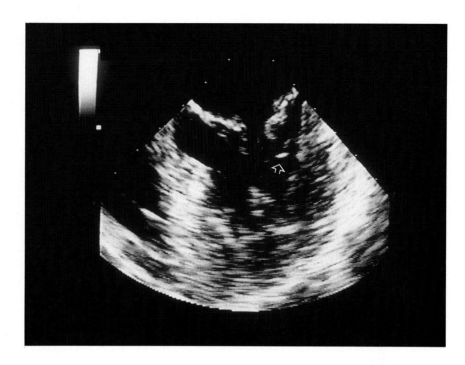

atrium during systole (Fig. 13-7) and are associated with marked prolapse of the affected leaflet; in this instance, the valve is said to be flail. Severely myxomatous valves, especially when the anterior leaflet is flail or when multiple major chords have ruptured, may not be amenable to repair.

In patients with recent endocarditis, vegetations may be attached to the leaflets or chords. These vegetations are more likely to be seen with transesophageal than with transthoracic imaging. Leaflet perforation and chordal rupture caused by endocarditis can often be repaired.

With rheumatic valve disease, thickening and/or calcification of the leaflets, restriction of leaflets, and a variable degree of shortening and thickening of the subvalvular apparatus may be identified. The ability to repair these valves depends on the mobility of the leaflets and chords and the degree of calcification.[21,22]

In patients with regurgitation due to coronary artery disease, the leaflets and chords appear normal. Ischemic mitral regurgitation is usually due to annular dilation resulting from left ventricular remodeling and enlargement after prior myocardial infarction. Regurgitation may also be caused by papillary muscle infarction in association with infarction of the

adjacent left ventricular myocardium, due to a lack of the normal tethering function performed by these structures. When the adjacent segment is aneurysmal, the dyskinetic wall motion may prevent proper coaptation of the valve by restricting the normal movement of the mitral leaflets during systole.[23] Papillary muscle rupture typically appears as a mass (papillary muscle head) that prolapses into the left atrium during systole, connected only to the leaflet by its attached chords (Fig. 13-8).

The leaflets and the subvalvular apparatus are repaired by a variety of techniques that depend on the underlying pathology and its severity.[24] Clefts are closed by direct suture repair. Holes are patched by pericardium. Calcific deposits are debrided by careful curettage. Redundant leaflet tissue is removed by quadrilateral resection with annular and leaflet reapproximation (posterior mitral leaflet) or by triangular resection (anterior mitral leaflet). Chordal support of the anterior leaflet is achieved by transposition of a normal chord and attached edge of the leaflet from the posterior leaflet; alternatively, prosthetic chordae may be used. Elongated chordae are shortened by incorporation into a papillary muscle. Torn chordae are resected. Fused chords are divided by careful incision. An elongated papillary

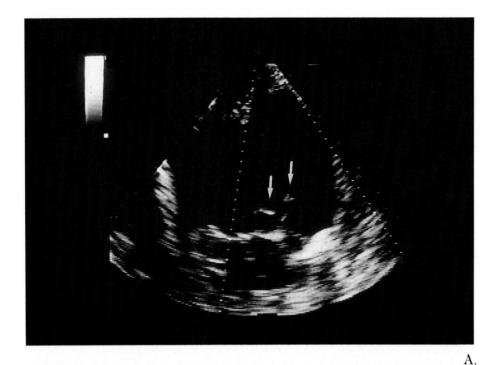

A.

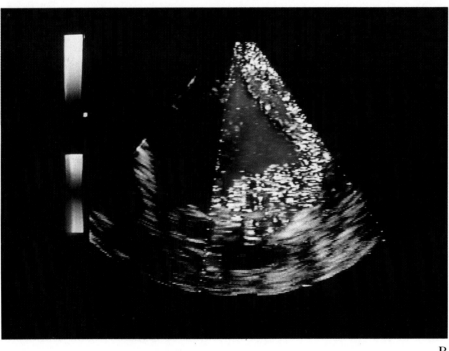

B.

Figure 13-7
Severely myxomatous mitral valve with flail mitral leaflet due to torn major chord (A). The flail anterior leaflet and attached chord (arrows) are seen within the left atrium during systole. The flail anterior leaflet was associated with severe mitral regurgitation directed along the free posterolateral wall of the left atrium (B). These findings were confirmed at surgery. The valve was not amenable to repair. Transesophageal view obtained in the transverse plane at the level of the left atrium. (From Czer and Maurer,[39] with permission.)

muscle is shortened by folding and securing with sutures. A ruptured papillary muscle may be reimplanted by suturing it to a normal papillary muscle or to the adjacent left ventricular wall which is not acutely infarcted.

After valve repair, the cause of residual regurgitation can often be identified by careful echocardiographic evaluation of the leaflets and chords. For example, continued prolapse despite ring annuloplasty may indicate insuffi-

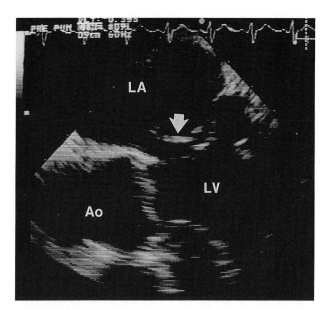

Figure 13-8
Ruptured papillary muscle (arrow) in a patient with severe mitral regurgitation after an acute myocardial infarction. The ruptured papillary muscle is imaged as an echogenic mass prolapsing into the left atrium (LA) during systole. Transesophageal view at left atrial level. Left ventricle (LV), aortic root (Ao). (From Czer, Siegel, Maurer, et al.,[40] with permission.)

cient chordal shortening. Residual regurgitation after repair of a cleft mitral leaflet may indicate inadequate closure of the cleft.

Systolic anterior motion (SAM) of the mitral leaflets and left ventricular outflow tract

(LVOT) obstruction have been observed in 4.5 to 6.0 percent of patients after mitral annuloplasty with a rigid Carpentier-Edwards ring, and occur most frequently in patients with redundant mitral leaflet tissue.[25,26] The rigid ring causes diastolic mitral flow to be directed against the interventricular septum (as with rigid prosthetic valves), with resultant anterior displacement of the posterior left ventricular wall and posterior mitral leaflet, causing both leaflets to obstruct the outflow tract during systole (Fig. 13-9). As with other types of SAM, there may be associated regurgitation, necessitating valve replacement. However, this condition can often be prevented by reduction of the excessive posterior mitral leaflet tissue.[24,25] SAM and LVOT obstruction have not been described following insertion of a flexible ring or after suture annuloplasty.

Papillary Muscles and Wall Motion
Several echocardiographic findings may be helpful in establishing ischemic heart disease as the cause of regurgitation. Thinning of the myocardium, atresia of the papillary muscles, and dyskinetic wall segments are indicative of prior remote infarction. Atretic papillary muscles are identified by their diminutive size and increased echocardiographic density on short-axis imaging (Fig. 13-10). Preoperative segmental wall motion abnormalities may be

Figure 13-9
Systolic anterior motion (SAM) of the mitral valve (arrow). This patient underwent ring annuloplasty but developed SAM with left ventricular outflow tract obstruction and severe mitral regurgitation, necessitating mitral valve replacement. Parasternal-equivalent long-axis view of left ventricle (LV), aortic root (Ao), and left atrium (LA) during systole (epicardial approach). (From Czer, Siegel, Maurer, et al.,[40] with permission.)

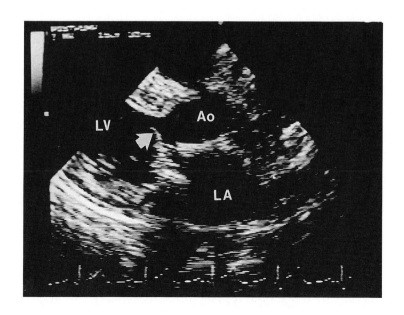

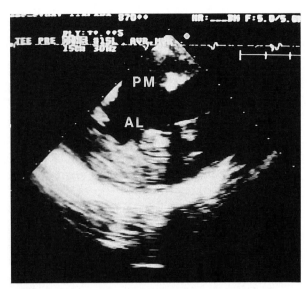

Figure 13-10
Infarction of posteromedial papillary muscle. Note the associated thinning of the inferoposterior wall. AL = anterolateral papillary muscle; PM = posteromedial papillary muscle. Transgastric short-axis view of left ventricle at papillary muscle level.

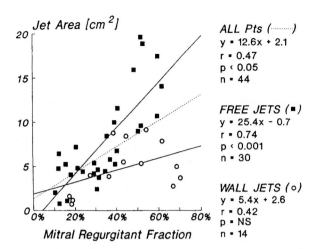

Figure 13-11
Coanda effect. Mitral regurgitant jets that impinge on the wall of the left atrium (open circles) have much smaller jet areas than do jets of similar regurgitant fraction that are directed into the center of the left atrium (closed squares). The solid lines represent the regression relationships for free jets (upper line) and wall jets (lower line), respectively, while the dotted line shows the regression relationship for all patients combined. (From Chen, Thomas, Anconina, et al.,[27] with permission.)

produced by reversible ischemia or infarction and by primary or secondary myopathic processes unrelated to ischemic heart disease. However, the postoperative finding of a new or worsening wall motion abnormality or lack of wall thickening in a patient with coronary artery disease indicates myocardial ischemia or poor myocardial preservation; such information is very useful for the intraoperative management of patients undergoing concomitant coronary artery bypass grafting.

Regurgitant Jet Direction and Origin

Eccentric jets that cling to the atrial wall (Coanda effect) have a smaller area than central (free) jets with similar regurgitant volumes and regurgitant fractions (Fig. 13-11).[27] Eccentric jets may represent severe regurgitation even though they occupy less than 40 percent of the left atrial area. Therefore, jet direction should be considered when grading regurgitation.

Eccentric jet direction provides corroborative evidence of structural leaflet abnormalities which may include leaflet prolapse, chordal elongation, chordal rupture, or papillary muscle rupture. For example, a jet directed laterally along the posterior wall of the left atrium is associated with anterior leaflet prolapse (Fig. 13-7). Similarly, a jet directed medially behind the anterior mitral leaflet is associated with prolapse of the posterior leaflet.

The origin of the jet in relation to the commissure is helpful in guiding surgical decision making in patients with regurgitation due to ischemic heart disease.[3,28] The mitral commissure may be divided arbitrarily into thirds: the inferior portion (adjacent to the inferior wall of the left ventricle); the central portion; and the superior portion (adjacent to the anterolateral wall of the left ventricle). The mitral commissure and the jet origin are imaged from the transgastric short-axis view, and by the transesophageal longitudinal view. We have found that ischemic mitral regurgitation usually originates from the inferior (42 percent) or the central (52 percent) portion of the commissure.[3,28] An example of a jet originating from the inferior portion of the mitral commissure is shown in Fig. 13-12. An example of a broad jet originating from all three portions of the mitral commissure is shown in Fig. 13-13.

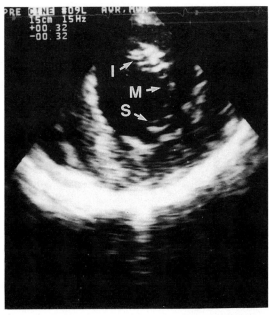

A.

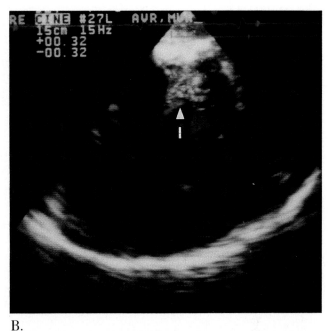

B.

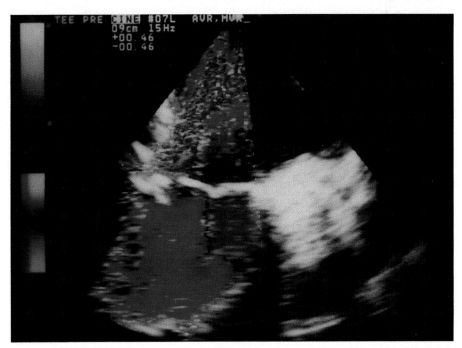

C.

Figure 13-12
Inferior commissural origin of mitral regurgitant jet. The inferior (I), middle (M), and superior (S) portions of the mitral valve commissure are identified on the transgastric view of the left ventricle at the level of the mitral valve (A); the regurgitant jet is clearly seen originating from the inferior portion of the commissure (B). In the transesophageal longitudinal view, the regurgitant jet is also seen originating from the inferior portion of the commissure (C).

Pulmonary Vein Flow Pattern

Pulmonary vein flow by transesophageal echocardiography provides useful information regarding regurgitant severity.[29] The normal pulmonary vein flow pattern consists of systolic and diastolic phases that are both directed toward the atrial cavity and have similar velocities (Fig. 13-14). With regurgitation, there may be blunting of systolic flow or flow reversal; flow reversal corresponds with severe regurgitation (Fig. 13-15). With eccentric jets, flow reversal may be more prominent in the pulmonary veins toward which the jet is directed. The same limitations that apply to V waves for evaluating regurgitant severity may apply to pulmonary vein flow.

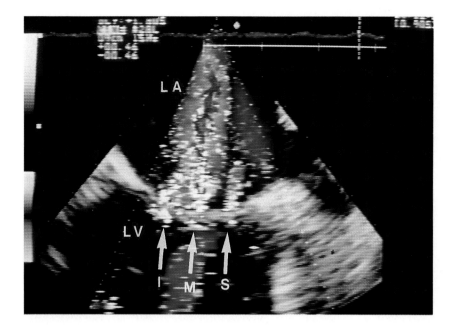

Figure 13-13
Multiple commissural origin of mitral regurgitation. Note broad jet of regurgitation originating from inferior, middle, and superior portions of mitral commissure in this transesophageal longitudinal view of the mitral valve.

Importance of Afterload

Systolic pressure has a significant influence on jet size and, therefore, evaluation of mitral regurgitation by Doppler color flow mapping must take left ventricular afterload into account. In 22 patients without intracardiac shunt or aortic valve disease, we studied the effects of phenylephrine infusion (mean dose, 150 μg) prior to cardiopulmonary bypass. The area, circumference length, and width of the left atrium and the maximal mitral regurgitant jet were measured by planimetry of color Doppler still frames.

In response to phenylephrine, the systolic arterial pressure increased significantly (from 108 ± 14 to 137 ± 17 mmHg, $P < .05$). Simultaneously, all jet dimensions also increased significantly (Table 13-1). On an individual basis, a systolic pressure increase was consistently associated with a jet dimension

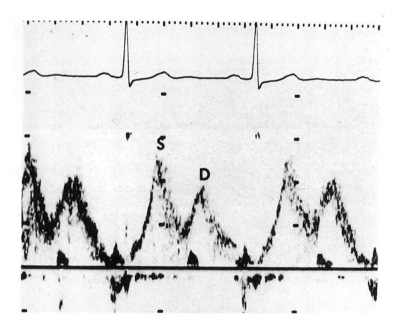

Figure 13-14
Normal pulmonary vein flow pattern. This pulsed-wave Doppler transesophageal recording of pulmonary vein flow in a normal subject shows the normal biphasic forward flow with systolic (S) and diastolic (D) flow components. (From Klein, Obarski, Stewart, et al.,[29] with permission.)

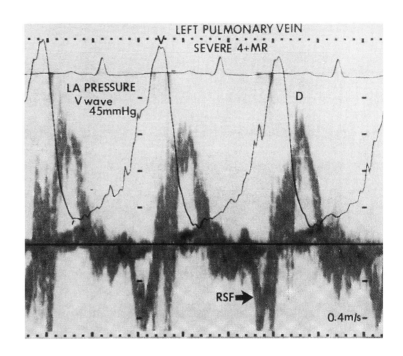

Figure 13-15
Pulmonary vein flow pattern with severe regurgitation. This pulsed-wave Doppler transesophageal recording of pulmonary vein and simultaneous direct left atrial pressure in a patient with severe (4+) mitral regurgitation demonstrates reversed systolic flow (RSF) in the left upper pulmonary vein. A large V wave is also noted, corresponding with the RSF in the pulmonary vein. (From Klein, Obarski, Stewart, et al.,[29] with permission.)

increase (Fig. 13-16). Similar findings were found when phenylephrine was administered after cardiopulmonary bypass.

Jet shape was measured by a circularity index (circumference squared, divided by 4 π

TABLE 13-1. Dimensions of Mitral Regurgitation Jet and Left Atrium Before and After Phenylephrine Infusion in 22 Patients

Dimension	Baseline	Phenylephrine
Jet:		
Length, cm	2.3 ± 0.9	3.5 ± 1.2*
Width, cm	1.2 ± 0.7	2.1 ± 0.7*
Circumference, cm	6.3 ± 2.9	10.7 ± 3.3*
Area, cm²	2.3 ± 1.8	6.5 ± 3.5*
Left atrial:		
Length, cm	6.1 ± 0.9	6.4 ± 0.7
Width, cm	4.1 ± 0.6	4.2 ± 0.6
Circumference, cm	18.4 ± 2.4	19.1 ± 1.8
Area, cm²	20.1 ± 5.1	22.1 ± 4.3
Jet-to-left-atrial ratio:		
Length, %	38 ± 15	55 ± 18*
Width, %	28 ± 18	49 ± 16*
Circumference, %	34 ± 15	56 ± 15*
Area, %	11 ± 8	29 ± 13*

*P < .05 compared with baseline value.
Values expressed as mean ± SD

times the area). This ratio is one for a circular shape, and for all other shapes is greater than 1. The circularity index was unchanged after phenylephrine infusion (1.58 ± 0.20 vs. 1.49 ± 0.27, P = NS), demonstrating that jets did not become disproportionately elongated. Thus systolic pressure had a significant effect on jet size, but not on jet shape.

It is important to realize that the relationship between regurgitant jet size and systolic pressure is not straightforward. A large increase in systolic pressure was not necessarily associated with a large increase in the jet area (Fig. 13-17). This should not be surprising; many physiologic variables may influence regurgitant jet size other than the systolic pressure, including atrial pressure, size and compliance, pulmonary venous compliance, regurgitant orifice size and geometry, and papillary muscle function. In addition, many technical factors may also influence jet size measurement, such as the gain setting, the pulse repetition frequency, imaging of low-velocity flows, differentiation of regurgitant from displacement flow, complexities in jet geometry such as multiple jets and vortex flow, approximation of regurgitant volume from the two-dimensional area, and temporal variation of jet size during systole.

Despite these limitations, changes in af-

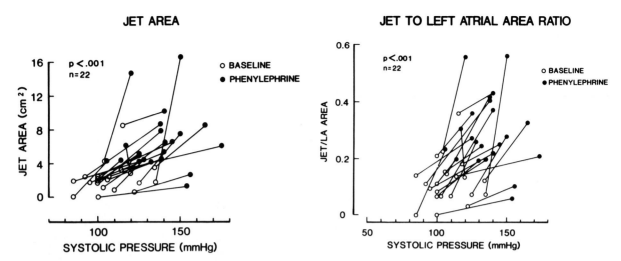

Figure 13-16
Afterload dependence of mitral regurgitation. An increase in systolic pressure (horizontal axis) produced an increase in jet area (left vertical axis) and jet-to-left-atrial area ratio (right vertical axis) in all except one patient (*P* < .001). (From Czer, Siegel, Maurer, et al.,[40] with permission.)

terload conditions may substantially influence the severity of regurgitation, as shown in Fig. 13-15. Care must therefore be exercised to match intraoperative systolic pressure to baseline or fixed reference levels when evaluating mitral regurgitation. If appropriate attention is paid to matching of the intraoperative systolic arterial pressure with that obtained during cardiac catheterization, very good agreement between angiographic and color Doppler evaluation of regurgitation has been achieved.[1,2]

Residual regurgitation after cardiopulmonary bypass should also be evaluated with hemodynamic conditions similar to the pre-

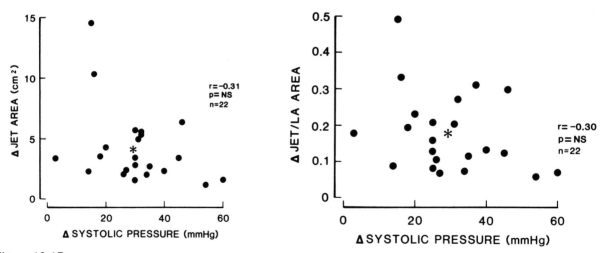

Figure 13-17
Relationship between the magnitude of increase in mitral regurgitant jet area and the amount of increase in systolic pressure. Small increases in systolic pressure (<20 mmHg) were associated with a large range of changes in jet area (left vertical axis) and jet-to-left-atrial area ratio (right vertical axis) so that no significant predictive correlation existed (*P* = NS). Thus, despite the association between increase in systolic pressure and increases in jet size (previous figure), the magnitude of increase in jet size could not be predicted from the magnitude of increase in systolic pressure. Asterisks indicate mean values. (From Czer, Siegel, Maurer, et al.,[40] with permission.)

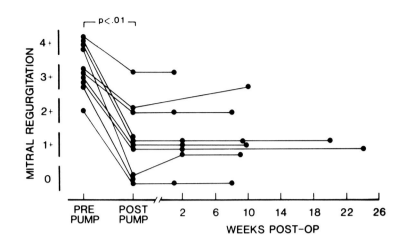

Figure 13-18
Longitudinal study of mitral regurgitation. Ten patients were examined before and after mitral valve repair by suture annuloplasty. There was no significant change in the grade of regurgitation after the initial postpump study: 2 (20 percent) changed by at most one grade and 8 (80 percent) had no change up to 24 weeks postoperatively. The initial postpump study was a good predictor of the long-term outcome after mitral annuloplasty. (From Czer, Siegel, Maurer, et al.,[40] with permission.)

pump study. If the systolic pressure is more than 15 mmHg below a prior baseline or fixed reference level, then phenylephrine should be administered to increase the systolic pressure to an appropriate level. In this way, the prepump and postpump studies can be compared under similar hemodynamic conditions.

Follow-up studies after mitral or tricuspid valve repair have demonstrated that there is no significant change in the grade of regurgitation from the postpump to subsequent postoperative evaluations (Figs. 13-18 and 13-19) unless there has been an intervening event. Thus the immediate postpump study is a good predictor of the long-term result after valve repair.

Valve Replacement

Homografts

Replacement of the aortic valve with a homograft is a technically demanding procedure. The structural and functional integrity of the homograft depends upon surgical skill and proper matching of the donor and recipient aortic annulus sizes. Only a few aortic annulus sizes may be available in hospitals without a large tissue bank of human aortic valves. Echocardiography can be used preoperatively or intraoperatively to determine aortic annulus diameter and therefore is helpful in selection of the proper size of homograft.[30] At the same

Figure 13-19
Longitudinal study of tricuspid regurgitation. Eighteen patients were studied before and after tricuspid valve repair by ring annuloplasty. There was no significant change in the grade of regurgitation after the initial postpump study, up to 22 weeks postoperatively. The initial postpump study was a good predictor of the long-term result after tricuspid annuloplasty. Tricuspid valve repair: ○ alone (n = 2); ● with mitral valve replacement (n = 16). (From Czer, Maurer, Bolger, et al.,[2] with permission.)

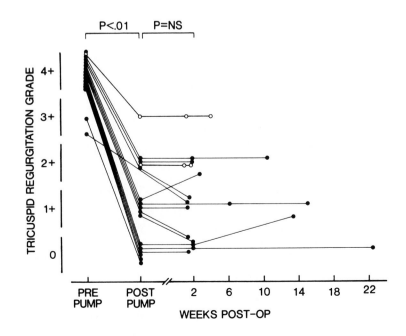

time, aortic root pathology and the competency of the other cardiac valves can be determined.

The annulus diameter is measured in the longitudinal plane immediately below the site of insertion of the aortic valve leaflets at the end of the left ventricular outflow tract (Fig. 13-20). A short-axis view may be used; however, care must be taken to avoid oblique views that foreshorten the annulus diameter or distort the annular dimensions. In heavily calcified valves, the insertion site of the leaflets may be difficult to determine and the annulus should be measured at the end of the left ventricular outflow tract. Measurements above the annulus (in the sinuses of Valsalva) are not accurate and frequently overestimate annulus size.[31]

Immediately after homograft replacement, regurgitation or stenosis may occur. The presence of either complication can be identified prior to chest closure by intraoperative Doppler echocardiography. Regurgitation is caused by stretching of the aortic commissures when the homograft is too small in relation to the native aortic annulus, while stenosis results from crimping of the homograft when an oversized graft is used.

Prosthetic Valves

The normal flow patterns of prosthetic valves have been established,[32–35] and these serve as the basis against which suspected abnormal prosthetic flow patterns can be recognized (see Chap. 6). Not infrequently, prosthetic valves have been explanted on the basis of Doppler echocardiographic findings and were later found to be normal.[34] Thus, late after valve replacement, proper interpretation of Doppler studies may avoid erroneous explantation of normally functioning valves. Moreover, immediately after valve replacement, intraoperative Doppler echocardiography has a role in selected patients, such as those in whom all or part of the native leaflet has been left intact during insertion of a prosthesis, in those with recent endocarditis, and in patients with connective tissue disorders, where valve dehiscence and malfunction may occur.

Normal regurgitation in the St. Jude valve consists of two converging retrograde jets if imaged in a plane parallel to the pivot guards, and two diverging jets around the edges of the leaflets with a central jet (from the coaptation line between the leaflets) if imaged in a plane perpendicular to the pivot guards. These jets are generally of low velocity with only short aliasing distances.[34] In the Medtronic-Hall valve, a single large central jet is seen with aliasing that extends quite far back into the receiving chamber, and peripheral jets without aliasing (see Chap. 6). Thus peripheral jets in Medtronic-Hall valves and all jets in St. Jude

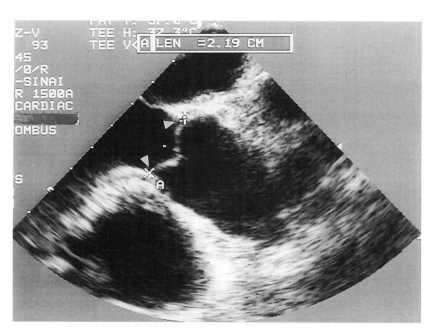

Figure 13-20
Measurements of aortic annulus diameter. The aortic annulus (arrows) is located at the base of the aortic leaflets, just above the left ventricular outflow tract. Transesophageal longitudinal view of left ventricle and aortic valve.

valves should be considered normal when minimal or no aliasing is present.

In the Björk-Shiley valve, peripheral regurgitant jets with short aliasing distances are seen at the periphery of the disk occluder. With normal bioprosthetic valves, only trace amounts of regurgitation are seen, arising from the coaptation lines between the leaflets. Early after valve replacement, very small jets of regurgitation may be seen which originate from the suture holes around a prosthesis; these disappear as the valve annulus becomes covered with endocardial or fibrous tissue.

In all mechanical valves, peripheral jets with significant aliasing distances represent strong evidence for pathological regurgitation.[34] In addition, if a highly aliased jet clearly arises from outside rather than within the annulus of the valve, a paravalvular leak is present and represents pathological regurgitation (Fig. 13-21).

Degeneration of a bioprosthetic valve may produce a flail leaflet, resulting in massive regurgitation into the left atrium.[32] Alternatively, prolapse of a leaflet may occur, producing an eccentric jet of regurgitation. Reverberations are often produced behind a prosthesis and may mask regurgitant jets; this is a problem when mitral prostheses are imaged

from the epicardial approach. Thus the transesophageal approach is preferred when evaluating mitral prostheses for regurgitation.

Antegrade flow through a St. Jude valve typically consists of three jets (Fig. 13-22). With caged-ball or caged-disk valves, flow is eccentrically directed. In bioprosthetic valves, a central flow jet is observed.[32] A common finding with mitral prostheses is that flow is directed toward the interventricular septum rather than toward the apex, as with native valves.

Doppler-derived velocities and gradients across normal prosthetic valves vary widely and are influenced by volumetric flow rate, particularly in smaller valve sizes.[35] It is important to recognize that Doppler gradients at high flow rates may be in a range ordinarily considered to reflect valve stenosis.[35] Moreover, certain valve designs, such as the bileaflet St. Jude and the caged-bill Starr-Edwards, produce localized high velocities within the valve and downstream pressure recovery during normal valve function. This phenomenon may cause the Doppler-derived gradient to exceed the catheter-derived gradient (the latter reflecting the recovered pressure) and is of particular clinical importance for smaller prosthetic sizes,

Figure 13-21
Paravalvular leak originating from the periphery of a mitral Björk-Shiley prosthetic valve. Transesophageal transverse view at the level of the left atrium.

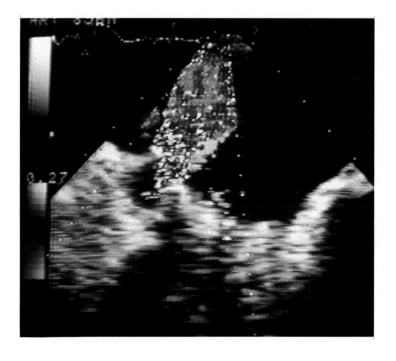

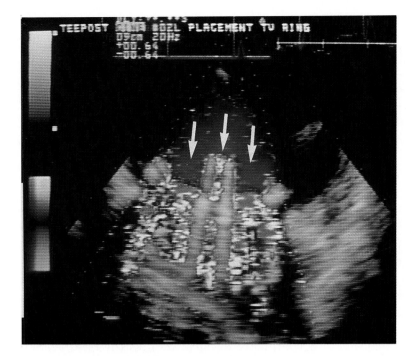

Figure 13-22
Antegrade flow pattern of St. Jude prosthesis. Three distinct jets are produced by this bileaflet valve. All three jets (arrows) are seen when the valve is imaged in a plane perpendicular to the open leaflets; if parallel to the leaflets, only one of the jets may be seen.

in which high Doppler gradients may be misinterpreted as indicating stenosis.[35] Other valve designs, such as the tilting-disk Medtronic-Hall and the bioprosthetic Hancock, do not produce a discrepancy between Doppler and catheter-derived gradients. Evaluation of prosthetic valve gradients is thus a complex process that must take into consideration valve design, valve size, volumetric flow rate, the presence of regurgitation, the location of Doppler interrogation in relation to the prosthesis, and in the case of aortic prostheses, the upstream velocity in the left ventricular outflow tract.

Ventricular Septal Rupture Following Myocardial Infarction

Rupture of the interventricular septum that occurs after an acute myocardial infarction creates a muscular septal defect with left-to-right shunting of blood flow between the ventricles. With inferior infarctions, the defect is often in the low septum, adjacent to the inferior wall of the left ventricle. After anterior infarction the defect is usually in the apical portion of the septum (Fig. 13-23). Multiple defects may also occur.

Intraoperative echocardiography is useful for identifying the precise location and number of defects. In addition, intramyocardial hemorrhage and edema may be identified by fracturing of the tissue and changes in the echocardiographic tissue density, respectively. Doppler color flow mapping can identify multiple shunts when all of the defects are not obvious echocardiographically.

Immediately after repair, color Doppler may identify small jets of high velocity that represent leakage through suture holes in the patch. On later follow-up studies, we have not seen these jets, suggesting that the small suture leaks are eventually sealed by clot formation or endothelialization. Larger leaks, and flow between two patches of a sandwich-type septal defect repair, are definitely abnormal and may indicate the need for revision of the repair.[36,37]

Aortic Dissection

Intraoperative evaluation of the aorta is most frequently required for aortic dissection. The descending thoracic aorta lies in close proximity to the esophagus and is easily imaged from the transesophageal approach (Fig. 13-1). The aortic root is also well seen, but the ascending and transverse aorta may be difficult to image due to interposition of the air-filled trachea. With a biplane transducer, acquisition of im-

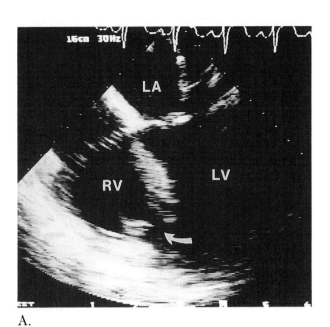

A.

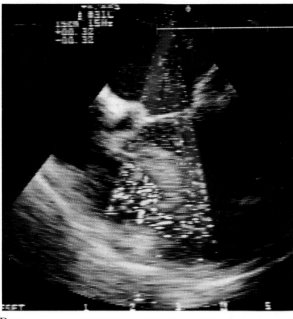

B.

Figure 13-23
Apical ventricular septal defect after anterior myocardial infarction. A channel (arrow) is seen between the distal interventricular septum and the apex of the left ventricle (LV). A left-to-right shunt was demonstrated by color Doppler. MV, mitral valve; LA, left atrium; RV, right ventricle.

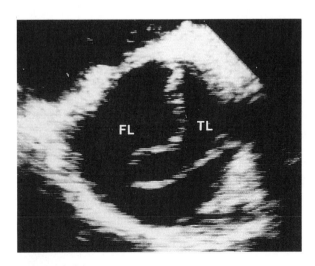

Figure 13-24
Dissection of descending thoracic aorta. The true lumen (TL) and false lumen (FL) are separated by the dissecting tissue. Transesophageal view in transverse plane. (From Czer, Siegel, Maurer, et al.,[40] with permission.)

ages in the longitudinal plane allows visualization of the transverse aorta; however, a "blind spot" in the ascending aorta may persist.

Prior to cardiopulmonary bypass, imaging should be performed to define the extent of the dissection (Fig. 13-24) and to locate the sites of blood flow entry into the false lumen. Since there may be multiple entry sites, a careful evaluation is mandatory; additional entry sites may cause further dissection if they are not recognized and treated. If the dissection extends below the diaphragm, epivascular imaging of the descending abdominal aorta can be performed through a minilaparotomy incision.[38] With types I, II, and IIR (retrograde) dissections, interrogation of the arteries is recommended.

After cardiopulmonary bypass, blood flow within the false lumen should be markedly diminished if all of the entry sites have been closed. Occasionally, some low-velocity swirling flow may be seen within the false lumen. If significant flow is seen, a careful search should be made to rule out additional entry sites.

Acknowledgments

The authors wish to thank Carlos Blanche, M.D., Alfredo Trento, M.D., Aurelio Chaus, M.D., Robert M. Kass, M.D., Sharo Raissi, M.D., Tsung Po Tsai, M.D., and Jack M. Matloff, M.D., of the Department of Thoracic and Cardiovascular Surgery; and John Bussell, M.D., Arnold Friedman, M.D., Harley Geller, M.D., and Errol Hackner, M.D., of the Department of Anesthesiology, whose patients were included in these studies. Special thanks to Michele De Robertis, R.N., for research and technical assistance, and to Liza Marcus for manuscript preparation.

References

1. Czer LSC, Maurer G, Bolger AF, et al: Intraoperative evaluation of mitral regurgitation by Doppler color flow mapping. *Circulation* 76:III-108, 1987.

2. Czer LSC, Maurer G, Bolger A, et al: Tricuspid valve repair. *J Thorac Cardiovasc Surg* 98:101, 1989.

3. Czer LSC, Maurer G: Intraoperative echocardiography in mitral and tricuspid valve repair. *Echocardiography* 7:305, 1990.

4. Melendez LJ, Chan KL, Cheung PK, et al: Incidence of bacteremia in transesophageal echocardiography: A prospective study of 140 consecutive patients. *J Am Coll Cardiol* 18:1650, 1991.

5. Steckelberg JM, Khandheria BK, Anhalt JP, et al: Prospective evaluation of the risk of bacteremia associated with transesophageal echocardiography. *Circulation* 84:177, 1991.

6. Dajani AS, Bisno AL, Chung KJ, et al: Prevention of bacterial endocarditis. Recommendations by the American Heart Association. *JAMA* 264:2919, 1990.

7. Maurer G, Siegel RJ, Czer LSC: The use of color flow mapping for intraoperative assessment of valve repair. *Circulation* 84 (suppl I):I-250, 1991.

8. Oury JH, Peterson KL, Folkerth TL, et al: Mitral valve replacement versus reconstruction: An analysis of indications and results of mitral valve procedures in a consecutive series of 80 patients. *J Thorac Cardiovasc Surg* 73:825, 1977.

9. Yacoub M, Halim M, Radley-Smith R, et al: Surgical treatment of mitral regurgitation caused by floppy valves: Repair versus replacement. *Circulation* 64(suppl II):II-210, 1981.

10. Oliveira DBG, Dawkins KD, Kay PH, et al: Chordal rupture: Comparison between repair and replacement. *Br Heart J* 50:318, 1983.

11. Adebo OA, Ross JK: Surgical treatment of ruptured mitral valve chordae: A comparison between valve replacement and valve repair. *Thorac Cardiovasc Surg* 32(3):139, 1984.

12. Perier P, Deloche A, Chauvaud S, et al: Comparative evaluation of mitral valve repair and replacement with Starr, Bjork, and porcine valve prostheses. *Circulation* 70 (suppl I):I-187, 1984.

13. Cosgrove DM, Chavez AM, Lytle BW, et al: Results of mitral valve reconstruction. *Circulation* 74 (suppl I):I-82, 1986.

14. Helmcke F, Nanda NC, Hsiung MC, et al: Color Doppler assessment of mitral regurgitation with orthogonal planes. *Circulation* 75:175, 1987.

15. Ormiston JA, Shah PM, Tei C, et al: Size and motion of the mitral valve annulus in man. *Circulation* 64:113, 1981.

16. Kay JH, Zubiate P, Mendez MA, et al: Surgical treatment of mitral insufficiency secondary to coronary artery disease. *J Thorac Cardiovasc Surg* 79:12, 1980.

17. DeVega NG: La anuloplastia selectiva, reguable y permanente. *Rev Esp Cardiol* 25:6, 1972.

18. Czer LSC, Maurer G, Trento A, et al: Comparative efficacy of ring and suture annuloplasty for ischemic mitral regurgitation. *Circulation* 86 (suppl II):II-46, 1992.

19. Carpentier A, Chauvaud S, Fabiani JN, et al: Reconstructive surgery of mitral valve incompetence. *J Thorac Cardiovasc Surg* 79:338, 1980.

20. Carpentier A, Deloche A, Hanania G, et al: Surgical management of acquired tricuspid valve disease. *J Thorac Cardiovasc Surg* 67:53, 1974.

21. Block PC: Who is suitable for percutaneous balloon mitral valvotomy? *Int J Cardiol* 20:9, 1988.

22. Nishimura RA, Holmes DR, Reeder GS: Percutaneous balloon valvuloplasty. *Mayo Clin Proc* 65:198, 1990.

23. Carpentier A, Loulmet D, Deloche A, et al: Surgical anatomy and management of ischemic mitral valve incompetence. *Circulation* 76 (suppl IV):IV-446, 1987.

24. Deloche A, Jebara VA, Relland JYM, et al: Valve repair with Carpentier techniques. *J Thorac Cardiovasc Surg* 99:990, 1990.

25. Mihaileanu S, Marino JP, Chauvaud S, et al: Left ventricular outflow obstruction after mitral valve repair (Carpentier's technique): Proposed mechanisms of disease. *Circulation* 78 (suppl I):I-78, 1988.

26. Schiavone WA, Cosgrove DM, Lever HM, et al: Long-term follow-up of patients with left ventricular outflow tract obstruction after Carpentier ring mitral valvuloplasty. *Circulation* 78 (suppl I):I-60, 1988.

27. Chen C, Thomas JD, Anconina J, et al: Impact of impinging wall jet color Doppler quantification of mitral regurgitation. *Circulation* 84:712, 1991.

28. Czer LSC, Maurer G, Bolger A, et al: Ischemic mitral regurgitation: Comparative evaluation of revascularization versus repair by Doppler color flow mapping. *Circulation* 76 (suppl IV):IV-389, 1987.

29. Klein AL, Obarski TP, Stewart WJ, et al: Transesophageal Doppler echocardiography of pulmonary venous flow: A new marker of mitral regurgitation severity. *J Am Coll Cardiol* 18:518, 1991.

30. Bolger AF, Bartzokis T, Miller DC: Intraoperative echocardiography and Doppler color flow mapping in freehand allograft aortic valve and root replacement. *Echocardiography* 7:229, 1990.

31. Czer LSC, Maurer G: Epicardial echocardiography and Doppler color-flow mapping in the adult patient, in de Bruijn NP, Clements FM: *Intraoperative Use of Echocardiography*, chap 9, p 157.

32. Czer LSC: Echocardiographic and Doppler evaluation of prosthetic heart valves, in Maurer G, Mohl W (eds): *Echocardiography and Doppler in Cardiac Surgery*, Igaku-Shoin, New York, p 109, 1989.

33. Baumgartner H, Khan S, DeRobertis M, et al: Discrepancies between Doppler and catheter gradients in aortic prosthetic valves in vitro: A manifestation of localized gradients and pressure recovery. *Circulation* 82:1467, 1990.

34. Baumgartner H, Khan S, DeRobertis M, et al: Color Doppler regurgitant characteristics of normal mechanical mitral vale prostheses in vitro. *Circulation* 85:323, 1992.

35. Baumgartner H, Khan S, DeRobertis M, et al: Effect of prosthetic aortic valve design on the Doppler-catheter gradient correlation: An in vitro study of normal St. Jude, Medtronic-Hall, Starr-Edwards and Hancock valves. *J Am Coll Cardiol* 19:324, 1992.

36. Maurer G, Czer LSC: Intraoperative Doppler color flow mapping, in Nanda NC (ed): *Textbook of Color Doppler Echocardiography*, Philadelphia, Lea & Febiger, 1989, p 258.

37. Maurer G, Czer LSC, Shah PK, et al: Assessment by Doppler color flow mapping of ventricular septal defect after acute myocardial infarction. *Am J Cardiol* 64:668, 1989.

38. Takamoto S, Kyo S, Adachi H, et al: Decision making in the treatment of aortic dissection by transesophageal and intraoperative Doppler color flow mapping. *Echocardiography* 7:348, 1990.

39. Czer LSC, Maurer G: Conventional and color Doppler intraoperative echocardiography, in Nanda NC (ed): *Doppler Echocardiography*, 2d ed, Philadelphia, Lea & Febiger, 1993, chap 37, p 427.

40. Czer LSC, Siegel RJ, Maurer G, et al: Transesophageal and epicardial color-flow Doppler echocardiography: Surgical repair of valvular, ischemic, and congenital heart disease, in Kaplan JA (ed): *Cardiac Anesthesia*, 3d ed, Philadelphia, Saunders, 1993, chap 12, p 386.

14

TEE Assessment of Left Ventricular Function for Intraoperative Monitoring

Hiroshi Watanabe
Jack Panopoulos
Yasu Oka

Introduction

The intraoperative assessment of cardiac function in patients undergoing cardiac surgery incorporates various established monitoring modalities. However, several limitations are attributed to conventional intraoperative monitoring systems.[1,2] The inability to visualize left ventricular and valvular anatomy, chamber volume, and flow dynamics represented the most important of these limitations. The introduction of transesophageal echocardiography (TEE) provides additional intraoperative information and enhances the assessment of left ventricular function during cardiac surgery.

Originally, transesophageal echo probes were limited to a single transducer permitting serial images from the transverse plane. The recent introduction of biplane probes incorporating an additional longitudinal transducer to a transverse transducer allows imaging of the heart in two orthogonal views. Information derived from biplane TEE can dramatically improve anesthetic and surgical management. Myocardial depression by anesthetic agents,

surgical intervention, and unphysiologic loading conditions are the most important causes of intraoperative left ventricular dysfunction.

TEE is an ideal method of monitoring left ventricular function and it permits early detection of regional wall motion abnormalities (RWMA) caused by myocardial ischemia. In this chapter, anatomy and view orientation of TEE are described first, then the methodology of evaluating global and regional left ventricular function. Examples of clinical cases that demonstrate the importance of intraoperative TEE monitoring in decision making by anesthesiologists, surgeons, and cardiologists are presented.

Anatomy and View Orientation of Left Ventricle (LV)

Anatomy[3]
The left ventricle (LV) is a bullet-shaped chamber with its apex directed anteriorly, inferiorly,

and leftward. It is surrounded by the lung and is contiguous with the diaphragm that separates the LV from the stomach inferiorly. The bicuspid mitral valve and tricuspid aortic valve are usually located at the base of the "bullet." The left ventricular wall is composed of the interventricular septum and the free wall with its two papillary muscles, the anterolateral papillary muscle (APM), and the posteromedial papillary muscle (PPM). The endocardial surface is irregular with numerous trabeculae carnae (Figs. 14-1, 14-2). The distribution of coronary blood supply to the LV is illustrated by simplified schemes[4] (Fig. 14-3). The normal heart has two coronary arteries. The left coronary artery begins as a main vessel that promptly divides into a left anterior descending artery (LAD) and a left circumflex artery (LCX). The left anterior descending artery courses along the anterior interventricular sulcus (area of cross oblique lines). This artery extends to

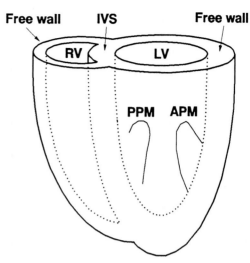

Figure 14-2
Left ventricle is composed of the free wall and the interventricular septum. Two papillary muscles originate from the anterolateral and posteromedial free wall. APM = anterior papillary muscle; IVS = interventricular septum; LV = left ventricle; PPM = posterior papillary muscle; RV = right ventricle.

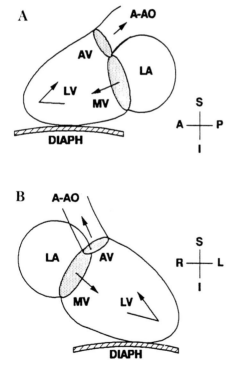

Figure 14-1
Configuration of left ventricle, viewed from left side (A) and anterior side (B). Arrows show bloodstream of left ventricle. A = anterior; A-AO = ascending aorta; AV = aortic valve; DIAPH = diaphragm; I = inferior; LA = left atrium; LV = left ventricle; P = posterior; S = superior.

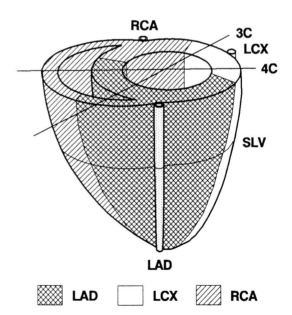

Figure 14-3
Distribution of the three coronary arteries of left ventricle. 3C = three-chamber view; 4C = four-chamber view; LAD = left anterior descending artery; LCX = left circumflex artery; RCA = right coronary artery; SLV = short-axis view of LV.

the apex, often looping over the apex, and perfuses the anterior two-thirds of the ventricular septum, a portion of the anterior right ventricular free wall, and the anterior left ventricular free wall including APM. The left circumflex artery turns laterally to the left and extends for a variable distance between the left atrium and ventricle in the atrioventricular groove. The left circumflex artery branches into the marginal artery that perfuses the lateral aspect of the left ventricle. The right coronary artery (RCA) courses along the posterior interventricular sulcus toward the apex (area of oblique lines). The right coronary artery divides into the posterior descending artery that perfuses the inferior one-third of the interventricular septum and the posterior left ventricular branch that perfuses a variable amount of the posterior inferior left ventricular wall including the PPM and most of the right ventricular wall.

View Orientation[4,5]

Left ventricular function is customarily assessed by gastric short-axis view (SLV) at midpapillary muscle (mid-PM) level by transverse (T) scan and long-axis view by longitudinal (L) scan (Fig. 14-4). The L-scans are obtained in seconds by switching from transverse to longitudinal modes (Fig. 14-5). The orientation of the L-scan is always orthogonal to the corresponding T-scan.

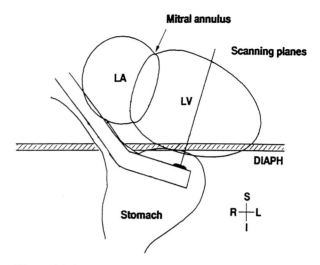

Figure 14-4
The optimal probe position to obtain transgastric view. LA = left atrium; LV = left ventricle.

Step 1: SLV at the mid-PM level is obtained with the probe tip positioned approximately 43 cm from the incisors in anesthetized patients, although this measurement may range from 38 to 55 cm.[6] Orientation of SLV image viewed on the screen is as follows: The inferior wall adjacent to the diaphragm is situated at the top of the screen, the anterior wall at the bottom of the screen, the lateral free wall of the LV on the right side, and the interventricular septum and right ventricle on the left side. The inner circle surrounded by the LV wall is the LV cavity. Anterolateral and posteromedial

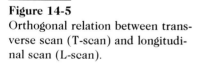

Figure 14-5
Orthogonal relation between transverse scan (T-scan) and longitudinal scan (L-scan).

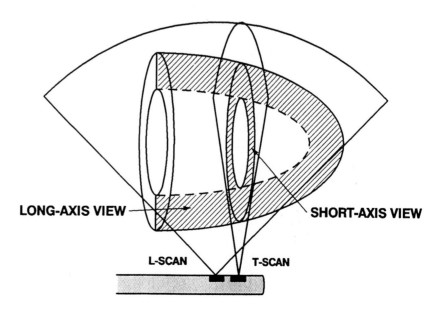

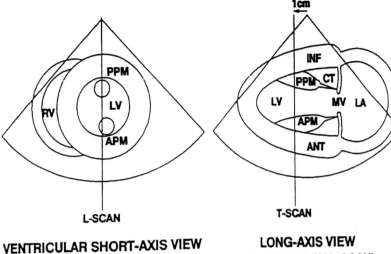

Figure 14-6
The schema of ventricular short-axis view in transverse scan (left) and long-axis view in longitudinal scan (right). ANT = anterior (wall); APM = anterior papillary muscle; CT = chordae tendineae; INF = inferior (wall); LA = left atrium. LV = left ventricle; MV = mitral valve; PPM = posterior papillary muscle; RV = right ventricle.

papillary muscles are most commonly found at 5 and 12 o'clock, respectively (Fig. 14-6). The endocardial edge is used for measuring the left ventricular volume and assessing regional wall motion.[7]

Step 2: Obtain transgastric long-axis view of LV by switching T-scan to L-scan. The apex is located at the left side of the screen, the left atrium on the right, the inferior wall and posteromedial papillary muscle at the top of the screen, and the anterior wall and anterolateral papillary muscle at the bottom of the screen (Fig. 14-7).

Step 3: Obtain M-mode using M-mark in B-mode of either T-scan or L-scan. M-mode reveals the inferior wall on the top and the anterior wall on the bottom side. LV cavity is seen between both walls (Fig. 14-8).

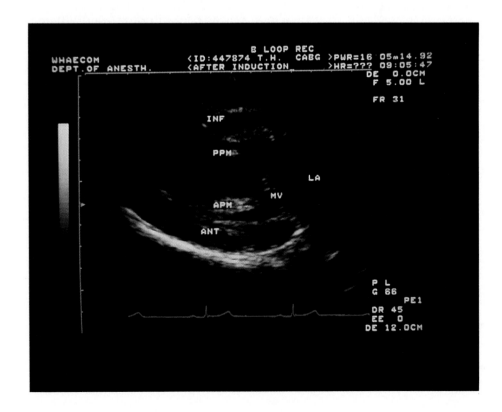

Figure 14-7
Long-axis view of left ventricle in longitudinal scan. ANT = anterior (wall); APM = anterior papillary muscle; INF = inferior (wall); LA = left atrium; MV = mitral valve; PPM = posterior papillary muscle.

Figure 14-8
The M-mode (left) is obtained by M-mark in B-mode (right). The M-mark is shown by the arrow from the top to the bottom in B-mode. AW = anterior wall; IW = inferior wall.

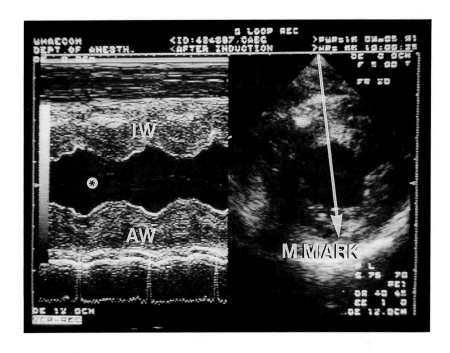

Evaluation of Left Ventricular Function

Global Systolic Function

TEE estimation of global systolic function complementarily adds more specific information to other routine hemodynamic variables such as pressures and cardiac output.[8] It enables measurement of LV dimensions and volumes, and ejection fraction can be obtained serially. Various methods of measuring left ventricular systolic and diastolic volumes have been used to obtain ejection fraction (EF).[9–11]

End-systolic area (ESA) and end-diastolic area (EDA) are obtained in B-mode, and percent fractional area change can also be calculated.[12] It is the indication of load-dependent cardiac performance.

Ejection Fraction

Two easy and reliable methods for determining ejection fraction are Teichholz's method and the area-length method. Teichholz's method is performed in the following manner[13] (Fig. 14-9):

1. Obtain SLV at mid-PM level.

2. Put M-mark in B-mode and position it so as to pass the maximal dimension of LV using the B-mode.

3. Freeze the M-mode image.

4. Measure the distance between the leading edge of the posterior endocardium and that of the anterior endocardium at end systole and end diastole.

End systole is the minimum dimension, while end diastole is at the peak of the R wave of electrocardiography (ECG).

End-systolic and end-diastolic volumes are calculated by inserting the end-systolic dimension (ESD) and end-diastolic dimension (EDD) in equation (1), and then ejection fraction, stroke volume, and cardiac output can be derived by inserting these volumes in equation (2). These calculations are performed by an on-line computer in the echo machine.

$$V = (7.0/2.4 + D) \times D^3 \qquad (1)$$

where V = volume
$\quad D$ = dimension

$$SV = EDV - ESV \qquad (2)$$
$$CO = (EDV - ESV) \times HR$$
$$\text{Percent EF} = (EDV - ESV)/EDV \times 100$$

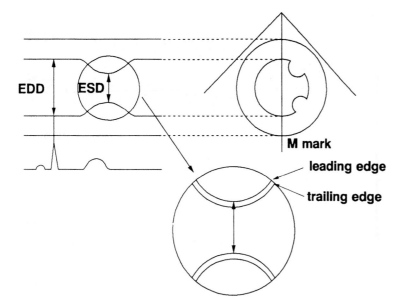

Figure 14-9
Diagram showing the method for measuring the left ventricular volume in M-mode. Dimensions are measured as the distances between the leading edge of the posterior endocardium and that of the anterior endocardium at end systole (at the peak inward contraction of the anterior wall or at the minimal dimension) and end diastole (at the peak of R wave). EDD = end-diastolic distance; ESD = end-systolic distance.

where SV = stroke volume
  ESV = end-systolic volume
  EF = ejection fraction
  EDV = end-diastolic volume
  CO = cardiac output
  HR = heart rate

Area-length method is calculated as following:

$$V = (5/6) \times A \times L \qquad (3)$$

where V = volume
  A = area
  L = length of long axis

After the area is calculated by tracing the inward perimeter of LV in short-axis view, the distance between basal and apex of LV in three- or four-chamber view is measured. The volume is then obtained by formula (3). This method is more accurate than the former, but it is not practical because the measurement takes a considerable amount of time. Accordingly Teichholz's method is often used for quick measurement.

Fractional Area Change (FAC)
The measurement of FAC is performed as follows (Fig. 14-10):

1. Obtain SLV at mid-PM level.

2. Synchronize views at end systole and end diastole of ECG.

3. Trace the endocardial edge of SLV at end systole and end diastole.

Percent fractional area change is calculated by the following equation:

Percent FAC = (EDA − ESA)/EDA × 100

where FAC = fractional area change
  EDA = end-diastolic area
  ESA = end-systolic area

The measurement of percent FAC correlated well with ejection fraction of radionuclide and angiography.[14]

There are pitfalls with these methods of determining ejection fraction. With Teichholz's method (single-plane, one-dimensional), ejection fraction may be underestimated when there are RWMA in the anterior or inferior wall and overestimated when RWMA are present in other areas or other levels of the LV wall. For fractional area change (single-plane, two-dimensional method) the measurements change with the ventilatory cycle and should be obtained at the same phase of the ventilatory cycle. Other methods such as the relationship of end-systolic wall stress (ESS) to end-systolic area (ESA) take several minutes for one mea-

Figure 14-10
Measurement of fractional area change. Trace line at end systole (right) and end diastole (left) for fractional area change. EDA = end-diastolic area (18.2 cm²); ESA = end-systolic area (7.58 cm²).

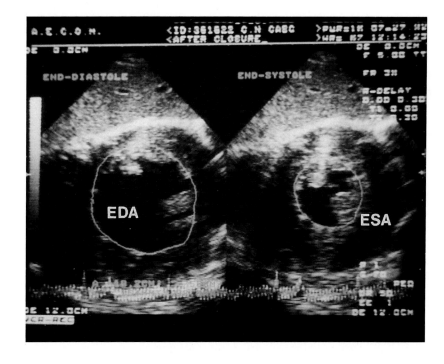

surement and may be impractical when continuous monitoring of regional wall motion in real time is mandatory.

End-Systolic Wall Stress (ESS) and ESS/ESA

End-systolic LV wall stress (ESS) is a good index of the interaction of afterload.[15,16] This is calculated by measurements of LV echographic end-systolic diameter and wall thickness and systolic arterial pressure or left ventricular systolic pressure. The formula is

$$ESS = P \times D/4h(1 + h/D)$$

where P = peak intraarterial pressure or
left ventricular systolic pressure

D = internal diameter of LV
h = wall thickness of the myocardium

Internal diameter (D) of LV and wall thickness of the myocardium (h) can be obtained by the measurement of echographic diameter and wall thickness in M-mode (Fig. 14-11), and intraarterial pressure (P) can be also obtained by a display of the arterial line in real time during operation.[17] Moreover, the ratio ESS/ESA is available for a load-independent index of contractility.[18] However, these need to be done as off-line evaluation, so that this is not practical as operative monitoring. In the near future, clinically useful on-line measurements of LV function and RWMA analysis will be available.[19]

Figure 14-11
Measurement of wall thickness (h) and internal diameter (D) at minimal dimension in systole in M-mode (left) using M-mark in B-mode (right).

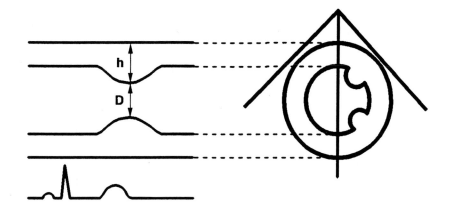

Regional Systolic Function

TEE detection of myocardial ischemia is determined by abnormality of regional wall motion and wall thickening. For quantitative analysis of RWMA, the American Society of Echocardiography recommends that the circumference of LV short axis of mid-PM level be subdivided into eight segments[20] (Fig. 14-12). The SLV at mid-PM level is the most important level for continuous monitoring of regional wall motion because this level of LV is usually perfused by three coronary arteries. However, when uniplane TEE is used, five other levels of LV [(1) mitral valve (MV); (2) chordae tendineae (CT); (3) high papillary muscle (high-PM); (3) low papillary muscle (low-PM); (5) apex] should also be scanned[7] (Fig. 14-13). With advent of biplane, basal and apical areas are easily evaluated by L-scan.

RWMA are evaluated in four categories[7] (Fig. 14-14): normal, hypokinesis, akinesis, dyskinesis.

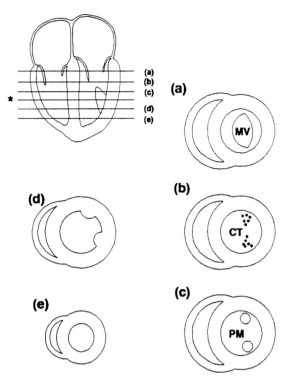

Figure 14-13
Five other levels of left ventricle excluding mid-PM level from basal to apex. * = midpapillary muscle level (mid-PM). Typical mid-PM level is shown in Fig. 14-12. CT = chordal tendinal level; MV = mitral valve level.

The motion of hypokinesis is normally directed, but the radius shortening and wall thickening are reduced while akinesis denotes absent motion and wall thickening during systole. Dyskinesis represents outward wall motion and wall thinning in systole.

Ischemic myocardium may also be assessed by measuring distances from epicardium to endocardium at end systole and end diastole.[21] This is obtained by the following formula:

$$\text{Percent WTh} = (\text{WTh}_{es} - \text{WTh}_{ed})/\text{WTh}_{es} \times 100$$

where

   percent WTh = percent wall thickening
      WTh_{es} = end-systolic wall thickness
      WTh_{ed} = end-diastolic wall thickness

Normal wall thickening is 40 to 80 percent.[22] However, it is difficult to obtain the fine epicardial border of the LV and thus there is inaccuracy in repeated measurements of WTh.[23] In our institution we presently use qualitative analysis of RWM and have noted the following: (1) Significantly more patients had TEE-

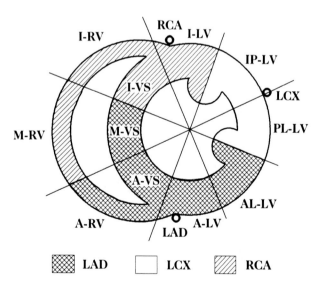

Figure 14-12
Segmental division of the left ventricle and coronary blood supplies for quantitative analysis at mid-PM level. A-LV = anterior left ventricle; A-RV = anterior right ventricle; A-VS = anterior-ventricular septum; AL-LV = anterolateral left ventricle; I – LV = inferior left ventricle; I-RV = inferior right ventricle; I-VS = inferior-ventricular septum; IP-LV = inferoposterior left ventricle; M-RV = mid right ventricle; M-VS = midventricular septum; PL-LV = posterolateral left ventricle.

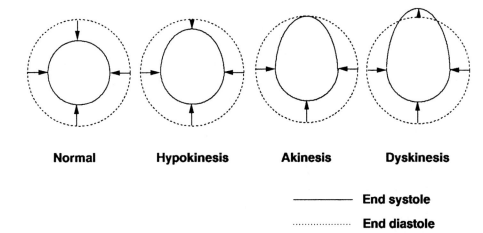

Figure 14-14
Classification of regional wall motion abnormalities.

Normal   **Hypokinesis**   **Akinesis**   **Dyskinesis**

———————— **End systole**

.... **End diastole**

defined ischemic episodes in the post-CPB period than in the pre-CPB period. (2) Poor graft and/or inadequate myocardial protection was strongly suggestive for post-CPB ischemia and was related to adverse outcome.

Thus TEE is a useful tool to enable us to detect problem areas at an early stage and to institute rapid and appropriate treatment to support and sustain patients.[24]

Difficulties in Obtaining SLV at Mid-PM Level

There may be pitfalls in obtaining a short-axis view at mid-PM level during cardiac surgery. The conditions are as follows:

1. When the heart is markedly dilated and lies transversely above the diaphragm.

2. When the diaphragm is elevated in the supine position and the heart lies transversely, especially in obese patients.

3. The stomach is pushed rightward by retention of gas in the intestine, splenomegaly, or abundant abdominal adipose tissue. Additional causes include air[6] in the stomach and esophagus, intestine, lung and chest tubes, etc., located between the heart and the transducer in the stomach.

All these pitfalls should be kept in mind when an optimal view is not obtained.

Diastolic Function

Diastolic function[25,26] is assessed by evaluation of mitral flow velocity patterns measured in the three-chamber view in transverse scan or two-chamber view in longitudinal scan using pulse-wave mode. The sample volume is positioned on the centerline of the inflow tract midway between the annulus and the tip of the leaflets. Mitral flow patterns obtained by Doppler echocardiography are illustrated in Figs. 14-15 and 14-16. Two negative peak waves are seen during diastole. The E wave occurs during early diastolic filling and the A wave occurs during atrial contraction. The following indices have been used to evaluate diastolic function of the left ventricle:

1. Peak E velocity/peak A velocity ratio

2. Integral area of E wave/integral area of A wave ratio

3. Acceleration time

4. Diastolic filling time

When myocardial ischemia occurs, peak E velocity decreases and peak A velocity increases, resulting in a decreased ratio. However, several factors including age, heart rate, rhythm, preload, position of sample volume, and respiration all affect the mitral flow pattern and thus Doppler-derived diastolic indices. Thus intraoperative evaluation of diastolic function is difficult and should be performed cautiously considering all these factors.

Mitral and Tricuspid Regurgitation Associated with Poor LV Function in CABG Patients

Mitral and tricuspid regurgitation is often associated with coronary artery disease (CAD) and

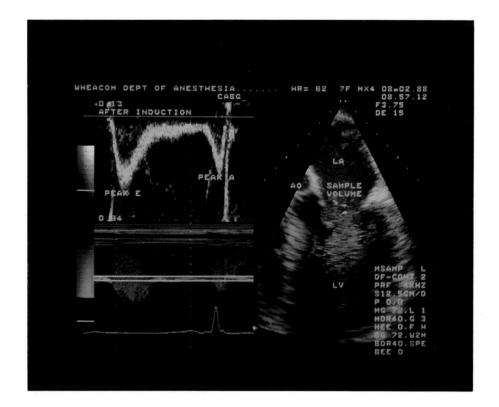

Figure 14-15
Transmitral flow with
PW mode. Mitral flow ve-
locity is measured in the
three-chamber view with
the sample volume posi-
tioned on the centerline
of the inflow tract, and
midway between the
annulus and the tip of
the leaflets. Two nega-
tive peak waves (E and
A waves) are seen. Note
that area of the E wave
is larger than that of the
A wave.

it is seen more frequently following CPB. Three-
and four-chamber views by T-scan and two-
chamber views by L-scan using CDI are used
for the evaluation. Detailed description is dis-
cussed in Chap. 13.

TEE Diagnosis and Decision Making During Cardiac Surgery

Eliminating or mitigating the factors that diminish left ventricular contractility can lessen
intraoperative risk, especially in high-risk patients. To achieve this end, the appearance
of altered LV function must be recognized
promptly. TEE affords anesthesiologists, surgeons, and cardiologists an ideal method for
monitoring intraoperative LV function. The
protocol for intraoperative TEE assessment of
LV function and the utility of perioperative
TEE in decision making at our institution is
presented. Upon arrival of the patient in the
operating room, the patient's chart is reviewed

to confirm that TEE is not contraindicated.
The incidence of contraindication in our experience is extremely rare. After routine hemodynamic parameters are measured, the patient
is induced with narcotic agents and muscle
relaxant and the patient's trachea is intubated.
The TEE probe is then inserted into the esophagus and connected to the echocardiographic
system and the echo view is continuously
monitored throughout surgery exept during
CPB. TEE evaluation of cardiac function during
cardiac surgery is usually determined at four
different stages.

Stage 1: After induction: from postinduction
to sternotomy
Stage 2: Pre-CPB: from sternotomy to CPB
Stage 3: Post-CPB: from initiation of weaning
CPB to chest closure
Stage 4: At the end of surgery: before leaving
operating room

Stage 1 represents the phase of the procedure
where views are easiest to attain and clarity is
at a premium. At this time, LV function is
assessed via the SLV at mid-PM level in the
T-scan. The L-scan is used for the evaluation

Figure 14-16
Parameters of Doppler measurements. DFT = diastolic filling time; DT = deceleration time.

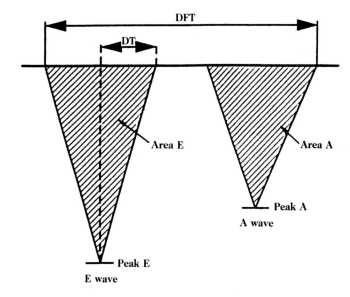

of the basal and the apical areas of LV. Mitral regurgitation due to ischemic changes may be detected via two- (L-scan) or three-chamber views (T-scan) and correlated with mitral flow velocity, wall motion abnormalities, and pulmonary artery wedge pressure.[27] TEE remains a more sensitive monitor for ischemic changes than ECG.[28] While evaluation of left ventricular function is the cornerstone of a thorough TEE examination, it is also necessary to evaluate other aspects of cardiac function. Of particular interest are the mitral valve, the aortic valve and aorta, the tricuspid valve, and the right ventricle, pulmonary vein, pleural cavity, pulmonary artery, and others. During stage 2, sternotomy, dissection of internal mammary arteries, periocardiotomy, and cannulations are performed. These various aspects of surgical preparation for CPB tend to obscure the clarity of stage 1 views. Thus stage 2 becomes somewhat difficult for detailed analysis and highlights the necessity of an expeditious echocardiographer. With the advent of retrograde cardioplegia, TEE may be useful in confirming the optimal position of the cannula in the coronary sinus when technical difficulty is present. During stage 3, changes in cardiac function detected by TEE fluctuate most dramatically as the patient is weaned from CPB. The correlation of hemodynamic data with TEE is invaluable to both anesthesiologist and surgeon in decision making. The function of

the LV and valves can be assessed immediately in real time and guide therapeutic interventions. TEE easily identifies hypovolemia in SLV and retained air bubbles in the three-chamber view of the heart. Confirmation of position of mechanical assist devices including intraaortic balloon pumps and ventricular assist devices may also be performed in real time. During stage 4, sternal closure may compress the LV or kink a grafted vein. TEE evaluation is of prime importance, and the effect of any of these detrimental effects on LV function or valvular function may be demonstrated rapidly and reliably in real time via TEE. It should be mentioned that echo views may often be unclear owing to acoustic shadows from a prosthetic valve, drainage tubes, and wires.

Case Presentation
The following six cases illustrate the utility of TEE for rapid assessment, diagnosis, and intervention.

Case 1: Hypovolemia after Weaning from CPB
The patient was a 49-year-old female with a past medical history of hypertension and the diagnosis of a dissecting aortic aneurysm (type 1). The ascending aorta was replaced with an artificial graft. When separating from bypass, BP was appropriate (101/62 mmHg). TEE revealed good LV function and adequate size

of LV (Fig. 14-17A). BP fell gradually (66/47 mmHg) as bleeding from graft site occurred. TEE demonstrated mild hypertrophy of LV and a very small LV cavity. Figure 14-17B illustrated a typical echo view of hypovolemia. Note kissing APM and PPM in the systolic phase. Bleeding at suture site was the reason for hypovolemia.

Case 2: Moderate to Severe Regurgitation Following CABS

The patient was a 76-year-old female with a past medical history of hypertension, unstable angina, and recent myocardial infarction. Mul-

tiple coronary artery grafts were performed. After CPB, rising pulmonary artery pressures were associated with moderate to severe mitral regurgitation (central) associated with poor LV function (Fig. 14-18A). Figure 14-18B illustrates reduction of mitral regurgitation with the infusion of dobutamine and nitroglycerin. Hemodynamics improved significantly, pulmonary artery pressure was decreased from 45/24 to 33/16 mmHg, and cardiac output increased from 3.4 to 4.2 liters/min.

It is not unusual to see transient regurgitation due to poor LV function after CPB in CABS

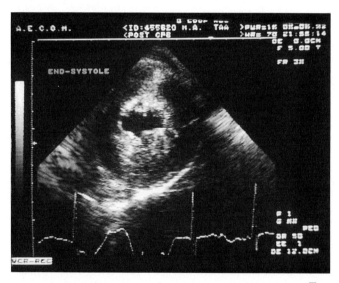

Top

Figure 14-17

A. The ventricular short-axis views of mid-PM level at end systole (upper) and end diastole (lower) immediately after CPB.

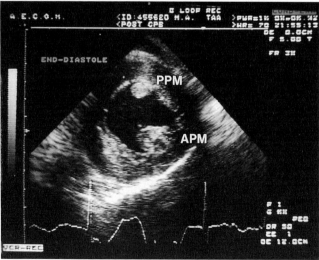

A.

Bottom

Figure 14-17

B. The same views as *A* during hypovolemia. Anterior (APM) and posterior papillary muscles (PPM) are very close to each other (arrows); the left ventricular cavity is very small at end systole (upper) and LV cavity at end diastole is much smaller than that of *A* (lower).

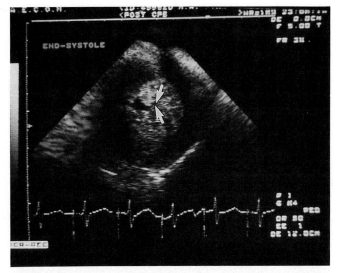

Top

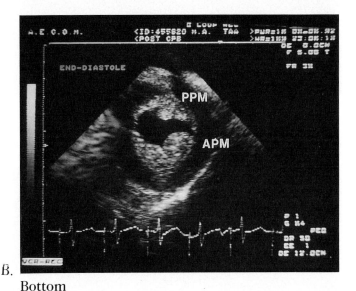

B.

Bottom

patients.[29] Rapid analysis and pharmacologic intervention can mitigate or reverse most of MR following CABG.

Case 3: RWMA of LV Following Mitral Valve Replacement

The patient was a 66-year-old female with a medical history of severe hypertension and mitral stenosis associated with congestive heart failure. Mitral replacement using a Medtronic-Hall valve was performed. After weaning from CPB, the patient was hypotensive. TEE showed normally functioning prosthetic valve in three-chamber view and trivial central regurgitation (normal for M-H valve) in color Doppler imaging (CDI), but a hypokinetic inferior septum was noted. ECG showed elevated ST segments in lead II. With confirmation that the valve replacement was successful, the presumptive diagnosis of air embolus in the right coronary artery was entertained. In this patient air was detected in the left atrium and left ventricular outflow tract (Fig. 14-19) and the air bubbles were thought to be completely eliminated by a venting tube by the end of CPB. However, residual air may have been existing in the heart. A further attempt to eliminate air was performed.

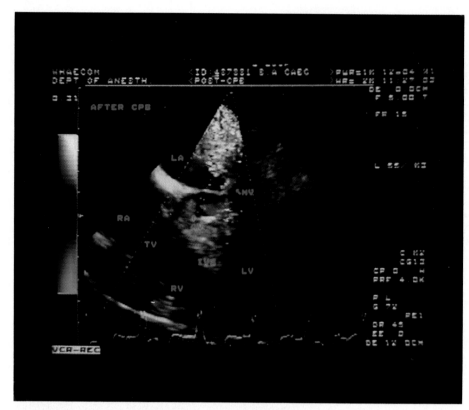

A.

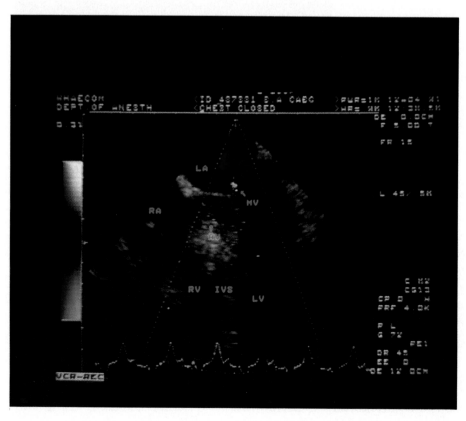

B.

Figure 14-18
A. Four-chamber view of post-CPB, showing moderate mitral regurgitation (mosaic pattern). AV = aortic valve; IVS = interventricular septum; LA = left atrium; LV = left ventricle; MV = mitral valve; RA = right atrium; RV = right ventricle; TV = tricuspid valve. *B.* The same view as *A* following the pharmacological intervention; no mitral regurgitation is detected.

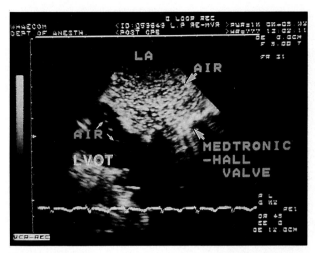

Figure 14-19
Three-chamber view at the end of CPB, showing air bubbles in left atrium and left ventricular outflow tract. LA = left atrium; LVOT = left ventricular outflow tract.

Regional wall motion in the inferior septum improved as well as ST segments returned to baseline and systemic BP increased from 75/49 to 95/55 mmHg. Air embolus in coronary arteries, especially in right coronary artery, is always a potential problem in open heart surgery, especially in the case of combined valve and coronary artery surgery.

Case 4: A Confirmation of the Optimal Position of Coronary Sinus Cannula and Evaluation of Left Ventricular Function Before and After CPB

The patient was a 68-year-old male, scheduled for CABS. He had a history of myocardial infarction 2 months prior to scheduled surgery. At pre-CPB period, cannulation of retrograde cardioplegia into coronary sinus was difficult; thus the optimal position of coronary sinus cannula was guided by TEE (Fig. 14-20). Inadequate myocardial protection caused by malpositioning of cannula may produce LV function. In this patient, RWM was normal in pre- and post-CPB.

Case 5: Rapid Detection of Poor Graft in CABS

The patient was a 62-year-old male with a past history of unstable angina, but good left LV wall motion (Fig. 14-21A). Single coronary artery graft to LAD with left internal mammary artery (IMA) was performed. After CPB, TEE detected persistent severe hypokinesis in the anterior and anteroseptal walls of LV associated with decreased systemic blood pressure (Fig. 21A, B). The surgeon immediately recognized poor quality of IMA graft and performed an additional vein graft to first diagonal artery. After weaning from second CPB, TEE showed improvement of the anterior wall motion (Fig. 14-21C). This was a typical case of rapid detection of poor graft, and TEE guided the surgeon to a successful operation.

Case 6: New RWMA Due to Kink of Grafting

The patient was a 48-year-old female with a history of old MI as well as recent MI,

Figure 14-20
Showing an optimal position of coronary sinus cannulas. Cannulas are seen as a line of strong echo in coronary sinus and balloon at the junction of right atrium and coronary sinus.

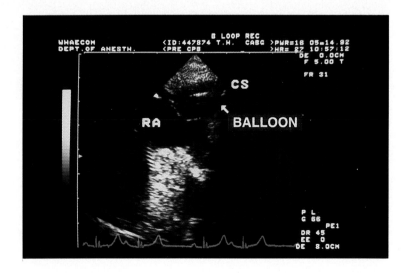

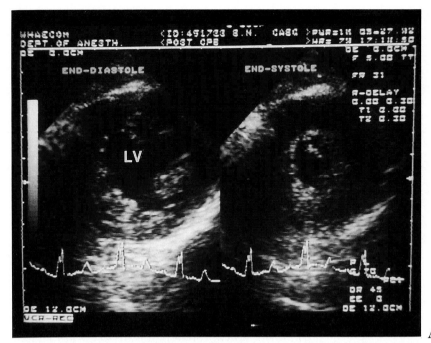

A.

Figure 14-21
A. The left ventricular contraction is normal at end systole and end diastole. LV = left ventricle. *B.* In the M-mode (left), delay in systolic contraction of AW motion is seen (arrows). * = LV cavity; AW = anterior wall; IW = inferior wall.

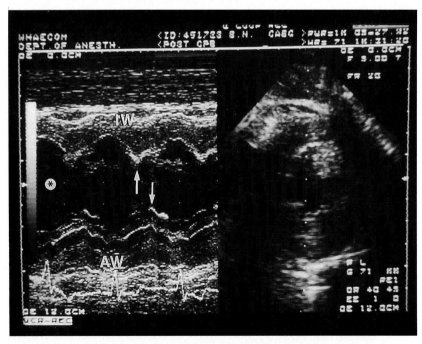

B.

hypertension, and unstable angina. Multiple coronary artery grafts were performed. Soon after CPB, regional wall motion was good (Fig. 14-22A, B), but at the time of sternal closure (45 min after off-CPB), anterior wall motion suddenly became severely hypokinetic (Fig. 14-22C, D). The surgeon found a kinked Ao-LAD graft. After rearrangement of the graft, RWMA returned to normal. Transient ECG change at V_5 and II leads appeared 15 min after new RWMA. Her postoperative course was unremarkable.

Figure 14-21
C. In the M-mode (left) using M-mark in B-mode, the contraction of inferior and anterior wall is seen normally. * = LV cavity; AW = anterior wall; IW = inferior wall.

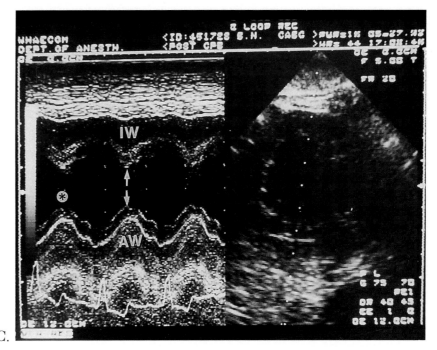

C.

Conclusion

The introduction of intraoperative TEE has provided valuable information for the clinical assessment of LV function and valve integrity and flow dynamics. In this chapter we have highlighted some important aspects of intraop-

erative TEE. An overview of this subject recently completed by Oka et al.[30] describes the topics presented here and details the myriad applications of TEE beyond LV function. Echocardiographically derived indices of preload, afterload, and contractility enhance our ability to assess the effects of various anesthetic and

Figure 14-22
Long-axis views of left ventricle in longitudinal scan, showing normal contraction at end systole (A) and normal dilatation at end diastole

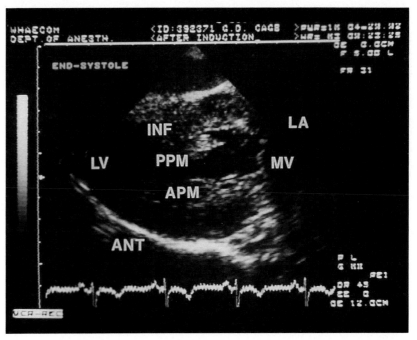

A.

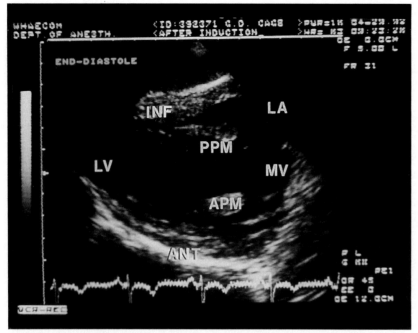

B.

Figure 14-22
B. INF = inferior (wall);
ANT = anterior (wall);
PPM = posterior papil-
lary muscle; APM = ante-
rior papillary muscle; LA
= left atrium; MV = mi-
tral valve; LV = left ventricle. Long-axis views of
left ventricle in longitudinal scan, showing the ab-
normal wall motion at
end systole *C.* and at
end diastole (*D*).

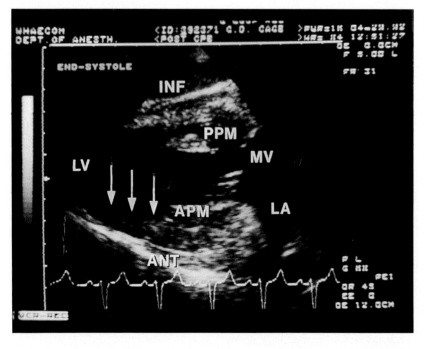

C.

Figure 14-22
Note the difference in wall thickness at end systole compared with *A*. At end diastole (*D*), it is almost the same as *B*. ANT = anterior (wall); APM = anterior papillary muscle; INF = inferior (wall); LA = left atrium; LV = left ventricle; MV = mitral valve; PPM = posterior papillary muscle.

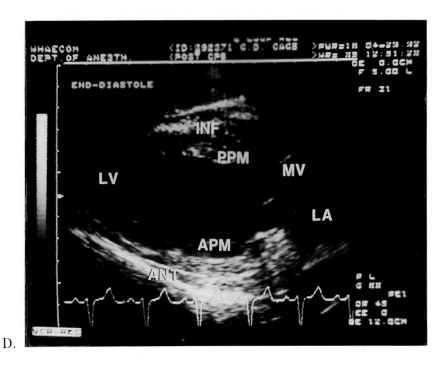

D.

surgical techniques on ventricular function. Early detection of RWMA, which are sensitive indicators of myocardial ischemia, may guide aggressive intervention for the reversal of such changes before damage to the myocardium occurs. As such, TEE has important applications as a clinical monitor and possesses a specific advantage over the routine hemodynamic monitors.

References

1. van Daele MERM, Roelandt JRTC: Intraoperative monitoring, in Sutherland GR, Roelandt JRTC, Fraser AG, Anderson RH (eds): *Transesophageal Echocardiography in Clinical Practice*. London, New York, Gower Medical Publishing, 1990, chap 12, p 1.
2. Lazar HL, Plehn J: Intraoperative echocardiography. *Am Thorac Surg* 50:1010, 1990.
3. Edwards WD: Applied anatomy of the heart, in Brandenburg RO, Fuster V, Giuliani ER, McGoon DC (eds): *Cardiology: Fundamentals and Practice*. Chicago, Year Book Medical Publishers, 1987, chap 4, p 47.
4. Seward JB, Khandheria BK, Oh JK, et al: Transesophageal echocardiography: Technique, anatomic correlation, implementation and clinical application. *Mayo Clin Proc* 63:649, 1988.
5. Curtius JM, Leischik R, Arnold G, et al: Biplane transesophageal echocardiography: Anatomical orientation and suggestions for "standard planes." *Am J Noninvas Cardiol* 5:65, 1991.
6. Orihashi K, Hong Y, Sisto DA, et al: The anatomical location of the transesophageal echocardiographic transducer in obtaining the short axis view of the left ventricle. *J Cardiothorac Anesth* 4:726, 1990.
7. Hong YW, Orihashi K, Oka Y: Intraoperative monitoring of regional wall motion abnormalities for detecting myocardial ischemia by transesophageal echocardiography. *Echocardiography* 7:323, 1990.
8. David DW, Protasio DL, Wyatt HL, et al: Early changes in regional and global left ventricular function induced by graded reductions in regional coronary perfusion. *Am J Cardiol* 39:537, 1977.
9. Kronik G, Slany J, Mosslacher H: Comparative value of eight M-mode echocardiographic formulas for determining left ventricular stroke volume. *Circulation* 60:1308, 1979.
10. Wyatt HL, Heng MK, Meerbaum S, et al: Cross-sectional echocardiography 2: Analysis of mathematic for quantifying volume of the formalin-fixed left ventricle. *Circulation* 61:1119, 1980.

11. Wyatt HL, Meerbaum S, Heng MK, et al: Cross-sectional echocardiography 3: Analysis of mathematic models for quantifying volume of symmetric left ventricle. *Am Heart J* 100: 821, 1980.

12. Haendchen RV, Wyatt HL, Maurer G, et al: Quantitation of regional cardiac function by two-dimensional echocardiography: 1. Patterns of contraction in the normal left ventricle. *Circulation* 67:1234, 1983.

13. Wyatt HL, Haendchen RV, Meerbaum S, et al: Assessment of quantitative methods for 2-dimensional echocardiography. *Am J Cardiol* 52:396, 1983.

14. Konstadt SN, Thys D, Mindich BP, et al: Validation of quantitative intraoperative transesophageal echocardiography. *Anesthesiology* 65:418, 1986.

15. Quinones AM, Mokotoff DM, Nouri S, et al: Noninvasive quantification of left ventricular wall stress. Validation of method and application to assessment of chronic pressure overload. *Am J Cardiol* 45:782, 1980.

16. Reichek N, Wilson J, Sutton MSJ, et al: Noninvasive determination of left ventricular end-systolic stress: Validation of the method and initial application. *Circulation* 65:99, 1982.

17. Brodie BR, McLaurin LP, Grossman W: Combined hemodynamic-ultrasonic method for studying left ventricular wall stress, comparison with angiography. *Am J Cardiol* 37:864, 1976.

18. Unpublished data.

19. Sklenar J, Jayaweera AR, Kaul S: A computer-aided approach for the quantitation of regional left ventricular function using two-dimensional echocardiography. *J Am Soc Echocardiography* 5:33, 1992.

20. Henry WL, DeMaria A, Feigenbaum H, et al: Report of the American Society of Echocardiography Committee on Nomenclature and Standards: Identification of myocardial wall segments. American Society of Echocardiography, 1982.

21. Guth BD, White FC, Gallagher KP, et al: Decreased systolic wall thickening in myocardium adjacent to ischemic zones in conscious swine during brief coronary occlusion. *Am Heart J* 107:458, 1984.

22. McDonald IG, Feigenbaum H, Chang S: Analysis of left ventricular wall motion by reflected ultrasound. *Circulation* 46:14, 1972.

23. Abel MD, Nishimura RA, Callahan MJ, et al: Evaluation of intraoperative transesophageal two-dimensional echocardiography. *Anesthesiology* 66:64, 1987.

24. Kato M, Nakashima Y, Levine J, et al: Does transesophageal echocardiography improve postoperative outcome in patients undergoing coronary artery bypass surgery? (in press).

25. Kitahata H, Hong YW, Goldiner PL, et al: Intraoperative left ventricular diastolic function using transesophageal two-dimensional color Doppler echocardiography (abstract). *Anesthesiology* 71(3A):A47, 1989.

26. Lawson WE, Seifert F, Anagnostopoulos C, et al: Effect of coronary artery bypass grafting on left ventricular diastolic function. *Am J Cardiol* 61:283, 1988.

27. van Daele MERM, Sutherland GR, Mitchell MM: Do changes in pulmonary capillary wedge pressure adequately reflect myocardial ischemia during anesthesia? *Circulation* 81:865, 1990.

28. Beaupre PN, Kremer PF, Cahalan MK, et al: Intraoperative detection of changes in left ventricular segmental wall motion by transesophageal two-dimensional echocardiography. *Am Heart J* 107:1021, 1984.

29. Kato M, Oka Y: Evaluation of mitral regurgitation during coronary artery bypass surgery by transesophageal color Doppler imaging. *Junkanseigyo (JPN)* 13:145, 1992.

30. Oka Y, Goldiner PL: *Transesophageal Echocardiography*. Philadelphia, Lippincott, 1992.

Index

Note: Page numbers followed by *f* indicate figures; page numbers followed by *t* indicate tables.